Series in Biomedical Engineering

Series Editor: Joachim H. Nagel

Series in Biomedical Engineering

Editor-in-Chief

Prof. Dr. Joachim H. Nagel
Institute of Biomedical Engineering
University of Stuttgart
Seidenstrasse 36
70174 Stuttgart
Germany
E-mail: jn@bmt.uni-stuttgart.de

The International Federation for Medical and Biological Engineering, IFMBE, is a federation of national and transnational organizations representing internationally the interests of medical and biological engineering and sciences. The IFMBE is a non-profit organization fostering the creation, dissemination and application of medical and biological engineering knowledge and the management of technology for improved health and quality of life. Its activities include participation in the formulation of public policy and the dissemination of information through publications and forums. Within the field of medical, clinical, and biological engineering, IFMBE's aims are to encourage research and the application of knowledge, and to disseminate information and promote collaboration. The objectives of the IFMBE are scientific, technological, literary, and educational.

The IFMBE is a WHO accredited NGO covering the full range of biomedical and clinical engineering, healthcare, healthcare technology and management. It is representing through its 58 member societies some 120.000 professionals involved in the various issues of improved health and healthcare delivery.

Previous Editions:

Spaan, J. et al: BIOMED, Biopacemaking, 2007, ISBN 978-3-540-72109-3

Sekihara, K., Nagarajan, S.: BIOMED, Adaptive Spatial Filters for Electromagnetic Brain Imaging, 2008, ISBN 978-3-540-79369-4

Madhavan, G., Oakley, B.; Kun, L.(Eds.): BIOMED, Career Development in Bioengineering and Biotechnology, 2009, ISBN 978-0-387-76494-8

Kanagasingam Yogesan, Lodewijk Bos,
Peter Brett, and Michael Christopher Gibbons
(Eds.)

Handbook of Digital Homecare

Springer

Prof. Kanagasingam Yogesan
Faculty of Medicine, Dentistry and Health Sciences
University of Western Australia
Director, Centre for e-Health
The Lions Eye Institute
2 Verdun Street
Nedlands
WA 6009
Australia
E-mail: yogesan@cyllene.uwa.edu.au

Drs Lodewijk Bos
International Council on Medical &
Care Compunetics (ICMCC)
Stationsstraat 38
3511 EG Utrecht
Netherlands
E-mail: lobos@ icmcc.org

Prof. Peter Brett
Aston University
School of Eng. and Applied Science
Chemical Eng. and Applied Chemistry
Birmingham
United Kingdom B4 7ET

Michael Christopher Gibbons
Johns Hopkins Urban Health Institute
2013 E. Monument St.
Baltimore MD 21287
USA
E-mail: mgibbons@jhsph.edu

ISBN 978-3-642-26069-8 e-ISBN 978-3-642-01387-4

DOI 10.1007/978-3-642-01387-4

Series in Biomedical Engineering ISSN 1864-5763

Softcover reprint of the hardcover 1st edition 2010

Typeset & Cover Design: Scientific Publishing Services Pvt. Ltd., Chennai, India.

Printed in acid-free paper

9 8 7 6 5 4 3 2 1

springer.com

IFMBE

The International Federation for Medical and Biological Engineering (IFMBE) was established in 1959 to provide medical and biological engineering with a vehicle for international collaboration in research and practice of the profession. The Federation has a long history of encouraging and promoting international cooperation and collaboration in the use of science and engineering for improving health and quality of life.

The IFMBE is an organization with membership of national and transnational societies and an International Academy. At present there are 53 national members and 5 transnational members representing a total membership in excess of 120 000 professionals worldwide. An observer category is provided to groups or organizations considering formal affiliation. Personal membership is possible for individuals living in countries without a member society. The IFMBE International Academy includes individuals who have been recognized for their outstanding contributions to biomedical engineering.

Objectives

The objectives of the International Federation for Medical and Biological Engineering are scientific, technological, literary, and educational. Within the field of medical, clinical and biological engineering its aims are to encourage research and the application of knowledge, to disseminate information and promote collaboration.

In pursuit of these aims the Federation engages in the following activities: sponsorship of national and international meetings, publication of official journals, cooperation with other societies and organizations, appointment of commissions on special problems, awarding of prizes and distinctions, establishment of professional standards and ethics within the field as well as other activities which in the opinion of the General Assembly or the Administrative Council would further the cause of medical, clinical or biological engineering. It promotes the formation of regional, national, international or specialized societies, groups or boards, the coordination of bibliographic or informational services and the improvement of standards in terminology, equipment, methods and safety practices, and the delivery of health care.

The Federation works to promote improved communication and understanding in the world community of engineering, medicine and biology.

Activities

Publications of the IFMBE include: the journal Medical and Biological Engineering and Computing, the electronic magazine IFMBE News, and the Book Series on Biomedical Engineering. In cooperation with its international and regional conferences, IFMBE also publishes the IFMBE Proceedings Series. All publications of the IFMBE are published by Springer Verlag.

Every three years the IFMBE hosts a World Congress on Medical Physics and Biomedical Engineering in cooperation with the IOMP and the IUPESM. In addition, annual, milestone and regional conferences are organized in different regions of the world, such as Asia Pacific, Europe, the Nordic-Baltic and Mediterranean regions, Africa and Latin America.

The administrative council of the IFMBE meets once a year and is the steering body for the IFMBE. The council is subject to the rulings of the General Assembly, which meets every three years.

Information on the activities of the IFMBE are found on its web site at: http://www.ifmbe.org.

Preface

Future of health care will be delivered at home.

ICMCC Board

Digital homecare is defined as the use of information and communication technologies to enable delivery and management of health care services at home. Due to various needs digital home care is becoming part of main stream health care delivery in most of the countries. This book on Digital Home Care covers all aspects of Digital Homecare, e. g. technologies; clinical applications; social, ethical and legal aspects; and future trends. It is certainly one of the important and fast growing areas in the fields of medicine.

We were motivated to publish this book due to overwhelming interest from our members who attended our annual conferences for text which explain adequately the concepts of digital homecare. This will be the first such handbook in the field.

We would like to take this opportunity to thank all the authors who have contributed to this book. The contributions from individual global experts from specific areas in the field make this book special.

We should also mention about the hard work done by the editors in specific our President, Lodewijk Bos. He was constantly pushed everyone to make this project a success even with his present health condition. Whenever he is healthy he sends e-mails to make sure that the progress of the book is in track. Without his encouragement and support this book would have been a dream.

The ICMCC Board

Contents

Digital Homecare – An Introduction

The Editors

Digital homecare is a phrase that is easily understood and can be described as a container expression. Assistive technology, telemedicine, mhealth, rehabilitation, are all contained within digital homecare. But it is impossible to find a proper definition of digital homecare. Looking for "digital homecare" in PubMed or Google Scholar delivers less than a dozen results. An important modern reference site like Wikipedia has no entry for it. There is a "lack of empirical evidence to support or refute the use of smart home technologies within health and social care, which is significant for practitioners and the healthcare consumer". [1]

In his chapter on standardization, Wouter Meijer says that digital homecare: "bridges the distance between the client/patient and his care providers, both in terms of spatial distance and in terms of distance in time. This new form of care enables the client/patient to remain at home, and yet receive good quality care. Another benefit of digital homecare is that it allows the demand for care to be satisfied at an affordable price."

So let's look at this apparently new form of care. It consists of three words: 'digital', 'home' and 'care' and three terms: 'digital home', 'digital care' and 'home care'. From this we can propose the following definition:

Digital Homecare is a collection of services to deliver, maintain and improve care in the home environment using the latest ICT technology and devices.

It is important to recognize the wide range of issues that are covered by digital homecare. This book, but also the various proceedings of the ICMCC Events [2] show anything from medication control to various forms of self-management, to telemonitoring or assistive technologies.

Digital homecare by default profits immensely from innovations in medical and care technology. The development of electronic health records will help to offer the patient/consumer and care provider(s) an overview of the results of delivered services as well as the output of various devices. Combined with the narrative input from the patient/consumer a solid foundation will be created that will bring forward a true participatory care.

Portability and miniaturization of devices as well as developments in wearable technologies (smart clothing) will strongly enhance their use and effectiveness. Of importance will also be new technological developments in the home environment (smart homes).). Latest disease management tools, messaging devices, and sensor technologies are increasing the ability to provide physiological monitoring on and

K. Yogesan et al. (Eds.): Handbook of Digital Homecare, BIOMED, pp. 1–4.
springerlink.com

around the patient's body from their own home. Some of these technologies include,

1) remote monitoring telehealth unit,
2) blood pressure/pulse device,
3) digital stethoscope,
4) pulse oximeter,
5) digital thermometer,
6) glucose meter,
7) peak flow meter,
8) Digital cameras,
9) ECG

Since the aging population is increasing but the number hospital beds are not increasing, it is ideal for patients to age at home with health care delivery provided at their door step. Patients can live better quality of life in the familiar environment and live longer with preventative care and self-management. The caregivers can be supported better handle the care of patients using telemedicine technologies. In addition to ageing population, patients with chronic conditions could benefit most from the digital home care, patients with hypertension, diabetes, heart failure and coronary artery disease, stroke, chronic pain, wounds, depression and mental health problems, dementia and palliative care and fall risk.

The care providers also benefit by keeping the patients at home and remotely monitor and care them. This will reduce the cost of delivery of care, increase the time available to accept new referrals and enable them to provide high quality care for the adults and pediatric patients.

Telemedicine in all its varieties is and will increasingly become a major part of digital homecare. Examples are telemonitoring chronic patients, teleconsultations for less mobile consumers, fall protection and alert services for the elderly and more recently areas like wound care.

Accessibility of digital resources is of growing importance, as care consumers as well as patients have a growing tendency to inform themselves about their (possible) conditions [3]. Whereas at the moment the focus is on the use of computers and their growing availability in the developed world, it is to be expected that television and more importantly cell phones will become major players in the field of digital homecare, especially in the lesser developed and developing countries.

As a new form of care, digital homecare is in essence the consequence of "the changing nature of health and medical practice itself [...]. This shift from acute, inpatient treatment to chronic, community based, guided self care and health risk management will demand unique advances from the information technologies." [4]

These advances from the information technologies are shaped by what is now called Health 2.0, "the combination of health data and health information with (patient) experience through the use of ICT, enabling the citizen to become an active and responsible partner in his/her own health and care pathway"[5] and make digital homecare into the main representation of patient 2.0 empowerment: "the active participation of the citizen in his or her health and care pathway with the interactive use of Information and Communication Technologies"[5].

With the upcoming importance of genomics, future developments like personalized medicine will most definitely become an important part of digital homecare.

Digital homecare benefits a very diverse "audience".

Due to an increasingly ageing population combined with a growing scarcity in professional resources the elderly are and will ever more be one of the largest target groups for digital homecare.

In addition to the ageing population, patients with chronic conditions could benefit most from digital homecare, like patients with hypertension, diabetes, heart failure and coronary artery disease, stroke, chronic pain, wounds, depression and mental health problems, dementia and palliative care and fall risk.

A third category of people that will seriously benefit from digital homecare are the disabled and those who can benefit from telerehabilitation programs. [6] [7]

All these categories can benefit from digital homecare "without limiting or disturbing the resident's daily routine, giving him or her greater comfort, pleasure, and well-being." [8]

Care providers also benefit from shifting the Point of Care to the patient's home and remotely monitor and care for them. This will reduce the cost of delivery of care, increase the time available to accept new referrals and enable them to provide high quality care for the adults and pediatric patients. [9]

References

[1] Martin, S., et al.: Smart home technologies for health and social care support. Cochrane Database of Systematic Reviews, Online (4) (2008) CD006412

[2] Medical and Care Compunetics 1-5. Studies in Health Technology and Informatics. IOSPress, Amsterdam (2004 – 2008)

[3] Fox, S., Jones, S.: The Social Life of Health Information. Pew Internet/California Healthcare Foundation, June 11 (2009), `http://www.pewinternet.org/~/media/Files/Reports/2009/PIP_Health_2009.pdf`

[4] Chris Gibbons, M.: Health inequalities and emerging themes in compunetics. Studies in Health Technology and Informatics 121, 62–69 (2006)

[5] Bos, L., et al.: Patient 2.0 Empowerment. In: Arabnia, H.R., Marsh, A. (eds.) Proceedings of the 2008 International Conference on Semantic Web & Web Services SWWS 2008, pp. 164 167 (2008)

[6] Manning, B.R.M., et al.: Active ageing: independence through technology assisted health optimisation. Studies in Health Technology and Informatics 137, 257–262 (2008)
[7] Botsis, T., et al.: Home telecare technologies for the elderly. Journal of Telemedicine and Telecare 14(7), 333–337 (2008)
[8] Chan, M., et al.: A review of smart homes- present state and future challenges. Computer Methods and Programs in Biomedicine 91(1), 55–81 (2008)
[9] Stachura, M.E., Khasanshina, E.V.: Telehomecare and Remote Monitoring: An Outcomes Overview. Adva. Med., October 31 (2007), http://www.viterion.com/web_docs/Telehomecarereport%20Diabetes%20and%20CHR%20Meta%20Analyses.pdf

Information Highway to the Home and Back: A Smart Systems Review

Prof. Bryan Manning (a), Prof. Luis Kun[1] (b)

(a) University of Westminster, London, UK
(b) National Defense University, Washington DC, USA

Abstract This chapter examines a range of issues emerging from the convergence of multiple technologies that, though they can radically assist and change the face of health and social care delivery, are critically dependent on their gaining acceptance by society to the point that they submerge into the fabric of daily life.
The main role of these technologies is to enable an evolutionary transition toward far more effective joined-up services and optimisation of scarce clinical and care resources. Interoperability is central to this spanning multiple levels starting with the full range of human, organisational, sociological and political dialogues; then moving to system and process interaction; and thence to data and information transfers, analysis and manipulation.
Behind all this lies the pressing demographic issue of ageing populations where the types of 'smart' services discussed will be needed to help the elderly stave off the effects of creeping impairment for as long as possible whilst continuing to maintain an active, healthy and autonomously lifestyle.

[1] Disclaimer: "The views expressed in this chapter are those of the author and do not reflect the official policy or position of the National Defense University, the Department of Defense, or the U.S. Government."

K. Yogesan et al. (Eds.): Handbook of Digital Homecare, BIOMED, pp. 5–31.
springerlink.com

1 The Global Village

1.1 Mobility

Over the last decades the growth of cheap and rapid travel has had a massive sociological impact, effectively shrinking the world - and as a consequence accelerating the creation of the global economy, and with it a heady mix of cross-cultural exchange. However on the darker side this increased mobility has created a ready vehicle for disease transfer and with it the need for the rapid transfer of knowledge to combat it.

Happily the Internet and the Information Super Highway provide the reach and means to access key medical information increasingly around the world. From a public health perspective global disease surveillance warnings and preventive measures can be "known" everywhere effectively instantaneously. Similarly discoveries at the leading-edge of medical research can reach the clinical "frontline" in the same way.

In the event of medical emergencies to individuals travelling the world rapid access to key information held on their electronic healthcare records [EHR] should be readily available to clinical staff engaged in treating them anywhere. This of course raises the issue of the need to update these records as treatment progresses to the point of their repatriation – and in particular with the problems of translation back into the "home" language.

Where individuals are emigrating either permanently or for a protracted period their records will need to be transferred to their new "home" domain without any loss of emergency access or content. This carries with it the need for "seamless" content transfer between "old" and "new" record systems as well as any language translation issues [1].

1.2 Identity

The validation of the identity of a patient, especially if they are unconscious, when access to their records prior to any clinical intervention is deemed necessary, can be decidedly problematical – especially if they are not carrying any recognised form of identification.

A potential solution to this problem lies in the use of biometric identifiers - however these need to be firmly linked to their "formal persona" registered with their national authority. Unfortunately this mechanism is not yet in place in many jurisdictions, who generally rely on passport/identity card photos or driving licences.

However as part of on-going work on international standards development for Identity Management and Biometrics a potential medium term solution has emerged. This would use DNA profiles, cross-checked with another biometric identifier [2, 3].

Such an approach would be dependent on current research to create a low-cost, portable "lab-on-chip" device that could rapidly process swabs becoming widely available worldwide. This would open up the possibility of using DNA phenotype variability within the basic twenty-two chromosomes, coupled with the additional two gender determinants, to provide a unique global reference coding for each individual [4].

1.3 Data Privacy

The use of DNA obviously has privacy implications that would need to be addressed to ensure overall cross-cultural acceptance and compliance with national legislation.

Key factors in this are firstly to ensure that the "formal persona" component alone may be used to as the reference source for person-related systems. By contrast the biometric identifier element needs to be separately secured, with access in response to clinical necessity limited to authorised personnel only, with such usage subject to audit.

Visibility and recognition of this separation is particularly important to maintain the trust and confidence of the public across jurisdictions, as is the need to emphasise the deliberate disconnection both within identity structures and between data records. So to must be the need for all to appreciate that on rare occasions some tightly controlled access must be allowed where national security is involved. Whilst DNA obviously has a significant part to play in forensic science applications, these should be dealt with a similar degree of access separation under the accepted constraints of the law of the nations concerned.

Informed Care

Whilst Web access to the very latest knowledge across the complete spectrum of medical and care professional expertise for care-givers and the recipients alike has considerable merit and potential for good, it needs to come with a "health warning"! The problem is that in such an unregulated global information supply system the content that it contains can range from exhaustively tested and extremely valuable, through to the highly dubious and downright wrong – often with little indication of its authenticity or integrity.

Although healthcare professionals are well versed in assessing and testing the validity of both source and content of new knowledge whether obtained by more traditionally published means or via the Web, the ordinary citizen is not – and can all too easily be persuaded to embark on a disastrous course of action. The key lesson to be learnt is that incomplete, incorrect, misinterpreted, misunderstood or misapplied information ultimately can kill as just as easily as the slip of a scalpel. The issue therefore is how best to protect all interested parties against such latent adverse events.

The core of this problem stems from the very nature of the Web - since anyone can set up a site and publish anything they wish - which is then accessible to all. In the absence of any global regulatory controls users need reliable means to help them assess the credibility of this content [5].

Much effort has been applied to resolving this issue particularly through a series of high level international meetings organised under the European Commission e-Europe and eHealth initiatives in collaboration with other nations. Faced with the need to support self-assessed user regulation, guidelines were established to enable bonafide information providers to either to self-certify or user appropriate certification bodies to confirm conformance to basic criteria. This information assurance approach is based on:

Transparency	Verifiable site provider	- credentials
	Objective clarity	- purpose/commercial interests
	Defined target audience	-clear levels of expertise
	Sources of funding	- sponsorship, etc.
Authority	Information sources	- date of publication
	Sources validation	- credentials and date confirmed
Privacy	Security/confidentiality	- policy/systems
	Personal data	- opt-in secure storage/release controls
Currency	Updating clarity	- date per item/page
		- regularity
Accountability	Oversight responsibility	- credentials
		- visibility of user feedback
	Responsible partnering	- certified code of practice linking
	Editorial policy	- content selection criteria
		- content credibility/ accuracy
		- supporting scientific rigour
		- ethical standards
Accessibility	Presentation quality	- search functionality
		- useability/readibility

2 Interoperability

The need to share information is self-evident in many, if not most, clinical and care circumstances – albeit with the codicil that this must be appropriate to the situation. However this conditional requirement necessitates its protection and precise control of access rights to it – especially where technology is concerned.

This leads directly to the major dichotomy between the need to know and share, versus the countervailing need to protect and keep private what may be critical information. The ultimate anomaly this presents can be illustrated by the presumption data protection legislation does not allow release details of the location of bed-bound or disabled patients to emergency services in the event of serious flooding – whereby protection of data can be set against, and effectively above the protection of life!

The need for effective interoperability necessarily exists at several levels - at that of human or organisational interaction; of patient information exchange; in process and systems interaction; and in terms of technological connectivity and interoperation. As a result it is all too easy for confusion to reign and generate hugely negative consequences.

At the clinical and care "frontline" the traditional non-inter-disciplinary "silo" traits imprinted on clinicians at the outset of their training mitigate against effective cross-disciplinary knowledge sharing. In this team working context interoperability relates to the holistic integration of practices, intellectual processes and operational constructs enabled by shared expertise and understanding. Without this "binding" effect the tendency is for individual practitioners to inadvertently undo each other's efforts – especially in community settings where close working contact is limited.

Where explicit patient information sharing is involved, the key considerations are broadly clinical "need to know" together with patient privacy and confidentiality of aspects of the on-going medical and social care records. Beyond the purely ethical issues, breaches of confidentiality can be especially "toxic" where serious damage can be done to the patient's relationships and their economic "health".

Processes and systems operate and interact at three distinct levels – firstly in terms of "frontline" professional clinical and care judgement and delivery; then in governance oversight through more formal procedural guidelines and constraints on practices used and to limit occurrence of adverse events; and finally as organisational and administrative procedures and controls, necessary to maintain corporate effectiveness.

Whilst these forms of human networking are central to any form of clinical and care service delivery, the rapid evolution of communications and computing technologies has the largely unadopted capability to facilitate major changes for the better in the way services are delivered. In the main the problem has been the significant failure by the administrators and technologists to recognise that regardless of the sophisticated functionality that they can provide – this is only an enabler for change.

However such change has to be perceived as beneficial in the first place. If it can be perceived as enabling and delivering radical improvement in personal professional capabilities and practice, coupled with a similar improvement in the quality of patient outcomes, it has a chance of adoption. Significantly it has to be desired, rather than imposed.

The aim of Compunetics – as a "system of systems" – is to help draw together these disparate strands into a cohesive interoperable holistic whole that maximises benefit to all concerned. As such it has to combine motivational psychology with the ability to facilitate enduring change; to support the processes of change together with the change of processes to deliver palpable benefits; to deliver valuable, highly valued knowledge and relevant information unambiguously to the point of need; and finally to create a reliable and resilient infrastructure that enable the whole complex entity to function smoothly and effectively. Its ultimate aim is thus to promote harmonious interoperability at all levels.

2.1 Development Initiatives

Currently there is no direct evidence of any significant attempt to tackle the multi-tier holistic interoperability issues outlined above. The nearest approach to this is the move to integrate Social Care and Primary Care within the UK NHS. However the effect is broadly to add a further set of "silos" alongside those that are already there.

The only other example was a collaborative venture in the USA some years ago [6], which aimed at drawing together an even wider community services network. In this case the aim was to focus particularly on disadvantaged and often dysfunctional family groups to establish their need and usage of available support across the main spectrum of service provision, i.e. Health and Social Care, Education, Welfare, etc.

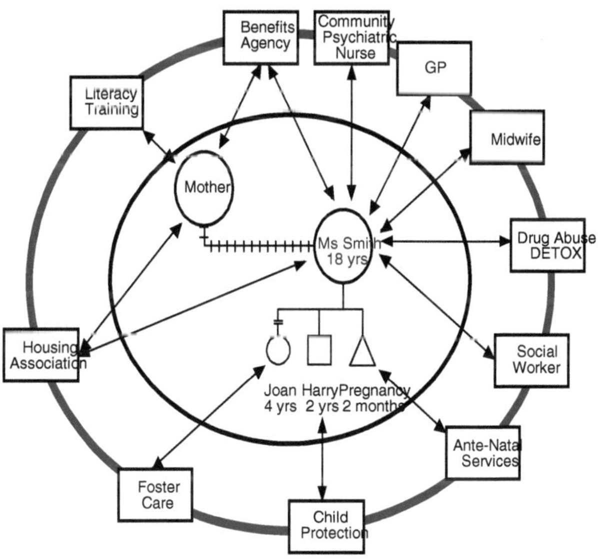

Fig.1 Genomap

The basis of this approach is illustrated [Fig.1] with a Genomap showing at its centre the dysfunctional relationships within this two generations of single parents, which are coupled with the services known to be involved as shown on the outer ring. The aim of this graphical outline was to act both as the interoperability coordination overview and a means of identifying relevant but missing services. These service "hubs" would in turn act as reference points to active and planned care pathways.

From an enabling technology perspective there is a considerable amount of ongoing activity within the European Union. This is set in the overall context of the European Interoperability Framework for Pan-European eGovernment services [PEGS] [7] which is underpinned by the following developmental streams:

European Interoperability Strategy	[EIS]
European Interoperability Framework	[EIF]
European Interoperability Architecture Guidelines	[EIAG]
European Interoperability Infrastructure Services	[EIIS]

It is interesting to note how the European Union defines interoperability within its PEGS document together with its overall high level context respectively as;

"Interoperability is the ability of disparate and diverse organisations to interact towards mutually beneficial and agreed common goals, involving the sharing of information and knowledge between the organizations via the business processes they support, by means of the exchange of data between their respective information and communication technology (ICT) systems"

It also goes on to explicitly observe what interoperability is NOT, namely:

Integration - changing and tighten coupling between systems
Compatibility - interchangeability of tools in a given context
Adaptability - changing tools by adding additional capabilities

The PEGS context is naturally focused on inter-state collaboration, as shown below as well as topographically [Fig.2].

"Cross-border public sector services supplied by either national public administrations or EU public administrations provided to one another and to European businesses and citizens, in order to implement community legislation, by means of interoperable networks between public administrations"

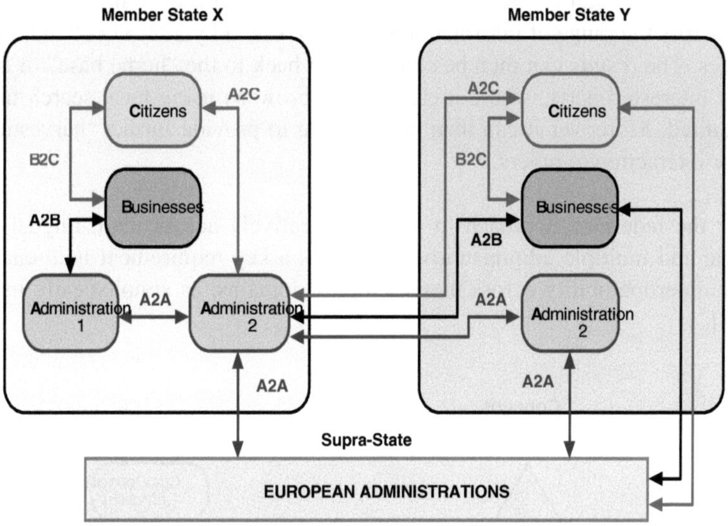

Fig.2 Primary Interactions

This topology is equally applicable to health care environments merely by a change in the "labels", as shown below:

A2A	Adminstration <-> Adminstration	= Care Organisation <-> Care Organisation
A2B	Adminstration <- > Business	= Care Organisation <-> Clinicians/Carers
A2C	Adminstration <-> Citizen	= Care Organisation <-> Patients
B2C	Business <-> Citizen	= Clinicians/Carers <-> Patients

Whilst this is the overarching programme several sector specific initiatives are already underway with the initial findings of an eHealthinterop initiative were published at the end of 2008. This sentence is awkward for a book that will probably be published after the date indicated. Suggest to revise the sentence as an initiative published at the end of 2008.

3 'Harvesting' Professional Knowledge

In this context a European Union funded project run by the CEN/ISSS (European Committee for Standardisation/Information Society Standardisation System) entitled e-Gov-share is equally applicable to the health and social care domain as it is in the multiplicity and diversity of eGovernment scenarios [8]. Its primary aim is focused on developing a federated systems approach to support inter-agency cross-border collation of information on any chosen topic - potentially fulfilling a vast range of highly focused user needs.

The process itself enables the 'harvesting' of relevant information from 'open' areas across the range of information repositories held by a set of collaborating authorities. The results can then be consolidated back to the "home base" of the particular interested party, where it can then be browsed using local search facilities as required. Moreover it can then be available to provide further 'harvesting' access or interaction to others.

For the federated approach to operate effectively across multi-lingual, multicultural and multiple administrative structures a key requirement is to enable semantic interoperability across these complex domains, as simplistically indicated [Fig.3].

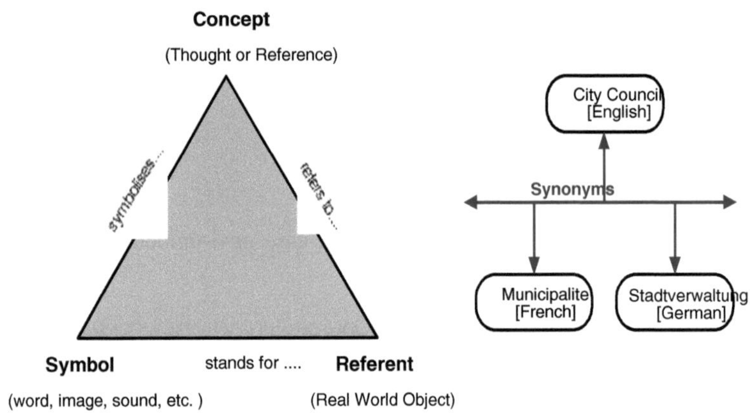

Fig.3 Semantic interoperability

Whilst this example shows "is equivalent to" synonym relationships, in reality many terms are not 100% identical being "is similar to" instead, often overlapping in their meaning with other terms. In order to cope with these problems the aim is to create a Terminological Resource Network (TRN) that acts as a term registry, and is being based CEN/CWA 15526 "European Network for Administrative Nomenclature".

The framework approach used maps the content of multiple Information Repositories and their associated Registries onto the generic ontology of the Shared Reference Model [eGovIM] providing a common platform from which content can be accessed. This is provided via an ATOM-based notification and exchange protocol transport layer to link accredited service users to their target sources [Fig.4].

The Semantic Reference Ontology combines and cross-indexes the terminologies used by individual Registries to enable interworking with service users without loss of intrinsic meaning. Initially it will focus on a range of resources types, including:

- Services
- Process Descriptions
- Standards & Interoperability Frameworks
- Documents
- Geographic Data

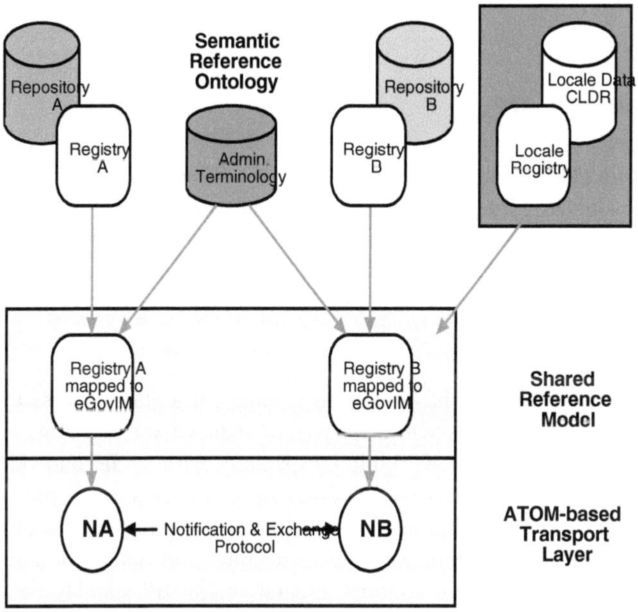

Fig.4 Architectural Framework Overview

An additional feature supporting the Shared Reference Model is the creation of a Common Locale Data Repository [CLDR] and associated Registry based in the main on sets of user preferences derived from Unicode TR35. Its objective is to act as the key reference taxonomy for linguistic, territorial and 'soft' cultural diversity issues.

4 Health Information Systems Interoperability

The e-Gov-share approach has fairly obvious potential applicability within national health and social care agencies not only to support professional knowledge acquisition and dissemination between agencies, but also as a means to share and exchange relevant patient data where deemed clinically or critically necessary.

This is particularly relevant in the latter case where a patient requires treatment whilst away from their home location, either abroad, or when relocating to another country permanently or for a protracted duration. In such cases European Telecommunications Standards Institute [ETSI] work on eHealth user profile coding and similar activities may be of use to rapidly obtain key information; to help in resolving legal issues; or even dealing with problems in semantic variability [9].

5 Community Care

The traditional provision of healthcare has centred on a medical model predominantly separated into a multiplicity of professional domains, together with a fairly rigidly tiered hierarchy of disciplines between them, across whose borders patients were interchanged as necessary and appropriate. Within these service "silos" the only shared feature of their practice has been a basic face-to-face patient contact and assessment approach [10].

However this stereotype has begun to change particularly across the community care-giving landscape, where these past boundaries are beginning to be superseded by multi-agency inter-working – especially with social and other support services. In many ways this is an overdue recognition that a full return to health and normality does not stop at the surgery door or the ministrations of the district nurse. Happily increased team working in hospital and out in the community is becoming a common theme – although mental health still tends to be kept somewhat at arms-length.

5.1 The Demographic Time-bomb

The recognition of the impact of the potential doubling of the percentage of the over 60s in the developed and developing world has been the subject of increasing concern and research activity for some time [Fig.5] [11]. Whilst the cost implications are obviously severe, they are likely to be exacerbated by the likely reduction in the number of professionals needed to cope with such an increase in demand, due to the long term trend of lowering birthrates.

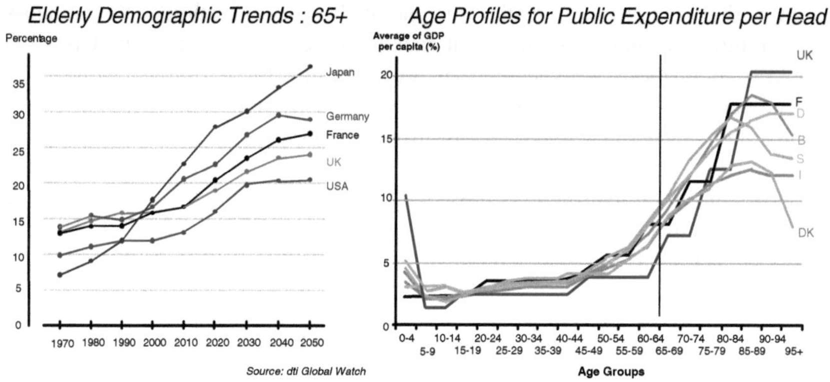

Fig.5 Elderly Demographic Change

The effect of a diminishing pool of available care professionals on service delivery will be bound to concentrate minds be on how to get more out of current processes. However although there are undoubtedly inefficiencies to be weeded out – especially by demolishing many outdated "silo-based" patterns of working – these alone are unlikely to stem the rising tide of demand, or release sufficient professional resource to cope.

In view of the scale these impending changes there appear to be two main options, namely:

- Alter the demand profile through lifestyle improvement
- Substitute use of technology for many resource intensive support functions

Ideally both should be combined with multi-agency, inter-disciplinary care process improvement. This would need to be based on the recognition that the elderly almost invariably suffer from a complex variety of "creeping" latent multiple co-morbidities that spread well beyond those of the purely medical model.

The lack of an equivalent set of "diagnostic" categories for the wider psycho-social, socio-economic problems that beset the elderly make it difficult to recognise and deal with them effectively – if at all. As in adult mental health treatment, these factors can act as semi-hidden "stressors" that compound, accentuate or trigger clinical conditions that need to be treated as an integral part of the whole care plan.

5.2 "Creeping" Impairment

Whilst ageing is frequently seen by the younger generations as an increasingly fraught medical condition, in reality it is one of slow degeneration of functionality based on impairments that often stretch back to earlier times in an individual's life cycle [12]. It is these weaknesses that are often the focus of increasingly frequently occurring medical problems – accentuated by a slowing degrading lifestyle that locks the elderly into a downward spiral of dependency.

In broad terms, impairment is most frequently dealt with by coping with the various inconveniences that it inflicts – as opposed to seeking to avoid or delay its impacts for as long as possible [Fig.6].

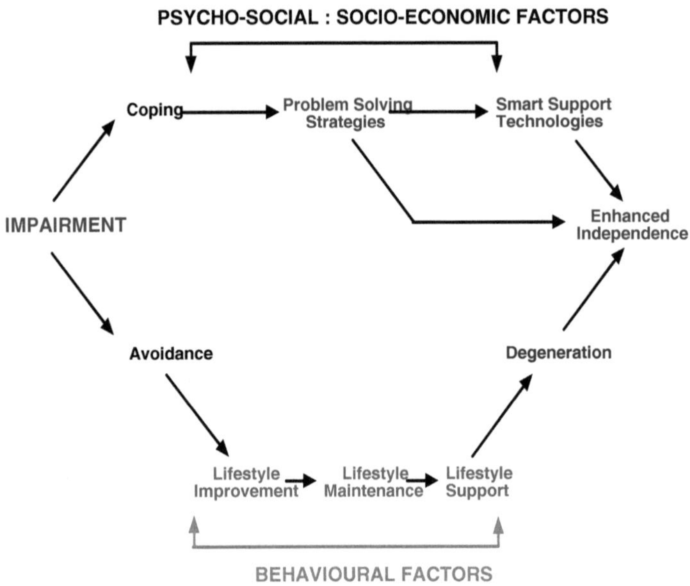

Fig.6 Ageing Influences

Paradoxically the vast amount of tacit knowledge of coping strategies to deal with their impairments employed by so many people – past and present – has never really been tapped. If collected, collated and mapped as self-care pathways for different situations it would not only provide a valuable resource for the impaired and the care professions alike, but also to focus the development and provision of Smart Support Technologies as more acceptable user-friendly aids to enhanced independence.

5.3 Self-Care Support & Lifestyle Improvement

The aim of helping the ageing to avoid or ameliorate "creeping" impairment is obviously a key factor in keeping them healthy and independent for as long as possible, as well as meeting and managing future demand on scarce resources.

However persuading them en mass to embark on personalised lifestyle improvement is dependent on understanding the many behavioural factors that have become in-built over long life-spans – and which will tend to negate any such moves. Initial research into this area indicates that the key factors that are central to achieving change toward increased self-care are motivation and personal control over content and rate of adoption of acceptable lifestyle change.

At the personal level motivation is dependent on assessing and balancing desirable benefits that may be attained against the risks entailed – particularly in terms of perceived levels of inconvenience that may be involved in their achievement. Equally important is that each individual concerned remains in control of their destiny – albeit with feedback and advice on how well they are achieving and conserving their target improvements.

Appropriately supported self-care depends an interaction between the individual and a remote support centre – either by mail, phone, or intuitive, easy to use computerised "smart" systems of various levels of sophistication.

Whilst this approach should obviously be tailored to individual needs, its generic core centres on the user regularly completing a self assessment pro-forma for processing by a support service centre. The results are then returned providing a current health status overview coupled with ongoing improvement options recommendations. These enable the user to consider the advice and incorporate it as, and if, desired into their own self-managed care plan and action it accordingly [Fig.7].

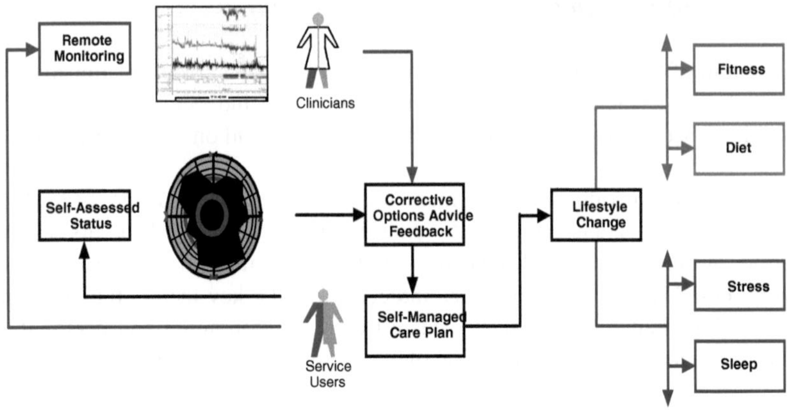

Fig.7 Supported Self-care

Selected lifestyle change options chosen by the user can be delivered as a series of incremental packs, whose contents vary dependent on required functionality – ranging from advice and guidance notes; to routines to be followed; plus a wide variety of devices and aids required to support certain routines/actions.

Feedback is provided is various forms to suit the users preferences and can be either in conventional report form, or various graphical format. A preferred display format is in the form of a "radar plot" with results plotted radially and linked to form a "scab" showing overall status – the aim being to shrink it back into a safe zone

This approach can be extended using various smart technologies to include remote physiological monitoring where clinically necessary. Typically this would use a range of diagnostic analysis techniques - such as measurement of heart rate variability and respiration – and provide appropriate advice either directly or through the patient's GP as circumstance dictate.

6 'Smart' Care Support

Surprisingly the Smart Home concept in various forms is now over twenty years old mainly stimulated by research initiatives funded by the European Union, particularly in terms both of the COST219 programme [13, 14] and Ambient Assisted Living Framework projects [15].

Here the main emphasis has been focused on technology – and in particular with a variety of variations on a basic telecommunications theme - to spawn topics such as telehealth, telecare, telemedicine, etc. Whilst this considerable effort has been expended on these developments, they have so far led to the promotion of a wide variety of largely incompatible commercial niche market systems designs.

In the UK the result has been that few companies have managed to secure anything like a dominant position in what has remained, until now, a relatively small and semi-dormant market. This lack of take-up is probably due to the unpreparedness of the elderly to spend savings on technology that they neither understand, nor believe that they need or could benefit from.

Although this has so far been a technology solution seeking to stimulate a market and then having fallen into the usual trap of failing to understand or research the perceptions and motivations of its target audience - its time appears to have come. The key difference is that its real market is the care service sector rather than the individual.

However this comes with the major caveat that for it to achieve its potential for good, care service providers, as ever, will have to find effective ways to overcome the tendency of its client base to reject any imposed solution to its problems out of hand regardless of it potential benefits.

A useful pointer to how to win acceptance comes from experience of a Scottish County Council as a result of a major revamp of their Elderly Services Department, in response to increasing overload. Originally they only provided a limited number of a basic Smart Home package comprising;

- "Lifeline" link and detector hub to monitor:
  - Smoke
  - Movement
  - Flooding
  - Temperature extremes
- Personal Alarm Pendant

These were only made available to those whose needs met a stringent assessment criteria. Despite the best of intentions this approach meet with a high level of either outright rejections, or begrudging acceptance and consequent low utilisation.

A subsequent research study revealed that a significant yet unexpected negative factor centred on the perceived stigmatisation of its recipients within their home community. This was successfully countered by the adoption of a "mainstreaming" approach whereby these packs are provided to all households once any resident reaches 66 years old [16].

The key lesson to be learnt from this is that much more needs to be understood about the ageing process from a psychological and behavioural point of view if the elderly are to be persuaded to engage and assimilate technological advances into their daily living culture.

6.1 'Smart Home' Systems

Whilst the idea of a basic "starter" pack is an essential building block, the variability in the range of individual user needs, desires and idiosyncrasies underlines the need for these support systems to be based on open systems architecture that can support an ever evolving range of functionality. Most importantly the elderly need to be given a clear perception of what benefits this functionality can bring them and how easy and intuitive it is to use - if they are to absorb it into their lifestyle culture.

In essence this service "market" needs to be user-led – albeit with careful caring mentoring support from the service provider. If it the technology push approach is used by the care service sector is followed, it is likely to fall on deaf ears and remain largely rejected.

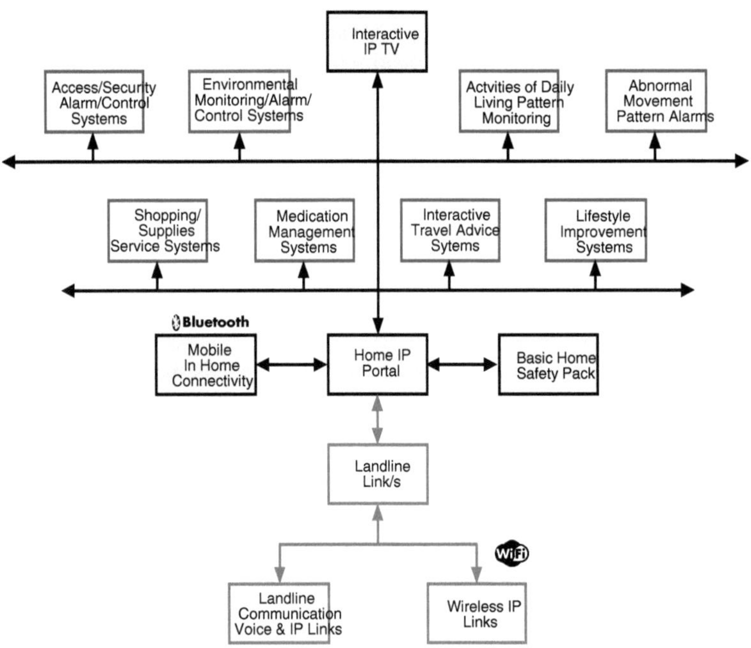

Fig.8 A Smart Home' Infrastructure

Currently existing installations are mostly alarm systems triggered by contact closures within a range of detectors that are hardwire linked – with exception of personal radio alarms - to a “lifeline” hub that communicates via a landline link to a remote alarm monitoring and response station.

With the rapid growth of IP broadband connectivity the existing hardwired approach can be largely superseded by an ever widening range of Bluetooth linked devices with much enhanced functionality and data transfer capabilities. The home alarm hub would be replaced by an IP portal providing multi-functional linkage with external services, with interactive control and communication primarily provided via an IP TV subsystem [Fig.8]

Whilst this opens up access to much enhanced service functionality, it also means that considerable amounts of personal data will be contained both within these networks and externally. As the elderly can be potentially more vulnerable than most of the population, system resilience, data security and personal privacy have to be in-built and set at a higher level than for the rest of the community.

As the enhanced levels of monitoring become more sophisticated and potentially beneficial in protecting the frail and allowing them to maintain their independence in their own home – with the confidence that support is always on hand brings to them. But it also radically raises the level of intrusion into their personal privacy [17].

This invasion of privacy is akin to that involved in clinical practice – except that in this case the privacy zone is external to the body concerned. It may well be that this should be protected using a variant of clinical ethically regulated in formed consent.

6.2 ‘Smart’ Wearables for a ‘Smart’ Environment

Despite the considerable benefits the “Smart Home” offers the ageing it also has a potential downside – in that increasing reliance on it can turn it into a “Smart Prison”!

However a solution to this dilemma lies in the convergence of leading-edge textiles design and manufacture with a combination of communications, computing and sensor technologies [18]. The stems from advances in the textiles field that allow both the integration of micro-electronics and conductive or optical fibres within fabrics, and that are also a capable of adapting their properties in response to external conditions or stimuli [19, 20].

Current research under the UK New Dynamics of Ageing programme is using this approach to develop a layered garment system that will function as a mobile communications platform, allowing the user to roam freely without loss of support service access [Fig.9] [21].

Working outward from the body surface the first layer incorporates a range of physiological monitoring devices, precisely located for maximum signal strength. These are linked back to a Bluetooth micro-module via conductive or optical fibres that are an integral part of this 3D knitted "Skinwear" for onwards transmission.

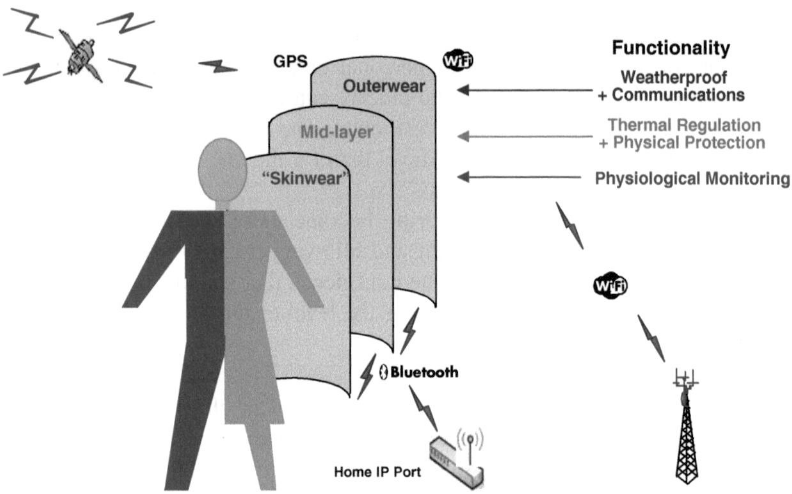

Fig.9 Smart Wearables – A Mobile Communications & Monitoring Platform

The next layer combines a variety of protective functionality whilst not compromising appearance or the style requirements of the wearer. Dependent on individual need garment may incorporate:

- autonomous self regulating thermal, moisture removal properties;
- textiles with intrinsic "memories" that accommodate abnormal "donning and doffing" movement whilst loss-lessly returning to their original shape
- materials that instantly change structure to absorb impact stresses.
- integral Bluetooth communications links as in "Skinwear"

The outer layer has all necessary weatherproof and thermal protection capabilities to deal with normal weather conditions, as well as acting as the mobile communications IP hub. Inter-layer Bluetooth communications traffic is transposed across to WiFi for external linkage via the hub.

Traffic within this layer is essentially identical to that of a distributed GPS-enabled mobile phone but minus the standard keyboard. The aim is to use the same approach pioneered in the Apple iPhone ideally with a flexible screen built into the forearm of the jacket. This allow the user to access a variety of map-based services to assist in travelling by public transport, roaming within the community, and locating required facilities in unfamiliar localities.

6.3 Help at Hand Anywhere

A further objective is to provide an open emergency channel link – similar to the "mayday" channel used by shipping until recently. This would replace the seemingly universally hated alarm pendant that is all too frequently is not being worn when an emergency occurs.

The incorporation of GPS provides the added benefit of being able to locate anyone who is incapacitated in anyway whilst away from home – especially those who rightly fear the day when memory loss or visual problems may strike and leave them stranded. In such circumstance their support service centre can either guide them home or call in help to collect them.

7 Embracing Change

Change is evolution by another name. In the healthcare service context it is primarily driven by social dynamics in terms of human interactions and life cycles, as well as by societal impacts and demands.

Treatment intervention processes advance in the same way through knowledge evolution, validation and dissemination and by subsequent interaction within the professions.

Behind the clinical scenes, computing and communications technologies that act as a key enabler in the collection, transfer, processing and distribution of information content continue to develop at an ever-increasing rate.

Currently these three domains generally remain in a state of semi-isolation, except where out of necessity they interact. As result these interactions are less than perfect as there is little on no one in a position to take a holistic view of what is inevitably an extremely complex and ever shifting situation. In the absence of such a perspective a range of well-intentioned initiatives are launched that tend to end up:

- meandering aimlessly through this maze ever seeking the way to their goals,
- causing loss of strategic impetus,
- duplicating effort and squandering scarce resources,
- siphoning off enormous sums of taxpayer funds to little effect,
- feeding mounting lost opportunity costs,
- failing to breakdown “silo” demarcation and secure effective interoperation
- hindering achievement of organisational goals, and mission objectives.

This needs to be clearly recognised to avoid continuing to court abject failure, which especially tend to centre on ICT-enabled projects with such monotonous regularity.

Since humans and their hugely variable idiosyncratic behaviours are the most obvious common factor, it is decidedly odd that this has remained largely ignored up until now.

7.1 Behavioural Compunetics

In attempt to resolve this dichotomy a new inter-disciplinary research subject has been created aimed as a convergence between:

- psychology of change;
- management science:
- process optimisation,
- risk management,
- benefits realisation;
- information management
- informatics

Initially the main thrust of this is focused on behavioural issues that have bedevilled and blighted so many healthcare initiatives.

The problem with change in human domains is that it generally works by accretion, slowly gathering acceptance and accelerating up to a tipping point after which it becomes the accepted norm. Unfortunately this slow, often stuttering, start at the outset is fuelled by an innate psychological reaction deeply imbedded in the comfort zone of the status quo, and coupled even deeper down in fear of the unknown.

The obvious counter to this is to focus on the motivational issues that open the way to acceptance. In broad terms these centre on the decision processes that inherently weigh the perceived scale of benefit against level of risk involved - from individual patient, carer and clinical interest perspectives, as well as those of the service provider organisations right through to those at the corporate level. However the codicil that is invariably attached to this is that desirable benefits must be achievable with minimum "pain" and problems to all those concerned.

In essence this comes down to determining how best to:

- present a cogent case for change
- win over the parties concerned
- gain a commitment adopt and implement the change whole-heartedly
- maintain the commitment through to securing the desired benefit/s

Whilst this is immediately recognisable as the exactly what a successful doctor -patient relationship is all about, it is surprising that this appears to be unrecognised as applicable in the wider sphere of care provision. In the circumstances the old clichés are somewhat apocryphal but apposite, i.e.:

"There are none so blind as cannot see"
"Physician heal thyself"

Although these are very basic antidotes, they point the way toward gaining a deeper understanding of the forces at work in highly complex and sophisticated organisations operating under great pressure in stressful life-and-death situations. In view of the enormous potential changes in the care-giving landscape that seem increasingly inevitable, the need will become ever more urgent to find an appropriate catalyst for change.

7.2 Process of Change and Change of Process

At its most basic virtually everything they we do or intend to do is a process. Almost invariably this involves a sequence of actions or events that can be mapped at a varying degrees of complexity as a source of reference for planning, modelling or analysis for whole range circumstances and situations.

A good example is a simplistic overview of some of issues involved in planning a process of change [22]. In this case the focus is how to move from the current "As Is" position to deliver the desired benefits of the intended "To Be" condition [Fig.10].

The starting point is the identification of benefits in the context of "downside" issues inherent in the existing situation in terms of:

- clinical practice constraints and deficits
- performance shortfalls and deficits

• knowledge transfer needs and change enabling requirements

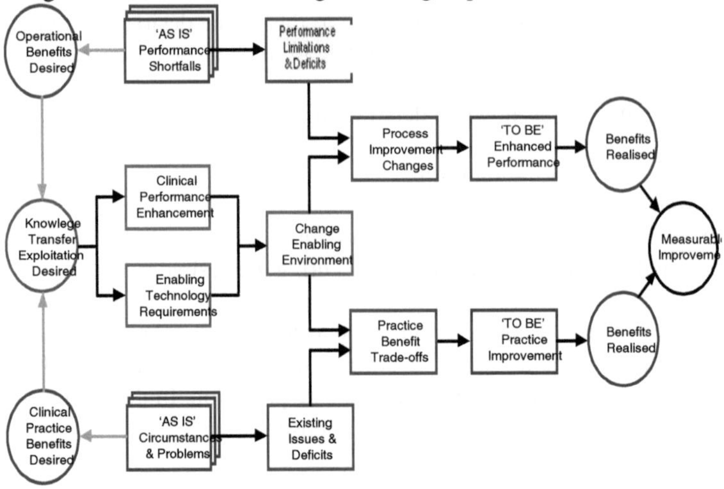

Fig.10 Benefits Realisation "Roadmap"

These in turn lead to identification of improvement requirements to deliver benefits via:

• clinical practice trade-offs
• support process changes

This concludes with the quantification and validation of the improvements achieved.

The important feature of this type of presentation - which is based on real cases – is its simplicity and avoidance of "technical" symbolism and semantics. This seemingly trivial point is particularly important particularly from a psychological point of view since clinicians and lay people tend to react strongly against what they perceive as demeaning use of "gobbledygook"!

7.3 A Whole Systems Approach

The key lessons to be drawn from this review is that radical change in the way health and social care is delivered is virtually inevitable, and that unless the problems of the current heavily blinkered "silo" oriented approach are dealt with quality of care may decline significantly.

The inference is that trends already underway are likely to radically shift care-giving away from a face-to-face patient contact, assessment, and treatment model to one that is likely to radically reduce "physical" contact and focus on trying to manage patient care increasingly via the Internet.

Whilst future circumstances may force the issue, the need is to manage change incrementally with sensitivity and considerable care. Achieving this needs a new way that help draw together the disparate components via a Whole Systems approach.

In essence this would firstly focus on the human domain issues through the development of Behavioural Compunetics techniques to engage all concerned.

Next would follow the development a "Systemic Management" approach that would act as a bridge between clinical/practice evolution and would guide supporting technology advances by working in far closer concert.

The final move would be to adapt the conventional Project Management approach to technology delivery to form a close back-to-back relationship with Behavioural Compunetics mentors to work together to support the change process.

References

[1] Annex B to eHealth-INTEROP Report in response to EU Mandate/403-2007: Patient and health practitioner identifiers. Ref DRAFT ESO_eHealthINTEROP_B0500_20080919.pdf, http://www.ehealth-interop.eu
[2] Manning, B.R.M.: Identity Framework. ISO TC215 WG1/WG4 Task Group Leader's Discussion Draft. Joint ISO/CEN Meeting. Goteborg (May 2008)
[3] Manning, B.R.M.: Human Identites. ISO TC215 WG1/WG4 Task Group Leader's Discussion Draft. Joint ISO/CEN Meeting. Istanbul (October 2008)
[4] BSI ISO/IEC 19794 series. Information technology. Biometric data interchange formats, http://www.bsi-global.com/en/Standards-and-Publications/Industry-Sectors/Biometrics/Biometrics/BS-ISOIEC-19795-series/
[5] HON Code of Conduct (HONcode) for medical and health Web sites. Health on the Net Foundation, http://www.hon.ch/
[6] Stosuy, G.A., Eaglin, J.P.: The Community Services Network: Creating an integrated Service Delivery Network - The Baltimore open systems laboratory model. New Technology in the Human Services 12(1-2), 87–98 (1999)
[7] European Interoperability Framework for Pan-European eGovernment Services - Draft for Public Comments – As Basis for Version 2.0 (15/07/2008), http://europa.eu.int/idabc/3761
[8] CEN/ISSS Workshop Agreement on Discovery of and Access to eGovernment Resource (WS/eGov Share), http://www.cen.eu/CENORM/sectors/sectors/isss/activity/egov_share.asp
[9] ETSI Specialist Task Force STF 352, Personalization of eHealth systems by using eHealth User Profiles. Terms of Reference (2008) (ToR352v04_HF_EC_eHea#27B739.doc)

[10] Kun, L., Coatrieux, G., Ouantin, C., Beauscart, R.: Improving outcomes with interoperable EHRs and secure global health information infrastructure. In: Medical and Care Compunetics 5. Studies in Health technology and Informatics, vol. 137. IOS Press, Amsterdam (2008)
[11] Commission of the European Communities [COM(2004) 356]: e-Health. - making healthcare better for European citizens: An action plan for a European e-Health Area, http://europa.eu.int/idabc/3761
[12] Manning, B.R.M.: Coping with increasing infirmity: Smarter smart support. In: Healthcare Computing 2008, Harrogate (April 2008)
[13] Towards an Inclusive Future. In: Roe, P.R.W. (ed.) Impact and wider potential of information and communication technologies, COST, Brussels, pp. 92–898 (2007)
[14] Roe, P.R.W. (ed.): Bridging the Gap? Access to telecommunications for all people. Presses Centrales, Lausanne.S.A (2001), http://www.tiresias.org/phoneability/bridging_the_gap/
[15] The Ambient Assisted Living (AAL) Joint Programme. AAL International Association c/o IWT Bischoffsheimlaan 25, 1000 Brussels Belgium, http://www.aal-europe.eu/
[16] Bowes, A., McColgan, G.: Smart technology and community care for older people: innovation in West Lothian, Scotland (August 2006) Age Concern Scotland ISBN: 1-874399-99-9
[17] Official Journal of the European Communities - Directive 2002/58/EC of the European Parliament and of the Council of 12 July 2002 concerning the processing of personal data and the protection of privacy in the electronic communications sector (Directive on privacy and electronic communications) L 201/37, http://eurlex.europa.eu/pri/en/oj/dat/2002/l_201/l_20120020731en00370047.pdf
[18] McCann, J., Hurford, R., Martin, A.: A Design Process for the Development of Innovative Smart Clothing that Addresses End-User Needs from Technical, Functional, Aesthetic and Cultural View Points. In: Proceedings of IEEE International Symposium on Wearable Computers, Osaka, Japan, October 18-21 (2005), http://www2.computer.org/portal/web/csdl/doi/10.1109/ISWC.2005.3
[19] Ibrahim, S.M., et al.: Fundamental relationship of fabric extensibility to anthropometric requirements and garment performance. Textile Research Journal 36, 37–47 (1966)
[20] McCann, J., Hurford, R., Martin, A., Davison, J., Cassim, J.: How can form and function become invisible in clothing design? A proposal for a design process 'tree' for functional apparel (2005); Include OS, London, April 5-8 (2005), http://www.hhrc.rca.ac.uk/programmes/include/2005
[21] Manning, B.R.M., McCann, J., Benton, S., Bougourd, J.: Active Ageing: Independence through Technology Assisted Health Optimisation. In: Medical and Care Compunetics 5. Studies in Health technology and Informatics, vol. 137, IOS Press, Amsterdam (2008)
[22] Manning, B.R.M., Benton, S.: The Safe Implementation of Research into Healthcare Practice. In: Medical and Care Compunetics 5. Studies in Health technology and Informatics, vol. 137. IOS Press, Amsterdam (2008)

Recommended Reading List

Mobility

- Annex B to eHealth-INTEROP Report in response to EU Mandate/403-2007: Patient and health practitioner identifiers.
  Ref DRAFT ESO_eHealthINTEROP_B0500_20080919.pdf
  http://www.ehealth-interop.eu

Interoperability

- European Interoperability Framework for Pan-European eGovernment Services - Draft for Public Comments – As Basis for Version 2.0 - 15/07/2008
  http://europa.eu.int/idabc/3761
- CEN/ISSS Workshop Agreement on Discovery of and Access to eGovernment Resource (WS/eGov Share)
  http://www.cen.eu/CENORM/sectors/sectors/isss/activity/egov_share.asp
- eHealth-INTEROP Report in response to EU Mandate/403-2007:
  Ref DRAFT ESO_eHealthINTEROP_v0500_20080919.pdf
  http://www.ehealth-interop.eu

Community Care

- e-Health - making healthcare better for European citizens: An action plan for a European e-Health Area. Commission of the European Communities [COM(2004) 356]:
  http://europa.eu.int/idabc/3761

'Smart' Care Support

'Smart Home' Systems

- Towards an Inclusive Future. Impact and wider potential of information and communication technologies. Edited by Patrick R.W.Roe, COST, Brussels. (2007) ISBN:92-898-0027.
  http://www.tiresias.org/cost219ter/inclusive_future/inclusive_future_book.pdf
- Bridging the Gap? Access to telecommunications for all people (Ed) Patrick R.W.Roe, Presses Centrales, Lausanne.S.A (2001)
  ISBN:1-96048-0209
  http://www.tiresias.org/phoneability/bridging_the_gap/

'Smart' Wearables

- Intelligent Textiles and Clothing. (Ed) Mattila H.R., Woodhead Publishing, Cambridge, UK (2006) ISBN: 978-1-84569-005-2
- Textiles for Protection. (Ed) Scott R.A (2005) Woodhead Publishing, Cambridge, UK. ISBN: 978-1-85573-921-5

Personalizing Care: Integration of Hospital and Homecare

Isabel Román[a,b], Jorge Calvillo[b,a], and Laura M. Roa[a,b]

[a] University of Seville

[b] Network Center of Biomedical Research in Bioengineering, Biomaterials and Nanomedicine (CIBER-BBN)

Escuela Superior de Ingenieros, Camino de los Descubrimientos S/N,
41092 Sevilla, Spain
isabel@trajano.us.es

Abstract. Hospital and homecare must be understood as a necessary conjunction to accomplish efficient personalized care. In this sense, the integration of hospital and homecare protocols and technologies should be considered from the moment that they begin to be designed. The proliferation of healthcare units and services complicates this task, as multiple administrative domains can be found, usually spread out in multiple technology domains, difficult to integrate. This hard integration requires a well defined middleware where heterogeneous and autonomous components must be included. The design of this middleware observing well accepted international standards is a cornerstone for the successful deployment. This chapter makes a review of the concept of personalized medicine, the main research trends in hospital and homecare and it finally proposes some approaches to design architectures providing healthcare scenarios and knowledge integration.

Table of contents

K. Yogesan et al. (Eds.): Handbook of Digital Homecare, BIOMED, pp. 33–52.
springerlink.com

Introduction: The concept of personalized medicine

The increase of life expectancy and consequent population ageing are changing healthcare delivery to new models that involve several factors, some of which can be listed as follows:

- The diseases model is evolving from acute and unique to chronic and multiple. The number of elderly patients grows. This kind of patient usually suffers from one or several chronic diseases that obviously need continuity in the care, in hospital and home, and the attention of several specialized healthcare suppliers.
- From the economical point of view efficient protocols and technologies for an effective homecare are crucial. Homecare could be cheaper than hospital care, but only if the involved technology is not expensive and the healthcare suppliers, as well as the patient and his/her possible carers, are correctly trained in the use of new technologies and in the protocols to follow.
- The interaction of patients and their carers grows when the care is moved to the home. Their perception about the evolution of their illness, quality of life, the received healthcare assistance … could be considered in a more efficient way.
- Healthcare is evolving from the merely healing point of view to the prevention and the improvement of the quality of life. Medicine is being personalized to the needs of a particular subject of care. Referring to homecare, this implies that interaction with care technologies must be personalized too.

Personalized medicine could be defined as the effective management of the available knowledge and the most adequate healthcare provision for a particular person in a specific moment and context. It is rooted in the hypothesis that diseases are heterogeneous, from their causes to their response to drugs. Each person's disease might be unique and therefore that person needs to be treated as an individual [1].

Although the term personalized medicine is frequently linked in the literature to biomedical technologies such as pharmacogenetics, pharmacogenomics, pharmacoproteomics, metabolomics, RNA interference, cell and gene therapies or nanobiotechnology, a more open concept of personalized medicine must include many other multiple sciences and technologies involved in healthcare provision. Since this concept is not exclusive of sick people, in addition to the care of pathologies, other aspects, as prevention, are also considered.

Numerous challenges must be addressed to make personalized medicine a reality and replace the traditional practice of medicine. Personalized medicine will imply radical changes in the pharmaceutical industry and medical practice, and it is likely to affect many aspects of society. The early stages of research including, but not limited to, diagnostic, disease monitoring, drug response and prognostic, will be linked with the later stages of clinical development. In the short term, clinical trials might be conducted in specialized units where detailed clinical, biological and genomic data are collected and integrated. Molecular, pharmacological, patient clinical data and best available evidence will be captured at various phases and integrated into a 'knowledge management system' that will consider all this knowledge and will assist the clinician in the delivery of quite personalized assistance.

In order to cover the most important aspects related to personalized medicine two main issues could be considered: personalization of care decisions and personalization of the interaction with the subject of care.

Personalized care decision can be described as a customized care plan for a particular subject. The consideration of all the circumstances about the subject of care must be combined with the best knowledge. As far as subject of care is concerned, the issues to be considered could be, among others: past history, genetic predisposition, environmental conditions, current symptoms, laboratory and other diagnostic test results and therapy response. Regarding the use of explicit knowledge of interest for the subject of care, the availability, confidence and understanding of the best current knowledge is essential, but also the capacity for generating new personalized implicit knowledge.

Personalization of the interaction with the subject of care is referred to several aspects. One issue that could be emphasized is the development of the best scenario for the care of a particular person, including the home, outdoor settings, the hospital or a combination of these. The use of the most suitable therapies, procedures, technologies and interfaces for a particular subject is fundamental too.

Protocols and technologies for personalized medicine

Personalization of care decisions

In traditional research techniques, the randomization process removes particular circumstances of individual cases and creates a knowledge gap between the evidence and future application instances. The consequence is that evidence based on any statistical approach is best applicable at the population level rather than at the individual level. But in personalized medicine it is necessary to manage individual, or instance-specific, knowledge. This refers to particular and contextualized facts and observations about individuals and it is very well applicable to real problems, because it uniquely identifies and precisely matches an application context. The hypothesis that the individual knowledge captured from a very specific context can be extrapolated to similar contexts and applied to individual problem solving supports a Case Based Reasoning (CBR) approach. Individual knowledge processing, or CBR, has become increasingly important for artificial intelligence applications and it is defined as the approach to solving new problems based on the solutions of similar past problems [2].

To increase the chances for a successful solution to a new problem, decreasing the knowledge gap and instantiation uncertainty, it is necessary a high similarity between contexts. The precision of context specification could be significantly improved with the use of the individual's molecular profiles and biomarkers. A biomarker is a specific biological trait in a subject, such as the level of a hormone or molecule, which can be measured for predisposition testing, disease screening and prognostic assessment, as well as to predict and monitor drug response [3]. Currently most used biomarkers are proteins, mRNA-expression profiling, single nucleotide polymorphisms and small molecules.

Emerging genomic and proteomic technologies are now resulting in the molecular sub-classification of disease as the basis for diagnosis, prognosis, and therapeutic selection. Bioinformatics assists in biomarker identification by providing integrated sources of genetic and genomic information associated with an array of potential biomarkers. These techniques, together with statistical advances, are needed to extract the most relevant data from the richness of molecular information generated by the new technologies. Another important aspect is an adequate validation of the enormous number of candidate biomarkers that will emerge from the studies. This will require access to large, and in some cases, prospective collections of well annotated clinical samples with appropriate consent and security issues addressed.

Molecular markers that predict the variation of the efficacy and toxicity of therapeutic compounds could be extremely useful in clinical trials, drug development and clinical practice, because they would allow the identification of patients who would benefit most from a drug. Pharmacogenomics can be defined as the application of whole-genome technologies for the prediction of the sensitivity or resistance of an individual's disease to a single drug or group of drugs. However, the discovery of these markers is not sufficient and the delivery of successful personalized medicine for completely individualized diagnosis, treatment and prognosis, will require the careful integration of biomarkers discovery and validation programs into drug discovery and clinical development programs [4,5].

Another key challenge for genetics is the study of polygenic diseases, where susceptibility to the disease results from the interaction of multiple genes rather than the action of a single gene. One of the key technologies is large-scale mRNA expression profiling by using oligonucleotide or cDNA microarrays. These devices enable the provision of complex molecular profiles of patient tissues. Bioinformatics tools help physicians to make sense of these profiles. The goal is to learn expression signatures that enable diagnosis or prognosis. This is a traditional problem in pattern recognition techniques such as data mining and artificial intelligence.

A relevant problem is that gene-to-sample ratios are typically in the hundreds hence there are far more genes on the arrays than patients in the study. A straightforward solution is extensive gene selection up to the point where fewer genes than samples are examined. It is important to note that gene selection introduces a bias in the diagnostic model, nevertheless access to the individual's information supposes an important increase of patients in the training set and reduces the need of gene selection improving the conclusions of studies [6]. Therefore, to realize the vision of personalized medicine, the agenda for medical and pharmaceutical research must include the assembly and integration of data from many sources on large numbers of patients. Clinical investigations should incorporate genotyping and molecular profiling technologies together with traditional clinical data collection and they should establish repositories of patient samples where possible. Of course, in this data-intensive scenario, where data sets are large and highly heterogeneous, there are crucial challenges to create knowledge from data such as representation of data that is suitable for integration or computational inference [7].

Environmental factors interact with genetic factors in a complex way for many diseases. This implies that, in addition to genetic and molecular information, context specification for efficient CBR must include these variables, like diet or lifestyle, as well as other relevant information. Linking genotypes to phenotypes is an important step to disease understanding and the combination of genome and biomarkers research with relevant personal information represents the substrate for the future personalized medicine [8]. Indeed, collections of patient cases are the focus of research in Electronic Healthcare Record (EHR) systems. Envisioned as complete collections of patient-specific data, the operational capture of genetic and molecular information during the delivery of patient care will create new opportunities to EHR enhancing CBR for decisions support. But despite the promising pilot studies, the integration of clinical and genomic information to support the delivery of patient care is not a routine yet. In their current state, EHR and other clinical information systems are not suited to the optimal management of patient-specific genomic information [9]. Genomic results have lifelong value and can affect decision making for family members. Different developments are necessary for the realization of the "genome-enabled electronic healthcare record" for care personalization, for example: improved tools to support the acquisition of genomic results as generated by molecular diagnostic and cytogenetic methods, ontologies appropriate for the description of all the multi-level clinically relevant concepts, from molecular to systemic, and applications capable of enabling clinicians to access and process the whole relevant knowledge to support their decision making. Finally, advances must be effectively transferred to the clinical environment.

Treatment and therapy decisions have been the focus in traditional healthcare approaches but new paradigms considered the importance of personalized prevention and recommendations. The ultimate goal of personalized medicine is to define disease at the molecular level so that preventive resources and therapeutic agents can be directed at the right population of people while they are still well. The challenge is to provide a suite of markers that can be used to assess one's lifetime risk of developing disease in the presence of various environmental variables and to provide the adequate recommendations for this particular person. The focus of medicine will be preventive. Lifestyle modifications and the use of prophylactic therapy will be recommended based on what is best for that patient to avoid chronic disease to which they could be susceptible. Patients will be more knowledgeable of their own health and risk profiles and more active in directing their own healthcare and will become more informed and demanding consumers [10].

The study of the pointed questions of life-science and the desire to collect and disseminate highly sensitive genetic and other personal information pertaining to biomedical research raise a number of important and non-trivial issues related to ethics, patient confidentiality as well as legal and social implications that must be considered in this new scenario. Even if anonymization is enforced, a specific person could be traced back either exactly or probabilistically, due to the amount of remaining information available. Governments must play an active role in addressing public concern over genetic information by, among other alternatives, drafting legislation to protect patients from discrimination by employers and insurance companies, or by encouraging pharmaceutical industry no to forget research in diseases that affect to little population.

The education and engagement of physicians and patients in this new paradigm is necessary too to be able to accomplish the diverse interdisciplinary challenges that are being faced nowadays and in the future. To widen the success of personalized medicine bioscientists and physicians need skills in biological and computer sciences.

Personalization of the interaction with the subject of care

The emergence of technologies that improve communications and human-machine interfaces provides the bases for pervasive computing, which enters the physical world and bridges the gap between the virtual and physical worlds. This concept could be best described by means of its three most important enabling technologies: ubiquitous computing, ubiquitous communication, and intelligent user-friendly interfaces [11].

- Ubiquitous computing refers to concepts such as the disappearing computer, in the sense that they are everywhere, and means integration of computing power and sensing into anything, including not only traditional computers, and devices, but also into everyday objects like furniture, household items or toys.
- Ubiquitous communication, in turn, means enabling anytime, anywhere communication of anything with anything else, not only people but also devices and any artefact. Central technologies in ubiquitous communication are ad-hoc networking and wireless communication technologies.

– Intelligent user-friendly interfaces enable natural interaction and control of the environment by the human "users", or inhabitants of the ambient environment. The interfaces support natural communication, take into account user preferences, personality, and usage context, and enable multisensory interaction.

Some researches use the term ambient intelligence, which refers to the presence of an environment that is sensitive, adaptive, and responsive to the presence of people or objects [12]. It aims to take the advances provided by pervasive computing one step further by realizing environments that are sensitive and responsive to the presence of people. The target is to make electronic devices disappear into the user environments, virtual devices are necessary to support a natural interaction of the user with the dissolved electronics. This new paradigm aims to improve people's quality of life by creating the desired atmosphere and functionality through intelligent, personalized, interconnected systems and services [13].

The application of pervasive computing and ambient intelligence technologies in healthcare environments is another cornerstone in personalized medicine, in the sense that these developments improve human/system interfaces making the system adapt to a particular user in a specific context, but not vice-versa. Interaction mode must be suited to the needs of the particular individual for which it is intended considering context, personal characteristics and even social and psychological aspects. This personalization is related to any user including patients, healthcare professionals and citizens in general.

One of the most important application areas for these technologies in healthcare is the support to independent living and wellness and disease management. The target population is composed by patients with chronic diseases and especially elderly people, a fragile patient who usually suffers numerous disorders, generally chronic. This population group could improve significantly their quality of life and the alleviation of risk at home or even outdoor by using personalized healthcare systems.

Considering the increase of life expectancy in developed countries, and the consequent population ageing, the health sector must face the challenges associated with a growing population group of elderly and comorbidity patients. Problems in supporting the quality of life in this ageing population must be solved. In addition to their increased levels of physical fragility and cognitive problems, elderly persons may also face various other problems, such as hearing and motor limitations, which could constrain their ability to interact with a computer system.

Of course, there is a huge variation in the skills and abilities of the subjects of care, and these may vary over time even for a single person. Adaptable and natural interaction, such as speech/audio and vision, gives users the possibility of developing useful and meaningful dialogues in different modes of communication and allows the switching between dialogue modes at any time smoothly and naturally [14].

Several technologies and researches are involved in such scenario. Microsensitive monitoring for environmental conditions and person's location permit the development of contextually aware systems that use rich predictive models of human behaviour from sensor data, enabling the environment to be aware of the activities performed within it. This helps the system to decide about the type of assistance to provide, to choose the mode and dialogue for interaction to "fit" the user's requirements and activity more appropriately and even to anticipate the user's preferences without conscious mediation. Developments in wearable or embedded sensors, and more generally measurement technology, make possible to monitor physiological parameters [15], such as pulse, skin temperature, and blood pressure, and lifestyle information in daily life and to trigger urgent assistance when necessary. Intelligent and suitable actuators could assist in different activities such as environmental control, medication administration or lifestyle recommendations to ensure the health and safety of the person including preventative healthcare opportunity [13].

Nowadays, interesting researches in the development of appropriate, non obtrusive and easy to wear and operate sensors and actuators can be accessible in the literature. RFID and computer vision are examples of technologies being considered in this context [16].

Ubiquitous communication based on mobile networks, different wireless technologies and mobile devices makes it possible to transfer and access of all kinds of information anywhere and anytime, and it is a key issue in the development of assistive healthcare technologies in home or even outdoor. Natural language and voice processing are other researches that could support pervasive computing.

In addition to this personalization for the patient, which offers people the ability to experience the benefits of sheltered housing from their own home, by giving them some control and flexibility over their private living arrangements, personalization for healthcare professionals interaction with the system could be improved with pervasive computing.

The coordination and collaboration among specialists with different areas of expertise, an intense information exchange, and the mobility of hospital staff, patients, documents and equipment imply that hospitals are convenient settings for the deployment of pervasive computing technology. Clinicians require access to complete patient information as well as medical knowledge for ''just-in-time'' and at the point of care. Ubiquitous computing techniques could provide accurate, timely and context-aware interaction with the global knowledge infrastructure to support the adequate decision-making [17].

Another important advance in the use of adaptable and natural interaction between the clinician and the system is the better perception from the patient viewpoint. For example, by using speech instead of the keyboard the interview with the patient could be done as a natural dialogue without the interferences that writing in a computer could represent.

Technologies and knowledge at home

Homecare is emerging as an adequate solution to meet population ageing and chronic assistance requirements and to make lighter the increase in healthcare cost. The ultimate technology advances allow healthcare delivery to be transferred from the hospital and clinic to the home.

Homecare is not only conceived to cure illness but promoting wellness in all the stages of life. The personalization of procedures, protocols and interfaces is especially relevant at home. The individual and his/her carers can participate in a more active way in health management and they are actively willing to receive feedback regarding health status and take part in the care process. For example, a diabetic subject could monitor his/her blood glucose values, store the results in a database and receive feedback such as an advice of changes in the diet to improve the blood glucose balance. Technology can meet people needs at home providing safety and independence. It can help in safety because remote monitoring systems, for example, can acquire vital signs and send an alarm call to the hospital without human intervention when an abnormal variation of them is produced. And independence is not obstructed thanks to the advances in miniaturization that allow the use of sensors which do not interfere with the activities of daily living.

Finally, the development of intelligent systems that learn behaviour patterns based on the subject's daily life or that monitor vital signs in real-time and process the results facilitates a more personalized care. The physician can know anytime the patient's conditions and not exclusively in the visit time. Furthermore, in an emergency case that requires a hospital visit, healthcare providers can access to the whole record of vital signs of the patient that comprises months or even years.

Main research fields in the homecare context

In recent years, many research groups around the world have paid attention to homecare and, as a consequence, new research trends are being developed ranging from wearable sensors to smart homes and assistance robotics. Each project tries to solve particular problems, such as elderly people living in their homes, patients suffering from cognitive impairments, for example Alzheimer disease, schizophrenia or brain injuries, or people who simply want to monitor their wellness.

Important issues to be considered in the home scenario are sensors and actuators, wireless communications or local information process. In most cases, the home is connected to an external system that provides professional assistance thanks to the information collected from home. This implies the need to consider network technologies to access these systems and technologies for an optimum management of the knowledge about the subject of care.

The use of wearable sensors for homecare is one of the most important research fields. Improvements in sensor technology and wireless communications allow sensors with a minimal form factor to be manufactured to measure a wide variety of physical parameters and they can be embedded within, for example, a ring or a wristwatch [18]. Their cost and power consumption are being reduced and this facilitates their introduction in the healthcare domain.

On the other hand, we can find smart homes projects which generally intend to monitor subjects with motor, visual, auditory or cognitive disabilities [19]. In each case, the home and its various electrical appliances have been fitted with sensors, actuators and/or biomedical monitors, so that several parameters can be analyzed from displacements in the home through a set of basic sensors to complete health monitoring system based on embedded sensors in the home furnishing and structures. Many projects in this field require an observation period (generally weeks or months) of the monitored individual in order to establish behaviour patterns. These records will allow observing deviations in the health status and evaluating some activities of the daily life such as eating, dressing, hygiene, etc.

Robotics is often associated with smart homes but it can meet different purposes. The robots in these homes can perform useful activities, for example, by easing the independence of elderly people, and/or serving as companions to ease the burden of social isolation. Although the use of robots is highly developed in the industry as effective workers, in the home environment this field is at an early stage but the increasing interest in introducing them in the home to solve specific situation will promote the development of assistive robots.

Technologies and infrastructures to solve particular problems

With the developments described above, many variables from individuals could be measured in their own environment, during daily activities, and to observe deviations in health status in early phases or to alert in emergency cases such as falls in the elderly. To achieve this, it is necessary to count on technologies and infrastructures which are able to monitor the patient's vital signs and to store and analyze those data to obtain results about the conditions of the monitored individual. Sensors and measurements are already available, but a complete health monitoring system is required. Many projects around the world have solved particular situations and developed specific technologies and they are an interesting initial point.

The approaches of solutions based on wearable sensors range from the biomedical sensors that monitor patients twenty-four hours per day to location systems that prevent elderly or cognitive disabled patients from getting lost.

Many projects are focused on working biomedical sensors into textiles, equipped with data storage and a wireless transceiver system. The data are automatically collected and sent to a central processing unit without the intervention of a third party. These systems are being developed in the form of a textile garment, a ring, a wrist-worn device, a chest belt, etc. Among the general physiological parameters that can be collected with them are ECG, temperature, blood oxygen saturation, blood pressure, breathing control and others [20]. More specific projects have been able to develop tools to measure the EEG for patients suffering from epilepsy and to alert of variations, to monitor patients with chronic obstructive pulmonary disease according to the patient's motor functions by using accelerometers, to quantify stress in terms of heart rate variability, to make automatic measurements of glucose for patients suffering from diabetes, etc [19].

All these systems can store a limited amount of data, but it is required that they can connect with an external system that stores and manages all the collected data. To achieve this, wireless technologies have been used because they allow developing tools with a high autonomy degree both indoor and outdoor. Reduction of power consumption, size and cost are challenges to improve these technologies.

The introduction of different kinds of sensors in the home environment has brought the development of intelligent and interactive homes. Among the most recent projects in this field we can find several different purposes to cover. On the one hand, we have the maximization of comfort that although it is not exactly a homecare target, it can promote the independence of elderly and disabled people. One of the most interesting projects focused on comfort tries to develop an adaptive house that uses neural networks to control temperature, heating and lighting by monitoring the environment and observing actions taken by the residents. The system attempts to economize energy resources while respecting the lifestyle and preferences of its inhabitants.

On the other hand, there are several projects that solve particular problems by using assistive technologies. For example projects aiming to enable elderly people to live at home by creating a smart and comfortable environment by using assistive technologies. Thus, the researches collect data about residents' health and physiological signs by equipping the bathroom with fully automated medical devices. The physical activity is monitored by placing infrared sensors in the rooms and magnetic switches in the doors. Other projects develop location systems to assist people suffering from dementia, systems that monitor human activity to detect unusual events, etc.

Finally, the application of robotics in the homecare has promoted some interesting projects usually focused on the disabled and elderly people. In this field there are developments of more autonomous chairs that can be controlled by residual movements of the patient, robots suitable for assistance to everyday tasks such as picking up objects from the floor or getting dishes from shelves, or assistive robots that act as routine activities reminders (eating, going to the bathroom, ...) and guide patients through their environment.

The challenges of homecare

Homecare is at an early stage but a complete revolution can take place in the short term. Until this happens, researchers must overcome different challenges that comprise technological, legal, commercial and ethical features.

First of all, identifying and satisfying the needs of the user is a major challenge in research and development on homecare technologies. Moreover, user acceptance is the key to successful diffusion among the general public. In this case, not only the subject of care must be taken into account but other actors such as the subject's immediate surroundings (family and neighbours, caregivers) and the manufacturers.

The reliability of measurement systems is an important problem related to homecare too. As the mobility, activity and vital signs of a monitored subject will be processed by algorithms to detect and signal dangerous situations, the accuracy of the input data is paramount. As for rehabilitation robots, these devices must be adapted to the handicap of the person requiring their services. The system should be easy to learn, reliable and user-friendly.

Another problem is the wide variety of communication networks that are nowadays available in the market and the lack of interoperability among different systems. This makes most of the projects to be isolated and that many efforts cannot be reutilized in other researches. It is necessary to establish the most suitable communication infrastructure for a given personal monitoring system.

In the development of effective homecare we can also identify legal and ethical issues because when it comes to distributed healthcare, a state has to protect its citizens from the possibility of malpractice. The barrier that separates the patient's home from the public vanishes and it is important to verify that the lines of communication are safe and secure. Furthermore, the transmitted data must be uncorrupted to ensure their correct interpretation and high quality care.

Future developments in homecare

Over the last twenty years progress in wired and wireless home networking, sensor networks, networked appliances, mechanical and control engineering and computers has been awesome. These advances continue taking place and they will not stop in the near future.

According to some authors, the next generation of wireless and network solutions will resolve many of the interoperability problems, changing the structure of homecare delivery systems. Besides, sensors will be smaller, cheaper and surely more and more powerful and this will allow applications more advanced and complicated. It will be possible to develop interface technologies of human intentions, feelings and situation, to improve system knowledge, and to enhance homecare systems in order to obtain a more personalized care.

Technologies and knowledge at the hospital

The situation

Nowadays traditional healthcare systems are being reviewed according to the need of improving the quality of care and to be more efficient. The usage of clinical computer systems for medical work in the hospital has shown that computer technology designed for the office is inadequate when used in a hospital setting because of the features inherent to this work: extreme mobility, ad hoc collaboration, interruptions, high degree of communication, etc. [21]. Hence, it is required to create new concepts of computer systems in a hospital environment.

Wireless technologies can solve these problems and change the healthcare model from a traditional hospital to an interactive hospital, where clinicians can access relevant medical information and can collaborate with colleagues and patients, with independence of time, place, and whatever they are doing.

Solutions of particular problems

There are some projects which aim at solving particular problems of medical work in hospitals. As in the case of homecare, each research group meets solutions focused on specific situations and in many cases, these solutions make the interoperability unachieved. In spite of that, many efforts should be considered as necessary steps in order to change all the healthcare system.

An example of particular problem which can be solved by developing new technologies is the basic clinical setting of the hospital where physician and nurses are required to move about the hospital in order to perform their activities. In case of emergency, this event makes necessary to call the clinician on duty usually by means of mobile phone with the time delay that it would mean. This situation is worse in patients hospitalized in Intensive Care Unit. To overcome these problems a wireless telecare system can be developed [22]. Recent innovations in wireless technologies now make it possible to equip healthcare professionals with personal digital assistants that enable access to a wide range of medical information over a wireless LAN in real-time.

Another research trend is the use of sensors to monitor hospitalized patients in real-time and the integration of systems in the patient's bed. Besides collecting all vital signs from the patient, we can equip the bed with various sensors that can identify the patient lying in the bed, the clinician standing beside it, or enhance the experience of a disabled patient with the use of assistive robots.

Challenges and future developments

Many challenges must be addressed to achieve the completely interactive hospital. First of all, it is required to develop an infrastructure which allows the deployment of heterogeneous clinical computer systems. The infrastructure must support clinicians to move around freely inside and outside the hospital, while maintaining their computational environment intact. Moreover, it must ensure the interoperability of the many different clinical systems in use at a hospital, providing basic mechanisms for developers of clinical systems to create highly integrated systems.

Anyway, the most ideal condition for a physician is to have in the point of care all the patient's clinical data, including medical records, laboratory test results, medication lists and so on. To achieve this, a comprehensive electronic health record that provides a common platform for the storage and retrieval of medical information needs to be in place. Furthermore, another challenge related to health information systems is the need of uniform integration and communication of data since different types of devices generate diverse formats of data. Therefore, the uniform integration is a serious challenge in the health domain.

Finally, the management of enormous amount of biosignal data collected by sensors in real-time is beyond the human capacity and it is required a machine abstraction of data to the effective handling of them. The automatic interpretation of the measured data will be a major problem too. Among the recorded data, the health system should detect abnormal findings and give warning messages to the responsible personnel. Information technologies are the key for the required reasoner systems but their development is far from being a reality.

Architecture for integration

A hard integration of devices and systems involved in the care of a subject is the cornerstone for an efficient management of the knowledge provided by all of them. This integration must ensure that knowledge management features consider any relevant information stored in any system, and that they could be implemented in every healthcare scenario. This implies that global access to knowledge and networking capacities are needed.

Several aspects make this hard integration difficult to be accomplished, but three factors could be specially remarked: there are heterogeneous technological domains, difficult to interoperate; there are different policies in the administrative domains; finally, the knowledge to integrate refers to very different semantic domains.

Management of technology by healthcare organizations

The structure of the individual health care centre, and particularly of the hospitals, is evolving from a vertical, aggregated organisation, towards the integration of a set of specialised departments, which are characterised by diverse logistic, organisational, technical and clinical requirements and aspects.

Until the 1970s, medical informatics researches were mostly focused on small and functionally limited applications for special departments of a hospital and were mainly dealing with 'departmental information systems'. From that moment they were already able to have broader views on such information systems, considering the information processing in a hospital as a whole; therefore 'hospital information systems' were considered too. Already starting in the 1990s and in this decade, researches and practical works are starting to focus on considering information processing in the healthcare regions, mostly in a rather global sense considering 'health information systems'.

The transition from local to regional and global architectures fortunately correlates with the intentions of many healthcare authorities to improve quality and efficiency of care through the development of adequate organizational frameworks that support patient-centered, not institution-oriented, shared care strategies. These strategies will include, among others, exploring networking care facilities in health regions, diagnostic and therapeutic telemedicine, as well as health monitoring and homecare [23].

Knowledge and business logic common to different sectors of the healthcare organisation shall therefore be integrated in a specific architectural layer of the underlying information system and shall be accessible through services based on public and stable interfaces. The ultimate objective of such a structure is to build an open federation of complementary heterogeneous systems, spread over the territory, individually autonomous but also capable of interworking to effectively meet different needs in the healthcare environment as care, social, research or administrative, increasing the overall effectiveness of the activities carried out.

Middleware approach

The goal of integration can be achieved through a unified, open architecture based on a middleware independent from specific applications and capable of integrating knowledge and business logic, and of making them available to diverse, multi-vendor applications. According to the integration objectives at organisational level, all aspects of the healthcare structure must be supported by the architecture, that must therefore be able to comprise all relevant information and all business workflows, structuring them according to criteria and paradigms independent from specific sectorial aspects, temporary requirements or technological solutions. The architecture is intended as a basis both for working with existing systems, allowing specific models to be integrated, as well as for the planning and construction of new systems [24].

Some questions arise in this new scenario: technical availability, quality of data, referential integrity, multiple types of data modelling, interfacing, quality of functionality, in particular concerning the support of healthcare processes and problems of transcription. Last, but not least, the ease of use of computer-based tools regarding data input and data usability for healthcare professionals in their daily work.

Standardization is crucial for integration. Standards already exist and will continue being defined for supporting specific requirements, both in terms of in situ user operations and with respect to communication procedures. Some healthcare middleware approaches are developed by standardization organizations, like CEN [24-26] or OMG [27]. Nevertheless, these architectures are domain specific and mainly based on the rigid description of information models and interfaces identified as fundamental in the healthcare environment. This paradigm makes difficult the integration of systems not compliant with these standards, needing the development of specific interceptors, or the inclusion of new facilities not considered when the standard middleware was described.

Some general architectures for distributed computing are focusing on the development of universal middlewares where any new service or application could be integrated easily. These are based on semantic techniques for the description of component's behaviour and the management of domain ontologies. Semantic Web and Semantic Grid are those where more research is current. The use of these technologies as the underlying middleware for health and medical systems could be crucial in the consecution of a global infrastructure that facilitate health knowledge management wherever and whenever it were needed. They key in these ontological strategies is close to artificial intelligence idea: the use of flexible ontology languages that provide the capacity to describe any concept and its relations with the others in a way that could be understood and managed by computers. The dual model approach, by the OpenEHR [28], is pioneering this idea in the healthcare domain.

This model is based on the ontological separation between a stable reference information model that covers invariant across the domain concepts, and formal definitions of variable clinical content in the form of archetypes and templates. The fix reference model is hardly implemented in the software that can "manage and understand" variable archetypes and templates. As a consequence, systems have the possibility of being far smaller and more maintainable than single-level systems. They are also inherently self-adaptive, since they are built to consume archetypes and templates.

OpenEHR results have been specially considered in the development of an important European Standard, the EN13606 that looks for an interoperable Electronic Healthcare Record. But for an optimum management of the care of a particular subject, all the knowledge had to be considered, and not only that included in the EHR. In this sense, the three-part European standard EN 12967-1,2,3 suites better with personalized medicine, indeed it has been developed as a middleware to integrate all the systems involved in a healthcare organization. It should be pointed that the methodology for the design of this middleware is ODP (Open Distributed Processing) [29-31], providing a layered approach to the definition of the middleware. For a better description of the relevant aspects to cover, the standard defines different workflows, covering special tasks as security, resources management, clinical information, activity management, etc. …

Looking for the global knowledge management needed in personalized medicine, some relevant innovations could be added to this standard, these are shown as contributions to EN12967's enterprise, information and computational viewpoints. Some of the more relevant contributions are:

The information viewpoint should be considered as an open and changing ontology and not as a fixed model. However elemental and invariable concepts can be considered as a basis of new ones, as in the dual model approach. This viewpoint might be expressed in some ontology language, as OWL [32], what will facilitate the evolution and incorporation of systems and the use of underlying open semantic middlewares as semantic grid. This ontology will evolve to include all the necessary concepts to provide the needed knowledge for personal healthcare, including concepts from very different levels, from cellular to systemic, and disciplines, from general knowledge as population studies or clinical guidelines to personal electronic healthcare record. The use of a standard ontology language, as OWL, will facilitate the incorporation of such heterogeneous concepts.

Semantic management workflow should be added in order to consider essential tasks for knowledge management as the management of ontologies, annotations, inferences and reasoning, etc… These facilities could be included in the underlying middleware if it is semantically enriched, providing a dynamic management of the information viewpoint.

Communication workflow could be added too, covering tasks related to connections between systems, as format conversion or the definition of communication protocols. Features for special communication needs between components inside the architecture could be considered here. This workflow is especially significant in the integration of hospital, home and outdoor scenarios. It includes, for example, considerations for the access network, connecting home to the middleware, or any other communication requirements. New generation networks are key technologies that should be considered here, since convergence is a main target in these networks and they are basic for the interconnection of healthcare scenarios.

In the computational viewpoint a language for the formal specification of ODP-based architectures and its extension to healthcare systems compliant with EN12967 could be introduced [33]. If it is expressed as ontology again, for example using OWL, this should facilitate the formal representation of any system using the whole ODP terminology in a very straightforward way. Some benefits with respect to previous formal languages are, for example, an easier management of relations between viewpoints, an easier use of reasoners for the management of ontology instances, to make the publishing, discovery, invocation and composition of components functionality in an automatic way. The management of proactive behaviour in the architectural components is facilitated too.

Discussion: benefits of integration

Healthcare systems are evolving from a disaggregated amount of heterogeneous and totally independent applications to global knowledge infrastructures that will support the personalized healthcare delivery in the future. Several issues are involved in this evolution including, among others, technical, social, ethical, legal and, of course, economic considerations.

Solving the integration among heterogeneous systems in a federated way and designing efficient knowledge management tools is the target of numerous present researches. Once a global knowledge management system is not a utopia, person-specific knowledge could be automatically combined with general medical knowledge and other tacit knowledge from the system to enhance the complete personalization of diagnosis and therapy.

New trends will be considered in healthcare delivery as personalized prevention and recommendations based on biomedical knowledge that includes patient genotype, phenotype and environmental conditions. The interfaces with the system will evolve from traditional keyboard/monitor and obtrusive sensors to more natural dialogues using devices embedded in the environment.

However, although technology improvement is facilitating the knowledge globalization it might have to be accompanied by regional, national and international strategies that should consider new trends like: the developments on global access to Healthcare Information, the extended use of this information, including research, new kinds of users, new types of data and health monitoring opportunities. Some conflicts will arise and will have to be solved, specially those related to ethical, privacy and confidentiality. Another immediate consequence is the need for appropriate education and training in order to have well-educated healthcare professionals or even health information and communication technologies specialists, with sufficient knowledge and skills to systematically process data, information and knowledge in medicine and health care. Interdisciplinary learning, research and daily work are essential to meet these challenges.

If appropriate infrastructure for the integration of patient management systems, biomedical applications, best evidence management and educational tools, are not in place, or if the different scenarios in healthcare are not considered in this infrastructure, then it will be difficult to realize the significant benefits forecast from the personalized healthcare approach.

References

[1] Ginsburg, G.S., McCarthy, J.J.: Personalized medicine: revolutionizing drug discovery and patient care. Trends in Biotechnology 19(12), 491–496 (2001)
[2] Pantazi, S., Arocha, J., Moehr, J.: Case-based medical informatics. BMC Medical Informatics and Decision Making 4(1), 19 (2004)
[3] Lutz, M.W., Warren, P.V., Gill, R.W., Searls, D.B.: Managing genomic and proteomic knowledge. Drug Discovery Today: Technologies 2(3), 197–204 (2005)
[4] Meyer, J.M., Ginsburg, G.S.: The path to personalized medicine. Current Opinion in Chemical Biology 6(4), 434–438 (2002)
[5] Ross, J.S., Ginsburg, G.S.: Integrating diagnostics and therapeutics: revolutionizing drug discovery and patient care. Drug Discovery Today 7(16), 859–864 (2002)
[6] Spang, R.: Diagnostic signatures from microarrays: a bioinformatics concept for personalized medicine. BIOSILICO 1(2), 64–68 (2003)
[7] Louie, B., Mork, P., Martin-Sanchez, F., Halevy, A., Tarczy-Hornoch, P.: Data integration and genomic medicine. Journal of Biomedical Informatics 40(1), 5–16 (2007)
[8] Lutz, M.W., Warren, P.V., Gill, R.W., Searls, D.B.: Managing genomic and proteomic knowledge. Drug Discovery Today: Technologies 2(3), 197–204 (2005)
[9] Hoffman, M.A.: The genome-enabled electronic medical record. Journal of Biomedical Informatics 40(1), 44–46 (2007)
[10] Ginsburg, G.S., McCarthy, J.J.: Personalized medicine: revolutionizing drug discovery and patient care. Trends in Biotechnology 19(12), 491–496 (2001)
[11] Korhonen, I., Bardram, J.E.: Guest Editorial Introduction to the Special Section on Pervasive Healthcare. IEEE Transactions on Information Technology in Biomedicine 8(3), 229–234 (2004)
[12] Boekhorst, F.: Ambient intelligence, the next paradigm for consumer electronics:how will it affect silicon? In: Solid-State Circuits Conference Proceedings, vol. 1, pp. 28–31 (2002)
[13] Aarts, E.: Ambient intelligence: a multimedia perspective. IEEE Multimedia 11(1), 12–19 (2004)
[14] Perry, M., Dowdall, A., Lines, L., Hone, K.: Multimodal and ubiquitous computing systems: supporting independent-living older users. IEEE Transactions on information technology in biomedicine 8(3), 258–270 (2004)
[15] Amigoni, F., Gatti, N., Pinciroli, C., Roveri, M.: What planner for ambient intelligence applications? IEEE Transactions on Systems, Man and Cybernetics, Part A 53(1), 7–21 (2005)
[16] Mihailidis, A., Carmichael, B., Boger, J.: The use of computer vision in an intelligent environment to support aging-in-place, safety, and independence in the home. IEEE Transactions on information technology in biomedicine 8(3), 238–247 (2004)
[17] Favela, J., Rodriguez, M., Gonzalez, V.M., Preciado, A.: Integrating context-aware public displays into a mobile hospital information system. IEEE Transactions on information technology in biomedicine 8(3), 279–286 (2004)
[18] Korhonen, I., Pärkkä, J., Van Gils, M.: Health monitoring in the home of the future. IEEE Engineering in medicine and biology magazine 22(3), 66–73 (2003)
[19] Chan, M., Estève, D., Escriba, C., Campo, E.: A review of smart homes – Present state and future challenges. Computer methods and Programs in Biomedicine 91(1), 55–81 (2008)

[20] Budinger, T.F.: Biomonitoring with wireless communications. Annual Review of Biomedical Engineering (5), 383–412 (2003)
[21] Bardram, J.: Hospitals of the future – ubiquitous computing support for medical work. In: Hospitals Workshop Ubihealth (2003)
[22] Bai, V.T., Srivatsa, S.K.: Wireless tele care system for intensive care unit of hospitals using bluetooth and embedded technology. Information Technology Journal 5(6), 1106–1112 (2006)
[23] Haux, R.: Health information systems - past, present, future. International Journal of Medical Informatics 75(3-4), 268–281 (2006)
[24] CEN /TC 251.Secretariat: SIS. EN 12967-1:2007. Health informatics - Service architecture - Part 1: Enterprise viewpoint (2007)
[25] CEN /TC 251.Secretariat: SIS. EN 12967-2:2007. Health informatics - Service architecture - Part 2: Information viewpoint (2007)
[26] CEN /TC 251.Secretariat: SIS. EN 12967-3:2007 Health informatics - Service architecture - Part 3: Computational viewpoint (2007)
[27] CORBAmed: OMG. Healthcare Domain Task Force standards, http://healthcare.omg.org/Roadmap/corbamed_roadmap.htm (accessed, March 2008)
[28] Archetype Definitions and Principles. OpenEHR Release 1.0.1., http://www.openehr.org/releases/1.0.1/architecture/am/archetype_principles.pdf (accessed, January 2009)
[29] ITU-T, Rec. X.901-Information technology – Open distributed processing – Reference Model: Overview (1997)
[30] ITU-T, Rec. X902-Information Technology-Open distributed processing-Reference model: foundations (1995)
[31] ITU-T, Rec. X903-Information technology – Open distributed processing – Reference Model: Architecture (1995)
[32] Ontology Web Language site, http://www.w3.org/2004/OWL/ (accessed, September 2008)
[33] Román, I., Roa, L.M., Madinabeitia, G., Reina, L.J.: A Standard Ontology for the Semantic Integration of Components in Healthcare Organizations. In: Bos, L., et al. (eds.) Medical and Care Compunetics 3. IOS Pres, Amsterdam (2006)

Standards for Digital Homecare

W.J. Meijer, M.D., partner in DiaDerma

Mailing address: Verlengde Fortlaan 82, 1412 EA Naarden, The Netherlands
E-mail address: meijer@ictus.nl

Abstract This chapter discusses requirements for digital homecare that are dictated by current international standards. The standards relate to services and devices.
For digital homecare **services,** standards concern quality assurance (quality management system and indicators), information management (quality of data and information), supporting systems (calibration, instruction and system integration) and organization. For organizing, the start is to define the needs of clients in terms of health and quality of life: independence, self-reliance, participation and self-determination. Next, processes must be described that lead to these goals.
Digital homecare **devices** (apparatus and software) are generally in the lowest risk class (Class I) according to: the amended Medical Devices Directive of the European Union. Requirements for CE-marking are: 1) a quality assurance system, 2) a risk analysis, 3) clinical evaluation and 4) post-market surveillance. Certification for ISO 13485 (quality management systems) and ISO 14791 (risk management) can assist in complying with the requirements.
Measures for implementation of standards in digital homecare are described.

Table of contents

K. Yogesan et al. (Eds.): Handbook of Digital Homecare, BIOMED, pp. 53–74.
springerlink.com

Why is standardization of digital homecare important?

Digital homecare is now finding its way into patients' and clients' homes. It is a new form of care provision. It bridges the distance between the client/patient and his care providers, both in terms of spatial distance and in terms of distance in time.

This new form of care enables the client/patient to remain at home, and yet receive good quality care. Another benefit of digital homecare is that it allows the demand for care to be satisfied at an affordable price.

So, the characteristics of digital homecare can be a benefit for the client/patient, as well as for the care providers. Yet, these very characteristics are also a cause of uncertainty for involved persons.

Digital homecare is an innovation. As with any innovation, the price for progress is uncertainty. There is uncertainty for care providers, clients/patients and providers of systems.

Care providers are not certain about guidelines and ethical constraints in cases where they do not see the client personally, but receive information at a distance.

For clients/patients there is uncertainty because their rights and roles in this new form of care have not been regulated. For instance, control of his (medical) information must be regulated in this context. However, in the international standards of ISO en CEN there is not yet a comprehensive normative document on digital homecare that formulates patient rights and roles.

Providers of digital homecare systems are uncertain about the choices that they have to make, due to the absence of a comprehensive standard. For instance, interconnectivity and interoperability of homecare systems with other communication systems are essential, but it is not yet clear which standards must be adopted.

Clearly, there is a need of a comprehensive standard that is internationally supported and that encompasses the whole area of digital homecare.

This chapter discusses requirements for digital homecare that are dictated by current international standards. It also describes aspects and requirements that should be covered by a new standard.

In this chapter the following areas for standardization in digital homecare are discussed:

1. at the level of services:
    a. client's goals and needs
    b. ensuring the quality of the services
    c. the quality of information
    d. managing supporting systems in the patient's home
    e. organizing the services
2. at the level of devices:
    a. standards for medical devices
    b. software.

Scope

Digital homecare comprises services and devices.

Services

Digital healthcare as a service concerns a wide variety of services.

The part of the services that relates to health care, is ,roughly speaking, Telemedicine. Telemedicine is defined as care process(es), in which at least one of the actors is an accredited healthcare practitioner, and in which the effect of distance is reduced by the use of information technology and data communications (NTA 8028). Since Telemedicine is a part of digital homecare, standards for Telemedicine are relevant for digital homecare.

For instance, the Dutch National Technical Agreement (NTA) for Telemedicine (NTA 8028), is a comprehensive standard for Telemedicine. In accordance with EN ISO 9001, EN ISO 9002 and EN ISO 9004, it has an orientation on processes. It describes quality aspects for the various involved processes: care processes, business processes (the related processes in the care organization) and information processes. In this chapter, these quality aspects are developed a step further for digital homecare.

Devices

For the devices that are employed in digital homecare, the main relevant standards are the amended Medical Devices Directive of the European Union (amended Directive 93/42/EEC) and EN ISO 13485. They are further discussed in the section 'Standards for medical devices'.

A question is whether an Electronic Health Record (EHR) must meet the requirements of medical devices, if it is used in digital healthcare. In our view, an EHR is a particular kind of software, namely a (collection of) database(s). If it is used in healthcare, it is a medical device by definition (see the section on medical devices). Thus, such an EHR has to meet the requirements for medical devices in general and in particular the requirements for software that are discussed in the section 'Software' in this chapter.

Goals

To ensure quality of digital homecare, standardization should aim at:

- (at the level of services) client centered and integrated services, integrated systems, appropriate organization and sustainable financing
- (at the level of devices) effectiveness and patient safety.

Client centered and integrated services imply that the needs of clients/patients are the starting point and that service providers cooperate to fulfil their needs.

Client's goals and needs

Clients' needs are broader than just the absence of disease.

Accordingly, in the Dutch National Technical Agreement (NTA) for Telemedicine, the NTA 8028, the goals of Telemedicine were defined broadly. Since Telemedicine is an essential part of digital homecare, these goals also hold for digital homecare. They include not only health, but also quality of life in non-medical terms as seen from the patient's perspective: 1) independence, 2) self-reliance; 3) participation in society and social life and 4) self-determination (autonomy through freedom of choice).

Client's control of data

In the Convention on Human Rights and Biomedicine, the members of the European Council have agreed on the right for private life and patient's rights on information as follows

1. *Everyone has the right to respect for private life in relation to information about his or her health.*

2. *Everyone is entitled to know any information collected about his or her health. However, the wishes of individuals not to be so informed shall be observed.*

Apparently, the patient's access to information about his or her health is regarded to be a basic right.

In the Netherlands, in the current standard on telemedicine, self-determination of the client/patient is one of the goals (NTA 8028). The patient's right of self-determination implies that he or she must have ultimate control over his own data (NTA 8028). The client/patient decides who, in which functional capacity within the care process, is entitled to access which data at which level ('reading') and is entitled to process it in some way: making additions, changes or possibly deleting ('writing') (NTA 8028).

In conclusion, there should be no barriers to the client/patient for the control and management of his own data. The healthcare provider must allow the client/patient access to his own data as quickly as possible and/or provide a copy of (part of) the record.

Ensuring quality of the services

The starting point for any improvement of quality are the needs of the parties involved (EN ISO 9000, EN ISO 9001, EN ISO 9004). The above mentioned goals, or needs of clients/patients must be central in quality assurance.

Quality management system

The responsible organization and providers must monitor, manage and where necessary improve the quality of the services are in a cyclical and ongoing process (EN ISO 9000, EN ISO 9001, EN ISO 9004). This can best be done by developing a quality management system based on indicators and criteria for quality.

Quality indicators

For quality measurement quality indicators have to be defined. Indicators relate to the desired outcome, or to the processes that are to lead to the outcome. Indicators must be relevant, simple, easily interpretable and easy to measure.

With the aid of quality indicators, the responsible organization can monitor the effectiveness and efficiency of care-related and logistic processes and report. The monitoring and evaluation of quality indicators also provide information for users (healthcare practitioners and clients/patients), healthcare providers, policy makers and healthcare insurers.

Managing information

In digital homecare, information is exchanged between various actors: clients/patients, caregivers and others, such as family carers. The quality of this information must be controlled.

The involved parties must make sure that adequate security measures have been taken to protect data, information and information streams.

A further discussion of security measures (is beyond the scope of this chapter. Here, only a few basic aspects will be mentioned.

Quality of data

With regard to data, generally accepted quality aspects are:

— availability. Data must be available for the user at the right place and at the right time. The fact that technology can never be 100% reliable makes it necessary to pay attention to the issue of continuity in the event of any failure or disruption;

— integrity. Information must have integrity, i.e. it must be reliable. Data must not be distorted or otherwise damaged by the information system;

— confidentiality. Data must be accessible for authorized persons only.

Quality of information

The above quality aspects relate to data. However, quality of data is not sufficient. Quality of information is equally important. Information means that data acquire meaning in a specific context, for a specific purpose. So, next to data quality, the quality of information should be managed, for instance:

— usability. The data must be usable for the purpose for which it is intended

— interpretability and analysability. The data must be unambiguous in relation to the purpose for which they are used.

Managing the supporting systems in the patient's home

Quality of patient's measurements

In digital homecare, there is a specific risk when the client/patient performs measurements (e.g. blood pressure) that were traditionally taken by a doctor or nurse.

Then, the healthcare practitioner must rely on the quality of the patient's actions but the quality thereof is not guaranteed by professional regulation or legislation. Specific measures then become necessary, such as regular checks and calibration of the patient's equipment and connections. Attention must also be given to correct use of the equipment by the patient.

In conclusion, quality demands on the user equipment and peripheral equipment used for digital homecare, information security at the workstation and the secure transport and storage of data, all form part of the overall security and safety of digital homecare.

System integration

Supporting systems must be adapted to the needs of clients/patients.

For instance, clients should not be exposed to many not-integrated systems. They get confused by a multitude of cables that enter their house to connect them with a multitude of systems, each of which has its own technical solution, its own interface with the client and its own usage manual (island solutions).

Accordingly, to promote integration of systems, a recent Dutch Vision Document (Bergeijk et al., 2008) makes a plea for an ´Entrance code for living related ICT applications and wideband services´. It aims at the user being in control and stimulating tele-applications. Dependency on one particular network company should be reduced and there should be more opportunity for new service providers. This can be achieved by disconnecting electronic connections from operational ICT applications (´Plug and Play in the house´) and standardization of the physical connections of instruments in the house by the use of open standards.

Organizing the services of digital homecare

It can be concluded that the above mentioned goals of digital homecare must be reached by activities in various fields. These fields cover 1) patient centered, integrated services, 2) managing the supporting systems, 3) information management, 4) quality assurance.

The activities need adequate organization. Organization is a key success factor for digital homecare. Organizing should aim at stimulating cooperation and management of processes.

Cooperation

One of the potential obstacles for digital home care is lack of coherence and cooperation. Cooperation between the various actors is to be organized.

Digital homecare involves various actors. The primary actors are the client/patient and his care providers. But equally important are those, such as manufacturers, who provide the instruments for them to benefit from digital homecare.

The performance of digital homecare depends on coherence and cooperation. For instance, when a diabetic patient measures his glucose levels himself, the patient must rely on the caregiver being available for feedback (Meijer and Ragetlie, 2007).

Failure in the cooperation between the actors may lead to suboptimal care, and even severe hazards. To avoid such risk, high demands must be made on all actors in the care process. Therefore, the responsibilities of the various parties can be set out in contracts or agreements.

Management of processes

According to ISO standards (EN ISO 9000, EN ISO 9001, EN ISO 9004), processes must be defined on the basis of the function that they perform in the achievement of the resulting situation (outcome) from the starting situation (input). Outcome is the desired final situation, i.e. the situation that fulfils the needs or requirements of the parties involved. The description must cover all processes and subprocesses that are necessary to achieve that desired situation. It should also set out the relationships between the processes and subprocesses, in terms of sequentiality and interaction; the output of one subprocess serves as input for a following subprocess (EN ISO 9004).

The responsibility for these subprocesses must be allocated to actors (actor is a person in a specific role in the process). In order to assure both quality and transparency, the roles and rights of the actors involved must be known and be clear, namely: what can be done, how and when (roles), and who may do what and when that may be done (rights) (NTA 8028).

Then, the entire process can be coordinated.

The rationale is to avoid the potentially disastrous consequences of unclear responsibilities. For instance, if no one is explicitly responsible for the continuity of the electric supply for electronic alarm systems, a discontinuity can occur leading to fatal results by a non-functioning alarm system. As another example, someone has to be responsible for the algorithms that determine whether the diabetic nurse should contact the diabetes patient who is being monitored by a digital homecare system.

It is essential that coordination and execution of the process should progress in accordance with predefined agreements and procedures.

At least the following questions must be answered:

- have procedures and protocols been written up and made known?
- has supervision been organized?
- is the person who processes the data, authorized to do so?

Standards for medical devices

Standards for medical devices are both product standards and process standards concerning management systems, quality management and risk management. For digital homecare, the most relevant requirements are in the Medical Device Directive 2007/47/EC of the European Union and in the standard EN ISO 13485 *Quality management systems - Requirements for regulatory purposes.*

The European Medical Device Directive 93/42/EEC

In the countries of the European Union, manufacturers of a medical device must meet the essential requirements of the Medical Device Directive 93/42/EEC as a condition to place the product on the European market and/or to put it into service. The goal of the Directive is safety and health protection of patients, users and, where appropriate, other persons, with regard to the use of medical devices.

On 5 September 2007, the amending European Union Directive for Medical Devices (2007/47/EC) has been published, which amends Directives 93/42/EEC on medical devices. All European Member States must apply Directive 2007/47/EC as national law from 21 March 2010.
The requirements in Directive 2007/47/EC have considerable consequences for manufacturers of medical devices. These implications will be discussed in the next sections. Firstly, the definition of medical device is discussed. Also, the essential requirements of the Medical Device Directive are dealt upon. Next, conformity with the Directive is described, with specific attention to EN ISO 13485 *Quality management systems - Requirements for regulatory purposes.* Finally, in the conclusion, the importance of the medical device standards for digital homecare is emphasized.

Definition of medical device

In the amended Directive 93/42/EEC, the definition of 'medical device' has been changed.

The first part of the adopted definition of 'medical device' in the amended Directive is: :

> ‘medical device’ means any instrument, apparatus, appliance, software, material or other article, whether used alone or in combination, including the software intended by its manufacturer to be used specifically for diagnostic and/or therapeutic purposes and necessary for its proper application, intended by the manufacturer to be used for human beings for the purpose of:
> — diagnosis, prevention, monitoring, treatment or alleviation of disease,
> — diagnosis, monitoring, treatment, alleviation of or compensation for an injury or handicap,
> — investigation, replacement or modification of the anatomy or of a physiological process,
> — control of conception,
> and which does not achieve its principal intended action in or on the human body by pharmacological, immunological or metabolic means, but which may be assisted in its function by such means (…).

In digital homecare, devices typically aim at prevention and monitoring and are therefore *medical* devices according to the definition. So, they will have to meet the requirements of the Directive.

The essential requirements in the Medical Device Directive

Full device-related quality assurance system

One of the essential requirements in the Directive is that manufacturers have to ensure application of the quality system approved for the design, manufacture and final inspection of the devices concerned. Application of the quality assurance system must ensure that the devices conform to the provisions of the Directive, which apply to them at every stage, from design to final inspection.

All the elements must be documented in a systematic and orderly manner.

For a full description of the requirements concerning the quality assurance system the reader is referred to the Directive (Directive 93/42/EEC amended by Directive 2007/47/EC), Annex II, that has been published on Internet.

EN ISO 13485

In order to facilitate compliance with the requirements concerning a quality system, the European Commission mandated CEN drafting requirements in a harmonized standard. Thus, CEN and ISO drafted the harmonized standard EN ISO 13485 which gives presumption of conformity with this essential requirement of the Directive concerning a quality assurance system. This standard is further discussed in the following section in this chapter.

Risk analysis and solutions

The devices must be designed and manufactured in such a way that, when used under the conditions and for the purposes intended, they will not compromise the clinical condition or the safety of patients, or the safety and health of users or, where applicable, other persons. Any risks which may be associated with their intended use must constitute acceptable risks when weighted against the benefits to the patient.

EN ISO 14971 is the standard for application of risk management to medical devices. It is further discussed in a following section on EN ISO 13485.

Clinical evaluation

Conformity with the requirements has to be based on clinical data. ('Clinical data' means the safety and/or performance information that is generated from the use of a device.) The evaluation of this data, the 'clinical evaluation', is to follow a defined and methodologically sound procedure based on:

1. either a critical evaluation of the relevant scientific literature currently available relating to the safety, performance, design characteristics and intended purpose of the device, where:
    a. there is a demonstration of equivalence of the device to the device to which the data relates, and
    b. the data adequately demonstrate compliance with the relevant essential requirements
2. or a critical evaluation of the results of all clinical investigations made
3. or a critical evaluation that combines the two previously mentioned evaluations.

The clinical evaluation and its outcome have to be documented and this documentation has to be included and/or fully referenced in the technical documentation of the medical device.

The clinical evaluation has to be in conformity with ISO 14155. This standard is now in revision.

The amended Directive puts a strong emphasis on post-market surveillance (see next section). The clinical evaluation must be actively updated with data from the post-market surveillance. Where post-market clinical follow-up as part of the post-market surveillance for the device is not deemed necessary, this must be duly justified and documented.

Where demonstration of conformity is an essential requirements based on clinical data is not deemed appropriate, adequate justification for any such exclusion has to be given.

Post-market surveillance

A particularly important requirement of the amended Directive 93/42/EEC is post-market surveillance: the manufacturer keeps up to date a systematic procedure to review experience gained from the devices in the post-production phase and updates the clinical evaluation.

If necessary, appropriate means must be implemented to apply any necessary corrective action and the competent authorities must be notified. Such actions are deemed necessary in the case of any malfunction or deterioration in the characteristics and/or performance of the device.

Classification

Depending on the intended purpose of the medical device, a medical device may be classified as Class I, Class IIa, IIb and III, with Class III covering the highest risk products. The higher the classification the greater the level of assessment required. Only for some medical devices in Class I a manufacturer is allowed to inspect his own product and place the CE-mark. In all other classes an authorized notified body has to do this task.

Digital homecare devices are classified in Class I as all non-invasive devices are classified in Class I, unless specific requirements apply. Since such specific requirements do not apply for most devices of digital healthcare, the devices are generally in class I. For further information on classification, the reader is referred to the amended Directive (Directive 93/42/EEC amended by Directive 2007/47/EC), Annex IX, that has been published on Internet.

Conformity with the (amended) Medical Device Directive

The EC declaration of conformity is the procedure whereby the manufacturer ensures and declares that the products concerned meet the provisions of the Directive that apply to them.

Technical documentation

The manufacturer must prepare technical documentation that allows assessment of the conformity of the product with the requirements of the Directive. The manufacturer must make this documentation, including the declaration of conformity, available to the national authorities for inspection purposes for a period ending at least five years after the last product has been manufactured.

CE-marking

To show that the device conforms with the requirements of the Directive, the manufacturer must affix the CE-marking visibly and legibly on the device. The CE-marking shows the conformity.

Guidance for the manufacturer to meet the requirements of ISO 13485

Two standards offer guidance for the manufacturer to meet the requirements of ISO 13485: EN ISO/TR 14969:2004 *Medical Devices - Quality management systems – Guidance on the application of ISO 13485:2003* and EN 1041:2008 *Information supplied by the manufacturer of medical devices.*

The guidance of EN ISO/TR 14969 can be used to better understand the requirements of ISO 13485 and to illustrate some of the variety of methods and approaches available for meeting the requirements of ISO 13485

EN 1041:2008 specifies requirements for information to be supplied by a manufacturer for medical devices in order to meet the essential requirements of the Directive. EN 1041 provides guidance on means by which certain requirements can be met.

Harmonized standards

In order to demonstrate conformity with the essential requirements of this Directive and to enable conformity to be verified, the European Commission stated that it is desirable to have harmonized European standards to protect against the risks associated with the design, manufacture and packaging of medical devices. The European Commission mandates the European Committee for Standardization (CEN) and the European Committee for Electrotechnical Standardization (Cenelec) for drafting and adoption of these harmonized standards in order to provide presumption of conformity with the clauses in the standard and the corresponding essential requirements in that Directive.

EN ISO 13485 Device-related quality management system

The main objective of EN ISO 13485 and the guidance on its application (EN ISO/TR 14969:2004) is to facilitate harmonized medical device regulatory requirements for quality management systems. Additionally EN ISO 13485 focuses on aspects of safety, effectiveness and meeting customer requirements.

EN ISO 13485 specifies requirements for a device-related quality management system. Furthermore, EN ISO 13485 requires that organizations shall establish risk management requirements, which must be thoroughly documented and conducted to all stages of the project's entire life-cycle, from design to final inspection. However, the standard refers to EN ISO 14971: 2007 *Application of risk management to medical devices* which provides manufacturers with a framework within which experience, insight and judgment are applied systematically to manage the risks associated with the use of medical devices.

The combination of increased regulation and technological advances forces manufacturers of medical devices to link their management system with enterprise-wide risk management programs. Manufacturers are increasingly requiring their sub-tier suppliers to attain EN ISO 13485 certification, because they aim to realize better products and better services.

EN ISO 13485 certification serves to combine the quality system requirements with the regulatory requirements process in order to improve company's efficiency, increase profits and open international doors to new markets.

Relation between Directive and EN ISO 13485

Harmonized standards (such as EN ISO 13485 and EN ISO 14791) help implementing the essential requirements of the Directive, but implementing them is not sufficient for meeting all the essential requirements of the Directive. (Every harmonized includes an Annex Z that provides the compliance with the specific essential requirements of the Directive concerned.)

Specifically, implementing EN ISO 13485 and EN ISO 14791 assists manufacturers to meet the requirements for risk and quality systems as required in Directive 93/42/EEC, but implementing them is not sufficient for meeting other requirements, such as clinical evaluation and post-market surveillance.

As soon as the standard EN ISO 13485 will be revised, the requirements of the amended Directive will be adopted and explained in the new EN ISO 13485 version of this standard.

Relation *EN ISO 13485 and EN ISO 9001*

The current version of EN ISO 13485 includes some requirements of EN ISO 9001, but also excludes some requirements of EN ISO 9001. Annex B of EN ISO 13485 explains the similarities and differences between all clauses of EN ISO 13485 and EN ISO 9001 and it also provides a rationale for these differences. A difference is the required amount of documented procedures; EN ISO 13485 indicates more specific requirements for control, inspection, validation and verification of processes.

Another important difference is the elimination of the terms 'customer satisfaction' and 'continual improvement' in the scope of EN ISO 13485 as they were not thought to be relevant in a standard whose objective is to facilitate the harmonization of medical devices regulations for quality management systems.

However, as pointed out above, in the amended Directive 93/42/EEC there is more emphasis on the requirement of post-market surveillance.

The increased emphasis on this requirement in the amended Directive has implications for the above mentioned differences between EN ISO 13485 and EN ISO 9001. The current version of EN ISO 13485 has been based on the old essential requirements of the Directive and therefore, the EN ISO 9001-terms 'customer satisfaction' and 'continual improvement' were less relevant.

In contrast, these terms will become more relevant because the new amended Directive requires that a the part of the quality system relates to post-market clinical follow-up and the results of this follow-up. Patient satisfaction is an issue in clinical follow-up and post-market surveillance has features of continual improvement. So, the EN ISO 9001-terms 'patient satisfaction' and 'continual improvement' become more and more important for medical device manufacturers.

Software

Digital homecare typically employs a combination of an 'apparatus' and software. In this section, requirements for the software will be discussed.

In digital homecare, there are two kinds of software. Firstly, there is ('embedded') software that is incorporated in an apparatus. This apparatus is a medical device (e.g. a pulsimeter). Naturally, such software must fulfil the requirements of the medical device wherein it is incorporated.

Secondly, there is software that is separate from the apparatus and is used in combination with the apparatus. Such software may have various functions such as transport of data from A to B, data storage and retrieval, data analysis, communication between persons and, last but not least, software for data control (e.g. access control, security). Such software is to be regarded as a medical device since it falls within the definition of 'medical device' from the amended Medical Devices Directive: '… any (…) software (…), whether used alone or in combination (…), and intended by the manufacturer to be used for human beings for the purpose of

- diagnosis, prevention, monitoring, treatment or alleviation of disease,
- diagnosis, monitoring, treatment, alleviation of or compensation for an injury or handicap (…)'.

Consequently, the software must meet the requirements of the amended Medical Devices Directive.

Software, which drives a device or influences the use of the device, falls automatically in the same class as the medical device and the corresponding requirements must be met.

The consequences of software being a medical device are considerable.

Firstly, the generic essential requirements of the amended Medical Devices Directive, as discussed above, must be fulfilled for software.

Secondly, software must conform with specific requirements: it has to be validated according to the state of the art taking into account the principles of development lifecycle, risk management, validation and verification (Annex I, Section 12.1a).

Next, these developments and validation principles must be applied to ensure availability, integrity and confidentiality of the information in accordance with current security standards such as ISO/IEC 27001.

Finally, speaking in even broader terms, these principles must be used to ensure the quality of software as specified by ISO/IEC 9126. The quality aspects of a software product can be divided into a number of categories, in accordance with

ISO/IEC 9126. The principal characteristics of the quality of software products are functionality, reliability, usability, efficiency, maintainability and portability (Table 1).

Table 1. Quality of software: characteristics and subcharacteristics

Characteristic	Subcharacteristics
Functionality	suitability, accuracy, interoperability, security, functionality compliance
Reliability	maturity, fault tolerance, recoverability, reliability compliance
Usability	Understandability, learnability, operability, attractiveness, usability compliance
Efficiency	time behavior, resource utilization, efficiency compliance
Maintainability	analysability, changeability, stability, teststability, maintainability compliance
Portability	Subcharacteristics of portability are adaptability, installability, co/existence, replaceability, portability compliance

These characteristics and subcharacteristics are relevant for digital homecare. For instance, interoperability is a subcharacteristic of functionality. It is defined as ´the compatibility of the software product to interact with one or more specified systems´. Digital homecare bridges distance and links actors at different locations, having different roles and responsibilities. So, systems must be interoperable so that the actors and the systems themselves can communicate with each other. This requires standardization (EN 13606, ISO/TR 16056, ISO/TS 16058, ISO 8348).

Conclusion for medical devices in digital homecare

Instruments, devices, apparatus and software for digital homecare fall within the definition of medical devices so the requirements of the (amended) Medical devices Directive 93/42/EEC should apply. Additionally EN ISO 13485 can assist manufacturers of digital homecare products to implement a quality management system and EN ISO 14971 can assist manufacturers to implement a risk management system.

These standards include requirements for medical device manufacturers and their sub-tier suppliers, specifically on the management of their processes, including post-market surveillance.

However, medical device manufacturers are not giving risk management its due gravity in their management systems (Steve Wichelecki, 2008).

It is essential that manufacturers and users are more aware of the harmonized standards that should safeguard quality and patient safety. Awareness is even more important since the trend is towards increasing regulation and mandatory CE-marking.

The future will be strongly influenced by the concerns of citizens and administrations on patient safety.

Implementing a standard

Implementation of a standard for digital homecare is a complex process. A thorough discussion of implementation is beyond the scope of this chapter. Only a few points will be made, to illustrate the kind of measures that must be taken to implement a standard for digital homecare.

Measures aimed at involved actors

Specific risks are ifnvolved when the patient is responsible for the performance of specific tasks that are traditionally performed by healthcare practitioners. Additional measures then become necessary, such as regular checks of the equipment and of the care consumer's connection; attention must also be paid to correct use of the equipment and the devices used by the care consumer to take measurements.

Measures concerning financing

Sustainable financing is a condition for sustainable digital homecare.

However, the structure of the reimbursement system in healthcare may lead to fragmentation and counteract integrated digital homecare. Creative solutions can be necessary to overcome these obstacles, as follows.

Just like in other markets, the value of the service can be expressed in monetary terms. One can assess the value that the service of digital homecare has for the client, in terms of monthly expenditure. (Also consider the potential contribution from relatives.)

Next, one could try to combine the monetary contributions from different sources (healthcare insurance, social welfare, municipality, etc.) as the income that can be spent for the service of digital homecare. If all involved parties cooperate in the interests of the patient, the result could be that the combined contributions are sufficient to pay for digital homecare.

Measures concerning organization

It is essential that the process of digital homecare is designed on the basis of any statutory requirements for the allocation and registration of the roles, rights and obligations of all actors concerned. Various documents of legislation and regulation can be relevant, depending on the country or region.

The responsibilities of the various parties can be set out in contracts or agreements.

Who is responsible for a standard for digital homecare

Society demands that for patients risks from care and medical devices is reduced as much as possible. Since digital homecare is a new form of care with new kinds of risks, there should be a new comprehensive standard for digital homecare.

A standard for digital homecare is to be considered as a regulating mechanism. It regulates the relations between those who are responsible for digital homecare on one side, and society on the other side.

A standard on digital homecare is preferably international for two reasons:

1. for manufacturers the market is international
2. patients are increasingly mobile and an international standard could stimulate uniformity and interoperability in data exchange across countries.

The development of a new international standard for digital homecare is the responsibility of stakeholders.

Stakeholders must assemble to develop and endorse a new standard. Stakeholders are providers of care services, providers of digital homecare systems, representatives of clients/patients and, perhaps most importantly, governmental bodies as representatives of their citizens. It is surprising that in the field of digital homecare relatively little contribution to standardization is made by governmental bodies. Possibly, this is so because governments prefer to make their own choices, and the long-term benefits of standardization are undervalued.

International standards should be developed in the context of official international standardization organizations, ISO and CEN.

In the Netherlands, an initiative to develop a new national standard for Telemedicine has been taken by the Netherlands Standardization Institute, NEN, and a group of stakeholders. The new standard is the sequel to the Dutch NTA 8028 and it will elaborate the quality aspects from NTA 8028 into specific quality requirements.

Also, at the time of writing this chapter, a proposal has been made by NEN to ISO to develop an international standard for digital homecare.

An international standard for digital homecare could build further on these building stones.

Availability of standards

It is important that there are no barriers to the use of standards that have been discussed in this chapter. However, both national standards and the international standards of ISO and CEN are generally not freely available but have to be paid for. In the field of digital homecare, the number of relevant standards is substantial. So, for many stakeholders this would result in a substantial investment that is avoided for financial reasons. This financial barrier hampers implementation of the standards. Eventually, this is detrimental to the quality of the services.

Authorities that are responsible for safeguarding the quality of digital home care, should promote free availability of the standards. In this respect, standards should be treated in the same way as legislation. Administrations of the different countries should cooperate to achieve free availability of standards, in the interest of the patient.

Acknowledgment

I am grateful to M.J.M. van 't Root, consultant NEN-Medical Technology for reviewing the part of the chapter concerning standards on medical devices and for giving many useful suggestions.

References

Bergeijk, A.E., van Kokswijk, J., Wijnen, E.: Visiedocument ICT-standaardisatie en Wonen Versie 2.0. NEN and Ministerie EZ (May 2008)

EN 1041:2008 Information supplied by the manufacturer of medical devices

EN13606. Health informatics – Electronic healthcare record communication – Parts 1-5

EN ISO 9000

EN ISO 9001:2008

EN ISO 9004:200O Quality management systems – Guidelines for performance improvements

EN ISO 13485:2003 Medical devices - Quality management systems - Requirements for regulatory purposes, 2nd edn.

EN ISO/TR 14969:2004 Medical Devices - Quality management systems – Guidance on the application of ISO 13485:2003

EN ISO 14971:2007 Medical Devices - Application of Risk Management to Medical Devices

European Council. Convention for the Protection of Human Rights and Dignity of the Human Being with regard to the Application of Biology and Medicine: Convention on Human Rights and Biomedicine. Oviedo, 4 IV (1997)

ISO/IEC 7498-1 Open Systems Interconnection – Basic Reference Model

ISO/IEC 8348 Open Systems Interconnection – Network service definition

ISO/IEC 9126-1:2001 Software engineering – Product quality – Part 1: Quality model

ISO 14155-1:2003 Clinical investigation of medical devices for human subjects

ISO/TR 16056-1:2004 Health informatics – Interoperability of telehealth systems and networks - Part 1: Introduction and definitions

ISO/TR 16056-2:2004 Health informatics – Interoperability of telehealth systems and networks – Part 2: Real-time systems

ISO/TS 16058:2004 Health informatics – Interoperability of telelearning systems

ISO 16484 Building automation and control systems

ISO/IEC 18028 Security techniques

ISO/TS 18308:2004 Health informatics – Requirements for an electronic health record architecture

ISO/IEC 27001:2005 Information technology - Security techniques - Information security management systems - Requirements

Medical Device Directive of the European Union: Directive 93/42/EEC amended by Directive 2007/47/EC, Official Journal of the European Union L 247/21, http://eurlex.europa.eu/LexUriServ/LexUriServ.do?uri=OJ:L:2007:247:0021:0055:EN:PDF

Meijer, W.J., Ragetlie, P.L.: Empowering the Patient with ICT-tools: the Unfulfilled Promise. The Journal on Information Technology in Healthcare 5(5), 313–323 (2007)

NTA 8028: 2007 Health Informatics – Telemedicine The Netherlands, Delft; NEN (2007)[i]

Wichelecki, S.: Understanding ISO 13485 Editorial, Quality Magazine (January 2008), http://www.qualitymag.com/Articles/Feature_Article/BNP_GUID_9-5-2006_A_10000000000000225133

[i] Endnotes

NTA 8028 is available in Dutch and in English and can be ordered at bestel@nen.nl or by phone +31(0)152690882.

Model-Based Methodology for the Analysis of e-Health Systems Diffusion: Case Study of a Knowledge-Centered Telehealthcare System Based on a Mixed License

Manuel Prado-Velasco[1,2*], Carlos Fernández-Peruchena[1], David Rubio-Hernández[3]

[1] Multilevel Modeling and Emerging Technologies in Bioengineering Group (M2TB), University of Seville, Spain

[2] I2BC, Innovation Institute for Citizens' Well-being, Malaga, Spain

[3] R&D division, SHS Consultores, Seville, Spain

Abstract There is an increasing need of solutions for the well-being of citizens within a current scenario featured by the aging of population, growth of chronic pathologies, higher demand of healthcare, and change of social models. Despite the proved reliability of ICT to provide efficient solutions to e-health, their diffusion is still very scarce.

This work presents a new integrative insight in the e-health diffusion problem by means of a mathematical model-based methodology. The model has been developed following an analogy to the chemical kinetics theory.

The outcomes obtained by the mathematical model agree with the results of experimental and theoretical studies about the diffusion of innovative information systems.

A knowledge-centered e-health system with mixed license model, based on a previous telehealthcare system published by some of the authors, is briefly presented in the last Section. It provides a business strategy that takes advantage of some of the concepts of the e-health diffusion model.

Introduction

The scarce diffusion of telehealthcare systems, wearable and smart monitors and biosensors, and other valuable applications of new technologies to improve the health care services in the different living scenarios of being humans has been recurrently claimed (Avison & Young, 2007; Coughlin & Pope, 2008; May et al,

* Corresponding author: Prof. Manuel Prado-Velasco, Graphic Engineering Dpt., University of Seville, Seville, Spain; E-mail: mpradovelasco@ieee.org.

K. Yogesan et al. (Eds.): Handbook of Digital Homecare, BIOMED, pp. 75–94.
springerlink.com

2005; Noury et al, 2007).

Paradoxically, there is an increasing need of solutions that limit the economical burden of the classic centralized public and private healthcare model within the current scenario, featured by the aging of population, the growth of chronic pathologies and neurological disorders, the increasing risk of pandemics, the higher demand of healthcare and quality of life, and the change of familiar models in industrial countries (Coughlin & Pope, 2008). The scenario in developing countries is different, notwithstanding some of the analysis and ideas that will be appointed in this chapter could serve as a basis to work. The chapter is focused to the first context.

Many studies in different areas have tried to know the reasons for this lack of success. An important suggested reason is the lack of a mature legal framework for the accountability in a distributed and high-technology-based healthcare system, which new organizational and social elements (May et al, 2005). The distance between e-health promises and reality of the majority of e-health systems is other relevant argued cause (Goldschmidt, 2005; May et al, 2005; Tanriverdi & Iacono, 1999). Near all commercial and even research systems present serious functional deficiencies, such as a poor interoperability and non-accomplishment of information standards and normalization of codes (Koch, 2006).

However, it is well-known that information systems (IS) present similar defects in nearly all domains, particularly at the beginning of the IS adoption and usage by the users and professionals. Indeed, information projects use to show a high rate of failures (Chin & Marcolin, 2001; Hohmann et al, 2003; Loebbecke et al, 2000), and even in those cases where adoption and subsequent business value of the target organization is improved, the deployment stage of the IS by first adopters is many times distressing. Some authors denote this pathological component of IS as the "dark side of IT projects".

Although important advances are being performed in the comprehension and solution of this situation in the e-health domain, in our opinion many of these studies present an uncompleted and even deformed perception of reality. A high number of articles show an excessive academic perspective that neglects aspects related to the market, business and behavioral paradigms, whereas industrial analyses tend to present a weak methodological and conceptual model. A recent and complete reflection regarding the growing distance between industry and academic, and even in the fragmentation of the IS research appears in (King & Lyytinen, 2006). An important conclusion from that source is the need to fuse design-science and behavioral-science paradigms to ensure the effectiveness of information systems. Coughlin and Pope point to a lack in the definition of user needs and markets, as well as how the services must be delivered to the home to provide digital care, as the causes for the poor diffusion e-health services (Coughlin & Pope, 2008).

Despite these obstacles, e-health systems have amply proved their capability and reliability to improve the users' wellness, keeping under control the economical burden of the socio-health system (Finkel et al, 2007; Haux, 2006; Marsh,

1998; Roe, 2007). This result justifies the efforts to achieve a wide deployment of e-health solution by building modern information and communication technologies (ICT) infrastructures in the public health sector of developed countries (Avison & Young, 2007; Goldschmidt, 2005).

The complexity of the minimal functional specifications required by the physician practice sites and hospitals, which is associated to the extension, high and variable semantic level, and the strong dependency of this one on the physician service (Prado et al, 2006a), together with the risk consequences on the patients' health of the uncompleted fulfillment of those requirements, is probably the most important barrier for e-health diffusion. Among the required functional specifications could be included the fulfillment of health information standards, the scalability to different populations and medical specialties, and the attention to the workflow, way of doing, and cultural factors (Demeester et al, 1998).

This chapter will present a new integrative insight in the e-health diffusion problem, by means of a model-based methodology. The model has been developed following an analogy to the chemical kinetics theory. The following section describes the proposed model, which is used subsequently to propose a methodology for the analysis of the e-health system diffusion success. An innovative e-health system designed in the framework of a business strategy (ISIS project) that takes advantage of some of the concepts of the new model will be succinctly presented.

Potential barrier for diffusion: an integrative academic and business model

We have developed a mathematical model for describing the success in the diffusion of e-health solutions, fusing business and technological requirements. This model is based on an analogy to the chemical kinetics theory.

We wish to describe the diffusion rate of e-health systems in physician practice sites (and the associated patient's homes) according to the functional specifications provided and required by each other, respectively, and to technological, industrial, organizational and socioeconomic factors. We formulate this problem by means of the following chemical reaction:

$$R + S \rightarrow P$$

The elements R and P refer to the non-diffused and diffused e-health systems into a type of physician practice sites, S, respectively. This chemical analogy is depicted in Fig. 1.

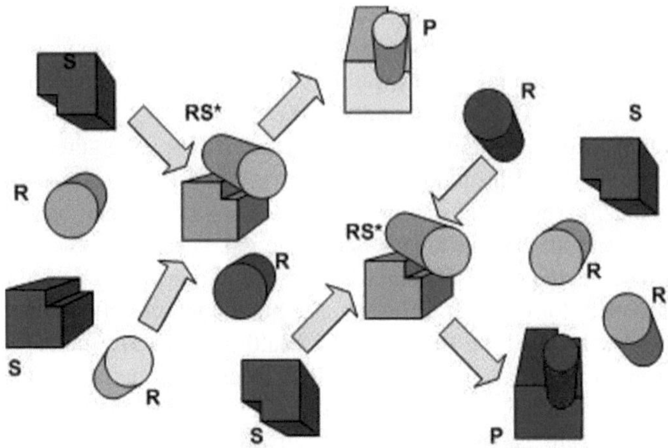

Figure 1: E-health IS (R), physician practice sites (S) and adopted IS (P). RS* forms refer to the transition-state (TS) complex of the reaction. Arrows are oriented according to direct reaction (diffusion of e-health systems).

In order to explain this analogy, we begin considering an e-health system as an information system (IS) that satisfies a particular set of functional specifications, *FS*. This set of *FS* can be reached using different technologies (*T*), license models (*M*), economical costs related to human and material resources (*C*), and organizational and opportunity factors (O). The influence of these factors in diffusion of IS has been recurrently studied (Chin & Marcolin, 2001).

An e-health system needs to meet a set of minimal functional specifications (FS_m) required by the type of clinics where it is intended to be adopted. As it has been reviewed in the Introduction, one of the reasons for the scarce diffusion of e-health systems is due to the extension and complexity of FS_m.

The *diffusion fraction* (*DF*) is defined as:

$$DF = \frac{N_P}{N_R N_S} \tag{1}$$

where N_R are the number of different e-health systems that compete to join to the substrates, *S*, which represent physician practice sites. N_S and N_P are the number of substrates and adopted e-health systems, respectively.

We can assume that *DF* is greater than 0, according to the necessity and reliability of the healthcare model provided by e-health solutions, as shown in the Introduction. However, *DF* is just the *equilibrium constant* of the chemical reaction aforementioned (Chang, 2002).

The feasibility of a reaction (thermodynamics domain) does not imply that reaction proceeds (Chemical kinetics domain). The later is measured by a second parameter, the total *equation rate*, or the rate in which reaction occurs (Chang, 2002; Monk, 2004). In terms of the elements described, we can define the *diffusion rate* (*DR*) as:

$$DR = -\frac{dN_R}{dt} = -\frac{dN_S}{dt} = \frac{dN_P}{dt} \tag{2}$$

The reaction is reversible, on account of the possibility of a physician practice site (S) for rejecting the use of a deployed e-health system (Hohmann et al, 2003). Considering that the *law of mass action* is based on a probabilistic argument: the rate of a chemical reaction depends on how often molecules of each species collide, which is proportional to the concentration or number of each one in sufficiently dilute mediums (Fowler, 1997), we can apply the chemical kinetics equation that derives from that concept to quantify the diffusion rate of e-health systems:

$$DR = kN_R^{\alpha} N_S^{\beta} - k\_N_P^{\gamma}, \tag{3}$$

where k and k_- are the rate constants of the forward (adoption) and reverse (rejection) reaction, respectively.

The order of the forward reaction, n, and reverse reaction, n_-, are:

$$\begin{aligned} n &= \alpha + \beta \\ n\_ &= \gamma \end{aligned} \tag{4}$$

If the reaction would proceed without intermediate steps, then:

$$\begin{aligned} \alpha &= 1 \\ \beta &= 1 \\ \gamma &= 1 \end{aligned} \tag{5}$$

This way n = 2 and n_- =1. However this is not our case. Intermediate steps are many times mediated by catalysts or substances that accelerate the rate of the reaction. Extending that concept to the problem of e-health diffusion, we can say that the exponents of the rate equation (3) depend on the mechanisms followed to implement and adopt the e-health system. It is a matter of fact that the capability to build and implement an IS compliant with a particular *FS* depends on the 4-ada [*T, M, C, O*] (Hohmann et al, 2003). This one defines the underlying mechanisms (intermediate steps) that control the conversion from a non-adopted to an adopted e-health system.

A better technology and license model, together with the reduction in economical cost and the improvement on organizational issues, facilitate the diffusion. Therefore, using the term *energy* in an generalized manner to proceed with the analogy, we can say that [*T, M, C, O*] affects to the *activation energy* that must be surpassed through the reaction path with the aim of reaching the product *P*. Figure 2 presents a classical energy diagram that shows the effect of intermediate paths reducing the activation energy from E_a to E_{ac} in the forward reaction (Monk,

2004). This is called *Potential Barrier Energy* (*PBE*) in this work.

A classical result in the chemical domain is that reaction rate, *DR*, and equilibrium position, *DF*, are independent. This is based on the following relationship between the equilibrium constant (*DF*) and the rate constants (Chang, 2002):

$$\frac{k'}{k'_-}\frac{k''}{k''_-}\cdots\frac{k''^{\cdot\cdot'}}{k''^{\cdot\cdot'}_-} = DF \tag{6}$$

where apostrophes in k and k_- refer to the rate constants of the intermediate reactions that define the path of the complete reaction.

As variables that exert an influence over *DR*, such as catalysts or temperature (energy) act equally on forward and reverse rate equations, *DF* does not depend on *DR*.

In practice, it is not necessary to calculate the value of all the rate constants, but only that of the slowest step, which is known as *rate-determining step* (RDS). Proceeding in this manner, *DR* is given by (3), and exponents depend only on the underlying steps (path of the reaction).

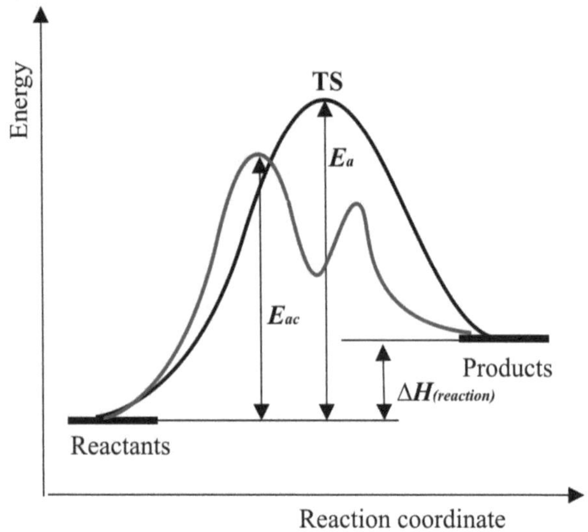

Figure 2: Reaction profile for an uncatalyzed reaction (upper single curve) and a catalyzed reaction which several intermediate steps. Diagram shows also the reaction enthalpy.

Considering that [*T, M, C, O*] controls the reaction path followed for achieving the diffusion of the e-health system, and assuming the validity of the probabilistic argument associated with the law of mass action in this domain, we can use this analogy to chemical kinetics and apply equations (1), (2), and (3) to quantify *DF* and *DR*.

Technically, we base on the *activated complex* theory, which is the kernel of the kinetics theory and catalysts (Fowler, 1997; Monk, 2004). This theory states that a *transient-state complex* (TS) is formed in any of the intermediate routes into the reaction path. This transient complex is very unstable and hence requires high energy to appear. However, some paths and catalysts reduce the energy requirements of the TS by modifying this transient complex in different ways. As a consequence, the ability to modify the reaction path affects the activation energy of the reaction (Fig. 2), which has been called *PBE* in our model of e-health diffusion. The TS complex forms have been presented in Fig. 1 with the superscript *.

The rate constants k and k_{-} depend on *PBE* and the energy of reactants by means of the Arrhenius equation (Chang, 2002; Fowler, 1997; Monk, 2004):

$$k = Ae^{-PBE/R_g K}, \tag{7}$$

and similarly for k_{-}. The variables R_g and K are the gas constant and temperature (in Kelvin), respectively, and A is a constant term. The energy of reactants is controlled by K. This equation has a structure very similar to the equation of Van't Hoff, but indeed it does not derive from it but empirically.

The *energy* (*E*) of the pool of e-health information systems (*reactants*) will depend on their functional specifications, that is, *E* depends on *FS*. The influence of the underlying mechanisms given by [*T, M, C, O*] on the value of *PBE* can also be considered as a modulation of the energy of the e-health system. This mathematical technique allows keeping the same *PBE* for all e-health competing systems, which is a necessary requirement to build a mathematical model for e-health diffusion based on the chemical analogy.

Hence, we can define $E = f(FS, [T, M, C, O])$, as the energy of the reactants, where *FS*, [*T, M, C, O*] refer to the *mean values of their Gaussian distributions*, in a similar way to the chemical kinetics domain (Núñez de Castro, 2001). Accordingly, the potential barrier energy, *PBE,* can be written by means of the *development cost function*, *DC*, as a function of a fixed reference 4-ada value $[T, M, C, O]_r$ and the required reference functional specifications FS_r:

$$PBE = DC(FS_r, [T, M, C, O]_r) \tag{8}$$

The modulation of the energy of the e-health system associated with [*T, M, C, O*] must be defined assuring that the exponent of the Arrhenius equation given by (7) is not modified when *PBE* is referred to the reference 4-ada $[T, M, C, O]_r$. Substituting the energy term of reactants, $R_g K$, by *E(FS)*, this condition can be written as:

$$\left.\begin{array}{l}\dfrac{DC(FS_r,[T,M,C,O])}{E(FS)}=\dfrac{DC(FS_r,[T,M,C,O]_r)}{f(FS,[T,M,C,O])}\\ f(FS,[T,M,C,O])=E(FS)\cdot f_E(T,M,C,O)\end{array}\right\}\Rightarrow$$

$$f(FS,[T,M,C,O])=\frac{DC(FS_r,[T,M,C,O]_r)}{DC(FS_r,[T,M,C,O])}\cdot E(FS)\Rightarrow \tag{9}$$

$$\boxed{f_E(T,M,C,O)=\frac{DC(FS_b,[T,M,C,O]_b)}{DC(FS_b,[T,M,C,O])}}$$

In equations (9) we have defined $f_E(T,M,C,O)$ as the term that modulates the energy related to *FS*, *E(FS)*.

The final (bounded) equation is as expected. That is, if the technology, *T*, facilitates the reach of *FS* with respect to the barrier (reference) technology, T_b, then the activation energy is reduced. This is equivalent to modulate (increase) the energy of the e-health system by a factor f_E that is inversely proportional to the activation energy associated with *T*, when *PBE* is kept equal to a reference value, according to (9).

The system can be simplified dividing the energies by the reference value of *PBE* given by (8). The resulting normalized energies and barrier potential of our mathematical model for e-health diffusion are:

$$\begin{aligned} e &= \frac{f(FS,[T,M,C,O])}{PBE} \\ pbe &= 1 \end{aligned} \tag{10}$$

In summary, equation (3) governs the diffusion (adoption) rate into a type of physician practice sites characterized by the required functional specifications FS_r of a set of e-health systems whose functional specifications, technologies, license models, resource costs, and organizational strategies have the mean values *FS* and [*T, M, C, O*].

The rate constants are given by the Arrhenius equation, where the exponential term is exp(-*e*), and *e* is given by (10). We denote it as *diffusion problem of type 1.*

A complementary problem is the description of the diffusion (adoption) rate of a particular type of e-health systems featured with the functional specifications FS_r and the mean value [*T, M, C, O*], into a set of physician practice sites, characterized by *FS* as the mean value of the required functional specifications. This second case can be addressed in the same way that the previous one, converting the variations of *PBE* associated to *FS* and [*T, M, C, O*] in modulations of the energy of the e-health systems. Rewriting equation (9) gives the following formulation for the energy $E = f(FS, [T, M, C, O])$, of the equivalent system:

$$\left.\begin{array}{l}\dfrac{DC(FS,[T,M,C,O])}{E(FS_r)}=\dfrac{DC(FS_r,[T,M,C,O]_r)}{f(FS,[T,M,C,O])}\\ f(FS,[T,M,C,O])=E(FS_r)\cdot f_E(FS,[T,M,C,O])\end{array}\right\}\Rightarrow$$

$$\boxed{f_E(FS,[T,M,C,O])=\frac{DC(FS_r,[T,M,C,O]_r)}{DC(FS,[T,M,C,O])}} \tag{11}$$

Therefore, this second case, denoted as *diffusion problem of type 2*, is governed by the same equations than the type 1, with the exception of the energy of the R reactants, $E = f(FS, [T, M, C, O])$, which is now given by (11). Note that the main difference between type 2 and type 1 diffusion problem is the dependence of f_E with respect to FS. That is, in the type 2 diffusion problem the modulation factor depends on the required mean FS of the physician practice sites.

A methodology to analyze the diffusion of e-health systems

We are going to present several cases that lead the definition of a first proposal for a model-based methodology of analysis of e-health systems diffusion, and throw light on the interpretation of the mathematical formulation.

Substituting equation (10) and (7) into (3) just at the beginning of the e-health diffusion ($N_P = 0$), considering a constant number of physician practice sites, N_S, and grouping constant terms, the following equation is obtained for DR:

$$DR = \underbrace{A_1 \cdot e^{-PBE/f(FS,[T,M,C,O])}}_{k_1} \cdot N_R^{\alpha}, \tag{12}$$

where A_1 and PBE are constants. The value k_1 is used afterwards.

The equation (12) is a simplified but interesting first case, since it shows the success of diffusion just at the beginning, avoiding any feedback between the number of adopted e-health systems (N_P) and the number of available practice sites (N_S). This feedback relationship is a well-known behavior of information systems (Hohmann et al, 2003). The equation (12) can be applied to the two types of e-health diffusion problems. It provides a relationship between DR and N_R, presented in Fig. 3, where k_1 is the apparent rate constant.

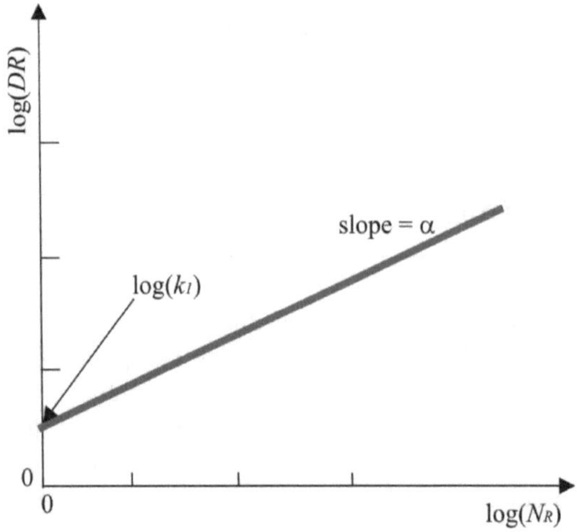

Figure 3: Diffusion rate as a function of N_R, in logarithmic scale.

For example, in the case of *type 1 diffusion problem*, Fig. 3 shows that the starting diffusion success into a type of practice sites featured by FS_r increases if the number of e-health solutions types grows. Under a *type 2 diffusion problem*, the same figure shows that the diffusion success at the beginning, for a particular e-health system deployed under a path given by $[T,M,C,O]$, increases if the number of types of practice sites (with different required functional specifications) grows. The latter is the meaning of N_R due to the conversion associates with equation (11)

.

The diagram of Fig. 3 can also be used to determinate empirically the order of the reaction, α, following a technique similar to that used in chemical area (Núñez de Castro, 2001).

A second and interesting case emerges when one tries to analyze the influence of the energy modulation factors in the starting *DR*, under the same conditions of the equation (12). We focus this case on a *type 2 diffusion problem*. Taking a constant number of practice sites types, the cited equation remains as:

$$DR = A_2 \cdot e^{-PBE/f(FS,[T,M,C,O])} \quad (13)$$

where A_2 is a constant that integrates N_R.

This equation is presented in figure 4, which shows the relationship between *DR* and the mean energy $E = f(FS, [T, M, C, O])$. This particular solution is explained in the following paragraphs.

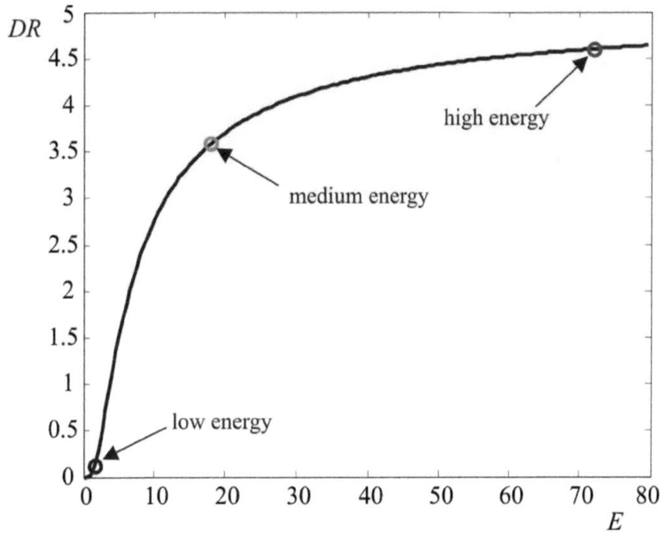

Figure 4: Diffusion rate as a function of the e-health energy under the conditions of equation (13). Marks (circles) on the curve show the influence of the license model and technology modulation factors of Table 1, as discussed in text.

According to equation (11), $f(FS, [T, M, C, O]) = E(FS_r) \cdot f_E(FS, [T, M, C, O])$. We are interested in studying the influence of the arguments that modulate the energy of the e-health system, $E(FS_r)$, with the aim of proposing a model-based methodology for analyzing the diffusion. We assume that f_E can be written in separated variables, as follows:

$$f_E(FS,[T,M,C,O]) = f_{EFS}(FS) \cdot f_{ET}(T) \cdot f_{EM}(M) \cdot f_{EC}(C) \cdot f_{EO}(O) \tag{14}$$

In addition, each one of the modulation factors, which depend on qualitative arguments, will be written as a function of a base coefficient, modulated in amplitude by correction factors with values lesser than 1.

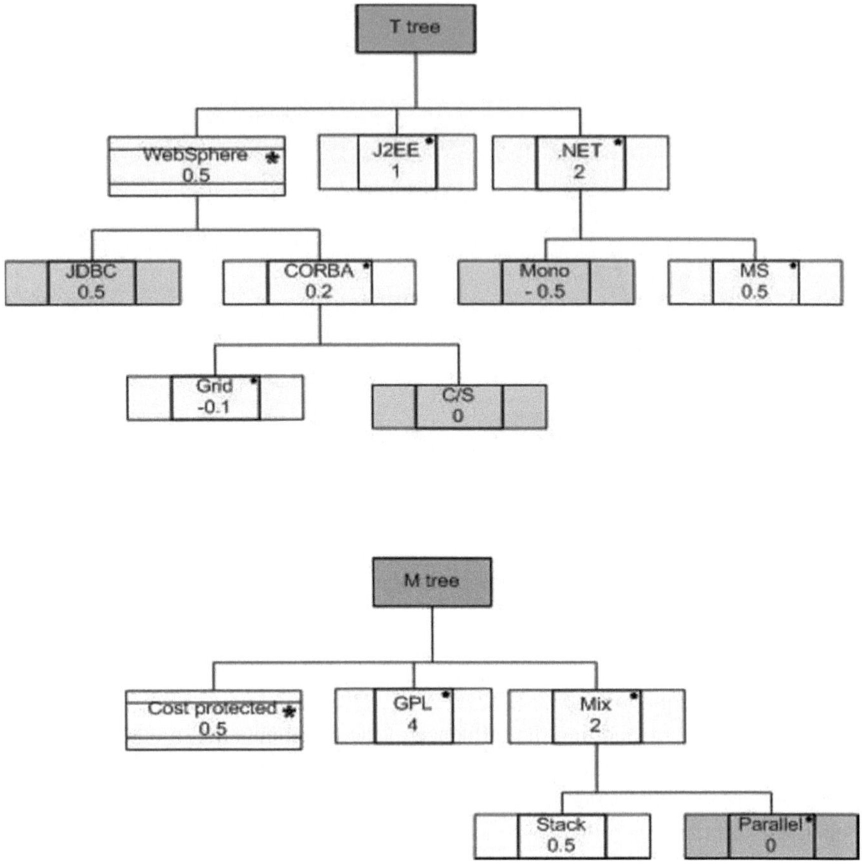

Figure 5: T and M trees presenting the base coefficients and correction factors, as explained in text. Technologies and license models have been indicated as an example, but their relationship to the node weights is shown only to clarify the study case.

The method is clarified by means of an example, which shows the influence of Technology (*T*) and the license model (*M*) on the diffusion rate.

The values of the base coefficients and correction factors of a simplified technology tree (a) and a license model tree (b) appear in Fig. 5. The equations for the associated modulation factors are:

$$\begin{aligned} f_{ET}(T) &= F_{T0} \cdot (1+\xi_{T1}) \cdot (1+\xi_{T2}) \\ f_{EM}(M) &= F_{M0} \cdot (1+\xi_{M1}) \end{aligned} \tag{15}$$

where ξ correction coefficients are lesser than 1.

T and *M* trees have three and two levels, respectively. They can be considered as classifiers trees. The first level is related to the base coefficients, which define the base technology, in the case of the *T* tree, or the base license model, in the case of *M* tree. The remaining levels must refer to particular variants of the parent node. As a consequence, the requirement $\xi \leq 1$ guarantees a proper selection of the base technologies and license models. Regarding the concept of energy and modulation factors as mean values associated with a Gaussian distribution, as the variance, σ^2, is not fixed, we can consider a very small value of σ for studying the influence of particular technologies and license models in *DR* by means equations (14) and (15). These equations propose a data-driven approach to set the energy function in the framework of the mathematical model developed in the previous Section.

The base factors and correction factors can be obtained using experimental data from diffusion success studies, as well as information regarding the reliability of different technologies and the other factors that modulate the energy. This type of knowledge concerns the field of diffusion research on innovative and information systems (Demeester et al, 1998; Hohmann et al, 2003; Loebbecke et al, 2000). Substituting (15) into (14), and then into (13), the following equation is obtained:

$$
\begin{aligned}
DR &= A_2 \cdot e^{-PBE/(E(FS_r)\cdot f_{EM}(M) f_{ET}(T) f_{EC}(C) f_{EO}(O))} \\
&= A_2 \cdot e^{-C/(E(FS_r)\cdot f_{EM}(M) f_{ET}(T))},
\end{aligned}
\tag{16}
$$

which can be fitted to the referred experimental data. A good method to guarantee the robustness of the fitted model is the identification of the $f_{Ei}(i)$ groups (equation (14)) as constant values in a first stage, comparing their resulting values to the base factors of equation (15) identified in second stage. If $f_{Ei}(i)$ are very far from their associated base factors, F_{i0}, the tree definition (classification) should be reviewed.

The value of *DR* for the three couples of modulator factors corresponding to a proprietary license model and a high development cost technology (low energy), a free license model (e.g. GPL) and a low development cost technology (high energy), and finally a mixed license model with an medium cost development technology (medium energy), whose associated values of base and corrector factors are presented in Table 1 and Fig. 5 (clearer nodes), have been shown in Fig. 4.

Those *DR* values have been computed with $A_2 = 5$, $C = 6$, and $E(FS_r) = 6$ (equation (16)). A_2 is the apparent rate constant and therefore its units depends on the equation order, *n*, whereas *C* and $E(FS_r)$ are given in energy units. Although *C* comprises several constant modulation factors in this example, it can be considered the apparent *PBE* of this e-health system diffusion problem.

Table 1: Weights of the nodes of the *T* and *M* trees, associated with the base and correction factors (nodes of trees in Fig. 5).

f_E	F_{M0}	ξ_{M1}	F_{T0}	ξ_{T1}	ξ_{T2}
Low Energy	0.5	0	0.5	0.2	-0.1
Medium Energy	2	0.5	1	0	0
High Energy	4	0	2	0.5	0

A conclusion of this second theoretical case presented in Fig. 4 is that the starting diffusion rate of an e-health system characterized by functional specifications FS_r, could vary between a value near 0 (low energy) and a maximum value A_2 that is reached asymptotically, as a function of the technology, license model, resource costs, and organizational factors. The asymptotic behavior of *DR* as a function of the energy suggests that a selection of [*T, M, C, O*] related to medium energy e-health system (see Fig. 4) is good enough to achieve a successfully diffusion.

We are also interested in the temporal evolution of adopted e-health systems, N_P. This is a well studied problem in the area of diffusion research of innovations (Chin & Marcolin, 2001; Hohmann et al, 2003; Loebbecke et al, 2000). However, the model presented in the previous Section provides a new perspective of the subject, filling a gap appointed by (Chin & Marcolin, 2001).

With that goal, we can develop the equation (3) for a *diffusion problem of type 2*, with a constant number of practice sites types (as the previous case), N_R. Firstly, in agreement with equation (6), we note that the Arrhenius equation for the forward and reverse reactions can be written as:

$$k = Ae^{-PBE/E} \qquad k_{-} = Be^{-PBE/E} \tag{17}$$

where *A* and *B* are constant terms.

Substituting (17) into (3), and following the previous nomenclature for the constant terms, the following equation for *DR* is obtained:

$$DR = e^{-PBE/f(FS,[T,M,C,O])} \cdot \left[A_2 N_S^{\beta} - BN_P^{\gamma} \right] \tag{18}$$

However the increase of N_P promotes an increase of N_S. This causal effect is well-known in the research on information systems diffusion (Hohmann et al, 2003). Taking $N_S = N_{S0} \cdot (1 + \zeta \cdot N_P)$, where ζ is called the *transmission factor*, and using (2), the equation (18) gives us the following differential equation for $N_P(t)$:

$$\begin{aligned}\dot{N}_p &= e^{-PBE/f(FS,[T,M,C,O])} \cdot \left(\underbrace{A_2 N_{S0}^{\beta}}_{A_3} (1+\varsigma N_P)^{\beta} - BN_P^{\gamma} \right) \\ &= e^{-PBE/E} \cdot \left(A_3 (1+\varsigma N_P)^{\beta} - BN_P^{\gamma} \right)\end{aligned} \tag{19}$$

This equation can be integrated for different values of the Arrhenius exponent, *PBE/E*, as well as the apparent (because N_R is constant) orders of the forward and reverse reactions, β and γ, respectively.

Figure 6 shows the temporal evolution of N_P given by equation (19) with $\zeta = 0.7$, $A_3 = 1$, and $B = 1$, for the indicated parameters. All the variables and parameters follow a homogenous units system.

It is very interested that the adoption curve follows an S-shaped form, in agreement with countless studies relative to the adoption of innovative products (Hohmann et al, 2003). However, this sigmoid pattern only occurs when reaction does not proceed in a linear manner (α, β ≥ 2). This outcome confirms that modulation factors or intermediate mechanisms associated to them have a clear influence on the diffusion of e-health systems. Our model provides a methodology to quantify the coupling between the positive and negative feedback mechanisms that characterize the sigmoid pattern (Aracil & Gordillo, 1997) of $N_p(t)$.

The figure shows also the influence of the *PBE/E* fraction on the diffusion rate. When the activation energy *PBE* is 5 times the mean energy of e-health systems, *E*, the diffusion rate is near zero. This result provides another perspective regarding the concept of failure in e-health systems adoption. It is interesting to note that the final value of N_P (null *DR*) can be calculated from (19) taking advantage of the equality γ = β to give:

$$N_p = \frac{1}{\left(\frac{B}{A_3}\right)^{1/\beta} - \varsigma} \tag{20}$$

Therefore, the equilibrium value for N_P is 3.33 for all the cases presented in Fig. 6, according to equation (20).

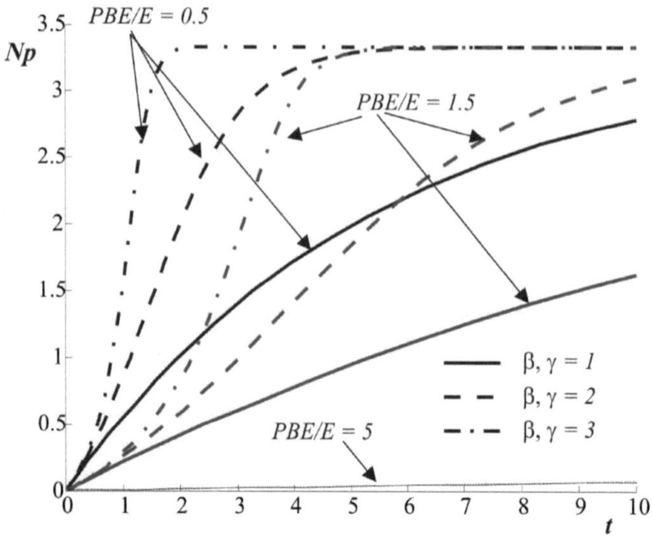

Figure 6: Temporal evolution of the adoption of the e-health systems, as a function of PBE/E and the reaction orders.

Description of an innovative e-health system

We have shown the strong influence of the modulation factors [*T*, *M* , *C* ,*O*] on the diffusion rate and success of an e-health solution. The present Section shows in a synthetic way an innovative e-health system that joins a novel knowledge-centered telehealthcare system designed by one of the authors (Prado et al, 2002; Prado et al, 2006b) with a free and open source software (FOSS) solution in e-health, within a business strategy (ISIS project). This one seeks a competitive e-health system able to manage wearable fall detectors placed in the place of care (POC) and seamlessly scalable to standard and new advanced added values around the Electronic Health Record (EHR).

This novel system follows a mixed license model, which starts with a GPL functional healthcare solution, validated in many physician practice sites. Advanced functions with proprietary and other types of license models are built over that base. This mixed license model, *M*, seeks to reduce the *PBE* value and this way to increase the diffusion rate, *DR*, as shown in Fig. 4. It refers to the *stack* type of license model appointed in the *M* tree of Fig. 5.

A simplified overview of the architecture of this mixed-license knowledge-centered telehealthcare system is presented in Fig. 7.

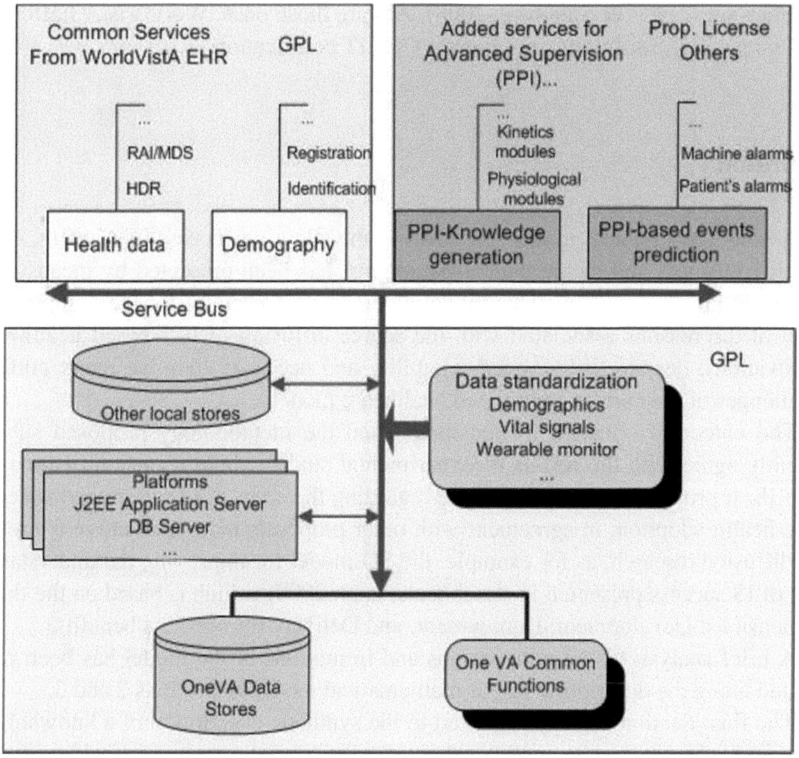

Figure 7: Block diagram of the computer architecture of the mixed license knowledge-centered e-health system. It is based on a simplified scheme of WorldVistA EHR FOSS solution, with GPL license, and a set of added values based on the Nefrotel concept of telehealthcare (right upper box).

According to the health and management functionalities, architecture's evolution, scalability and portability issues, evaluation and feedback from many physician practice sites, and the CCHIT (certification commission for Healthcare Information Technology) compliant, the WorldVistA EHR FOSS system was preliminarily selected as the GPL e-health system over which advanced functions like real-time and personalized knowledge generation (Prado et al, 2002) could be implemented.

A more detailed description of the concept of personalized knowledge generation and the derived telehealthcare architecture in the renal domain appears in (Prado et al, 2002; Prado et al, 2005; Prado et al, 2006b).

Many sources describe with detail functions and the computer architecture of the WorldVistA EHR solution (www.worldvista.org). An interesting report comparing several FOSS EHR systems selected also WorldVistA together with other ones on the basis of the fulfillment of a set of criteria that include open-source license, demonstrated clinical data-management capabilities, design for ambulatory care, compliant with HIPAA security, and implemented in at least ten physician practice sites (Faus & Sujansky, 2008). Among those ones, WorldVistA EHR was the unique FOSS solution compliant to CCHIT certification.

Summary

A new mathematical model for studying the adoption success in e-health, integrating business and technological paradigms, has been presented by means of a chemical kinetics analogy. This model emerges as a response for the comprehension of the reasons associated with the scarce diffusion of ICT-based healthcare innovations, despite their proved reliability and necessity to solve many current challenges of the current centralized healthcare model.

The outcomes obtained by the model and the methodology proposed subsequently agree with the results of experimental studies about diffusion of innovative IS. It provides a new perspective regarding the concept of failure and success in e-health adoption, in agreement with other proposals more qualitative from the IS diffusion research, as for example, the 3D-model for improving the understanding of IS success presented in (Loebbecke et al, 2000), which is based on the three dimensions: Development, Deployment, and Delivery (of business benefits).

A brief analysis of the assumptions and limitations of the model has been presented along the description of our mathematical model in Sections 2 and 3.

The final Section has been devoted to the synthetic description of a knowledge-centered e-health system, which takes advantage of the integrative view of this study. The new e-health system facilitates the deployment of the IS due to the null cost of the GPL base and common services, allowing the addition and research in very advanced non-free services, as it is the real-time knowledge generation and short-term prediction mediated by PPI components (Prado et al, 2002; Prado et al, 2003) or an advanced system for detecting falls by means of wearable human movement monitors (Prado-Velasco et al, 2008).

The paradigm underlying the PPI-based knowledge generation is associated with initiatives whose objective is to provide tools and services to share and model the human physiology dynamics under a multilevel approach. These initiatives are under the Systems Biology umbrella. Accordingly, the briefly presented e-health system provides a business strategy to take advantage of the synergy between systems biology and e-health (Prado et al, 2005). This synergy is recently beginning to be considered a reliable approach to reach the objective of a really personalized and predictive medicine (Hood, 2008).

Acknowledgements

This work has been partly supported by the "Ministerio de Industria, Turismo y

Comercio", "Acción Estratégica de Telecomunicaciones y Sociedad de la Información, Avanza I+D", within the National Plan for Scientific Research, Development, and Technological Innovation, under Grants TSI-020100-2008-64 (ISIS) and TSI-020301-2008-15 (Tratamiento 2.0).

References

Aracil, J., Gordillo, F.: Dinámica de sistemas (Systems Dynamics): Alianza Editorial, Madrid (1997)

Avison, D., Young, T.: Time to rethink health care and ICT? Commun. ACM 50(6), 69–74 (2007)

Coughlin, J.F., Pope, J.: Innovations in health, wellness, and aging-in-place. IEEE Engineering in Medicine and Biology Magazine 27(4), 47–52 (2008)

Chang, R.: Química [Chemistry], Séptima Edición edn. McGraw-Hill, Mexico (2002)

Chin, W.W., Marcolin, B.L.: The future of diffusion research. SIGMIS Database 32(3), 7–12 (2001)

Demeester, M., Guillen-Barrionuevo, S., Millet-Roig, J., Traver, V., Mocholi-Salcedo, A.: Culture and the deployment of health care telematics applications. In: Engineering in Medicine and Biology Society, 1998. Proceedings of the 20th Annual International Conference of the IEEE, vol. 1233, pp. 1234–1237 (1998)

Faus, S.A., Sujansky, W.: Open-Source EHR Systems for Ambulatory Care: A Market Assessment. In: California Healthcare Foundation, p. 6 (2008)

Finkel, S., Czaja, S.J., Schulz, R., Martinovich, Z., Harris, C., Pezzuto, D.: E-Care: A Telecommunications Technology Intervention for Family Caregivers of Dementia Patients. Am. J. Geriatr Psychiatry 15(5), 443–448 (2007)

Fowler, A.C.: Enzyme kinetics. In Mathematical Models in the Applied Sciences, vol. 9, pp. 133–144. Cambridge University Press, Cambridge (1997)

Goldschmidt, P.G.: HIT and MIS: implications of health information technology and medical information systems. Commun. ACM 48(10), 68–74 (2005)

Haux, R.: Health information systems - past, present, future. International Journal of Medical Informatics 75(3-4), 268–281 (2006)

Hohmann, L., Fowler, M., Kawasaki, G.: Beyond software architecture: creating and sustaining winning solutions. Addison Wesley, Reading (2003)

Hood, L.: Systems Biology and Systems Medicine: From Reactive to Predictive, Personalized, Preventive and Participatory (P4) Medicine. In: Personalized Healthcare through Technology, Vancouver, Canada, August 20-24, IEEE, Los Alamitos (2008)

King, J.L., Lyytinen, K. (eds.): Information Systems. The State of the Field. John Wiley & Sons Ltd., Chichester (2006)

Koch, S.: Home telehealth–Current state and future trends. International Journal of Medical Informatics 75(8), 565–576 (2006)

Loebbecke, C., Powell, P., Levy, M., Martin, A.: Conceptualizing Information System Success: Towards a 3D-Model. In: First Gulf Conference on Decision Support Systems, Kuwait, pp. 1–7 (2000)

Marsh, A.: The Creation of a global telemedical information society. International Journal of Medical Informatics 49(2), 173–193 (1998)

May, C., Mort, M., Mair, F., Finch, T.: Telemedicine and the 'Future Patient'? Risk, Governance and Innovation. In: Economic & Social Research Council, p. 3 (2005)

Monk, P.: Physical Chemistry: Understanding our Chemical World. John Wiley & Sons, West Sussex (2004)

Núñez de Castro, I.: Enzimología [Enzymology]: Ediciones Pirámide, Madrid (2001)

Prado-Velasco, M., del Río-Cidoncha, M.G., Ortíz-Marín, R.: The Inescapable Smart Impact detection System (ISIS): an ubiquitous and personalized fall detector based on a distributed "divide and conquer strategy". In: Personalized Healthcare through Technology, 30th Annual International Conference of the IEEE Engineering in Medicine and Biology Society, Vancouver, British Columbia, Canada, August 20-24 (2008)

Prado, M., Roa, L., Reina-Tosina, J., Palma, A., Milán, J.A.: Virtual Center for Renal Support: Technological Approach to Patient Physiological Image. IEEE Transactions on Biomedical Engineering 49(12), 1420–1430 (2002)

Prado, M., Roa, L., Reina-Tosina, J., Palma, A., Milán, J.A.: Renal telehealthcare system based on a patient physiological image: a novel hybrid approach in telemedicine. Telemed J. 9(2), 149–165 (2003)

Prado, M., Roa, L.M., Reina-Tosina, J.: Hybrid and customized approach in telemedicine systems: an unavoidable destination. In: Bos, L., Laxminarayan, S., Marsh, A. (eds.) Medical and Care Compunetics 2, vol. 114, pp. 238–258. IOS Pres, Amsterdam (2005)

Prado, M., Roa, L.M., Reina-Tosina, J.: Methodological issues for the information model of a knowledge-based telehealthcare system for nephrology (Nefrotel). In: Medical and Care Compunetics 3, pp. 96–107. IOS Pres, Amsterdam (2006a)

Prado, M., Roa, L.M., Reina-Tosina, J.: Viability study of a personalized and adaptive knowledge-generation telehealthcare system for nephrology (NEFROTEL). International Journal of Medical Informatics 75(9), 646–657 (2006b)

Roe, P.R.W. (ed.): Towards an inclusive future Impact and wider potential of information and communication technologies, p. 329. COST, Brussels (2007)

Tanriverdi, H., Iacono, C.S.: Diffusion of telemedicine: a knowledge barrier perspective. Telemed J. 5(3), 223–244 (1999)

The Consumerisation of Home Healthcare Technologies

Ade Bamigboye, B.Sc (Hons), M.Sc, MBA

Wireless Matters

Abstract Though widely promoted as needing to play a significant role in future healthcare systems, Digital Homecare could serve to complicate situations for patients and care providers unless it becomes much easier to create, deliver and manage the complex mix of technology, support and services that are appropriate to a patient at a specific time. Any holistic approach to Digital Homecare must be able to support a patients' Physiological, Physical, Emotional and Environmental care needs. Furthermore, solutions must meet the requirements of patients' family and friends who will need to take on much more participative supporting roles if Digital Homecare is ever to be deployed on a scale that will alleviate stretched healthcare resources and save the millions of dollars that studies claim can be saved. In all but the simplest of systems the patient gateway is a key technology component. Intelligent Gateways are critical to driving mass adoption of Digital Homecare. Without them, Digital Homecare solutions will remain the niche, high end technology applications that they are today functioning only in un-integrated silos. Current and future participants in the Digital Homecare sector should focus on developing more intelligent gateways to ensure mass adoption.

Table of contents

K. Yogesan et al. (Eds.): Handbook of Digital Homecare, BIOMED, pp. 95–116.
springerlink.com

Introduction

Custodians of healthcare systems accept that the ongoing demographic and lifestyle changes occurring in populations across the world are severely testing their ability cope. The elderly are living longer and are tending to remain at home either because of the lack of affordable care home facilities or because they feel more comfortable in familiar environments. The lifestyle of the younger generation is causing healthcare problems that would not previously have been noticed until much later in their lives. In between these extremes, there are the "worried well" who may also place a demand on the services of healthcare professionals even if they are least in need. These combined set of pressures has created an imbalance between the availability of healthcare professionals and demand for their services. The shortage of healthcare resource is global and affects specialists as well as generalists. In clinical practice, the effects are felt across primary, secondary and tertiary care. In the community, the lack of domiciliary carers combined with dispersed families who have in the past provided a lot of informal care is also a huge problem for people dependent on receiving care at home. It is not only patients that are affected. It is additionally their family, friends and employers who need to find some way of continuing to manage their own lives whilst providing ongoing care as best that they can.

An increasing number of healthcare professionals now believe that future healthcare systems that are aimed at supporting patients outside of dedicated healthcare facilities need to be implemented on a much wider scale than they are at present and that this needs to be done now rather than may years into the future. There is a firm belief that only steep step changes in the provisioning of healthcare at home will make any relevant impact and that technology has got to play an increasingly significant role. A technology led step change is desirable for many reasons but a significant reason is that once perfected, technology can be replicated quickly and solutions distributed widely. It will also require, rather than hope, that patients adopt and fully engage with newer models of receiving healthcare services once they have left the security of dedicated healthcare facilities. The new model of home healthcare delivery will require a greater degree of supported self-management and in this context, the requirement is that patients must understand that whilst some aspects of their care will become more impersonal and remote, the greater interest is in continuing to be able to provide a high quality of healthcare to all that require it.

Analysing the literature for either the reported number of patients that could benefit or the amount of hard cash that could be saved by deploying Digital Homecare and comparing these to actual deployments, Digital Homecare is very much a niche market. The key generic issues are high equipment costs, difficult technical integration, and a lack of clarity over which equipment to use as well as open debates relating to standards and the ethics of this approach to delivering healthcare services. These all contribute to the lack of widespread use. Country specific issues are also a contributory factor. In the USA the question of reimbursement is critical. In the UK where much of the healthcare is provided by the State Funded NHS it is a question of proving real value for money and determining how to fund it.

Overview of Digital Homecare

Digital Homecare can be defined as any combination of Digital Technologies installed in a home environment to enable delivery and management of health care. In this context Digital Technology means any combination of software, hardware and communications configured to provide the appropriate functionality for the patient and the carers who support them. Substantial advances across all of these technology areas over the last 10 years has driven rapid innovation in products and services that can easily be used in the healthcare sector. This is visible in the increased range of products and services designed for personal rather than professional use. Innovation is enabling the creation of such a broad range of solutions so that apart from on-going improvements to first generation Telecare and Telemedince products, emerging products and services now include

- healthcare portals that offer advice, diagnostics and networking for a wide range of conditions
- digital health vaults such as those available from Google and Microsoft that enable users to store and manage their own medical records and can receive data from a wide range of readily available medical devices
- devices from consumer product manufacturers that are either designed for a specific healthcare application or that find a role in this market such as gaming company Nintendo whose Wii product is now seeing use in physical and cognitive therapy

Digital Homecare solutions should aim to make available all of the functionality identified in Table 1.

Table.1 Scope of functionality in Digital Homecare

Digital Home Care Functionality	**Description of Functionality**
Condition Management	Assist patients to comply with a prescribed or recommended regime of treatment and care. This will include sending reminders when medication is due or when data needs to be collected. An additional element of functionality is sending messages of encouragement when pre-set goals are reached.
Assistance with activities of daily living	Help users who have physical impairments to perform tasks around the home that would otherwise require the presence of another person. This will include managing heating and lighting, opening and closing doors, manipulating switches and engaging in communications.
Monitoring	Performing regular collection of data to be used for analysis and planning. Analysis can be used to identify adverse trends and adjust care regimes or implement preventative measures.
Emergency Management	Determine and set in motion all appropriate response protocols when any emergency situation is reached. Appropriate data can be transmitted in a timely manner to all of the right persons or groups.
Advice, Educate and Coach	Translate raw medical data into coherent non-medical language that is to be used as the basis for automated communication with consumers. As different consumers will have different levels of understanding Digital Homecare solutions must be capable of multi-level communication.
Information Management	Users will expect that agencies have all the relevant up to date information so it is necessary to ensure accurate recording and timely distribution data and information to all of the relevant agencies. Possible recipients will include General Practitioners and other Clinical Personnel, Pharmacies, Carers, Friends and Family

Negative Aspects of Digital Homecare

Though widely promoted as needing to play a significant role in future healthcare systems, Digital Homecare could serve to complicate situations for patients and care providers unless it becomes an easy, cost effective matter to create, deliver and manage the complex mix of technology, support and service that is appropriate to a patient at a specific time.

From the consumer's viewpoint, one of the biggest concerns is the potential increase in physical isolation from the care team although this can be mitigated to some extent through the use of technologies such as Video over IP, Social Networks and mobile phones. Additional problems relate to how difficult the technology is to use.

From the healthcare service providers' viewpoint there is an increased workload as well as the possible misuse of equipment and data to deal with. Both of these can easily lead to situations that are harmful to the consumer. The increased workload to health service providers arises as a result of the requirement for training professionals to be able to assess and specify appropriate solutions, managing the vast amounts of data generated and responding to alerts arising from deployed solutions.

Digital Homecare for the Patient's Support Network

Digital Homecare solutions will also have to meet the varied requirements of the patients' extended carer network - family and friends - that will also be required to take on much more participative roles. Members of a patients' extended carer network who may in the past have been used to carrying out tasks such as collecting medication, providing reports to the patients' clinician, providing mentorship and support are likely to see this role extended. In this new role they are likely to get involved in helping patients to understand and select appropriate solutions, install, maintain and use the equipment to help with care and care planning. The technology will need to provide authorised users with secure and controlled access to patient data and status reports. For users who are not members of a professional healthcare group there will be very different levels of confidence in dealing with healthcare issues. The technology will need to be able to present data and analysis in many different ways, be very clear, well understood and provide the users with confidence when using the equipment.

Even with all of these technology challenges and in spite of the still huge resistance from many quarters, technology driven solutions have been proven to be beneficial and now needs to be made easily accessible, address a much wider range of healthcare issues and be deployed on a much larger scale. In this, there is an implied degree of consumerisation that is not common even in the most advanced healthcare systems and it is to this that we now turn.

Defining Consumerisation in Digital Homecare

A strict definition of a consumer market is one in which products and services aimed at a mass market are purchased by consumers rather than professionals. Factors that distinguish consumer oriented products and services from professional products are that consumer products are accessible by the wider market, affordable and well understood so that deep expertise is not required before the consumer can enjoy the utility. If the current generation of Telecare and Telemedicine services are judged by these benchmarks, they can not be described as ready for the consumer market.

In the marketing sense, Digital Homecare solutions would be categorised as "Consumer Durables" alongside other household electronic appliances such as DVDs and TVs. Whilst there is no argument to suggest that Digital Homecare needs to be deployed on as wide a scale as these products, in the context of Digital Homecare, to consider consumerisation is to consider how the equipment, facilities and services that are typically available in dedicated healthcare facilities can be "scaled down" for use in domestic environments. This means that the physical size of the equipment must fit comfortably in the average patient's home, must be very robust and easy for the patient, their family and carers to use. At the same time the products must offer a high level of functionality and be supported by the same type of services and expertise that would be found in a dedicated healthcare facility. In real terms for example, how can a multi-parameter monitoring device which has been designed for high volume use and to integrate with a hospital's IT system be redesigned and repackaged to monitor patients at home, capture data and deliver this to remote systems used by professional carers to perform diagnosis and deliver advice ? and all of this of course has to be delivered within a reasonable price. One can say that consumerised Digital Homecare has the following characteristics:

- ❑ Consumers (patients and their guardians) can buy direct from suppliers but are able to consult a recognised body of expertise for advice on what would be an appropriate solution
- ❑ Products fit well with the consumers environment and are easy to use
- ❑ Consumers take responsibility for using and managing equipment correctly
- ❑ Professional carers acting as licensed advisors can explain the benefits and use of appropriate solutions and train consumers within a couple of hours
- ❑ Products based on clearly defined standards which are widely supported by professional groups
- ❑ There are a number of suppliers in the market ensuring long term market development, best pricing and innovation, product choice and options

The need for consumerisation

Modern thinking on home healthcare is that it is not just about patients living longer at home even when diagnosed with chronic illness. It is about a better quality of life for the patient as well as their family and carers. For friends and families, technology that connects, monitors and informs in a way that they can understand regardless of their level of knowledge or confidence is good. The common theory is that patients fair better when being cared for in a familiar environment. Several research reports, testify to the fact that a better quality of life can be achieved when patients are at home, can be monitored and given appropriate support and response when required. Improvements in quality of life can occur on several levels but the key impact is where patients develop a much greater degree of confidence to get on with activities of daily living in the knowledge that there is support system in operation that is capable of monitoring conditions, pre-empting potential problems and organising rapid response as appropriate.

Digital Homecare can provide this through performing automated checks and notify carers of adverse trends even before the patient has a chance to call for assistance. This is in contrast to even a few years ago when patients with chronic illness would expect, resources permitting, to reside in a care home surrounded by professional staff, 24 x 7 x 365 to receive this level of monitoring. The relatively low cost of consumer electronics helps to make this a reality.

The increased interest and wider acceptability of Digital Homecare is also being driven by the increasingly easier access to medical and health information that can be understood by non medical people as well as self-help guides. Certain demographics are also more motivated to achieve healthier lifestyles and this has stimulated the growth of people seeking solutions for monitoring aspects of their physiology even when not diagnosed with any problems. These so called "worried well" are being increasingly well served with a range of products and services.

System Benefits of Consumerisation

Because patients with long term chronic illnesses utilise the majority of resources in any healthcare system, early installations of Digital Homecare have tended to be aimed at this group of patients. This group often has clearly defined management and monitoring requirements and it has been easier to make a business case for the deployment of expensive and largely experimental technology. In these cases, the key benefits derived from being able to deploy Digital Homecare are to maintain or increase the intensity of monitoring without further straining the system.

Further down the continuum of care benefits are derived from the ability to monitor, predict and pre-empt episodes that if not corrected would become more chronic in nature and hence expensive to treat.

Current State of Digital Homecare

The way in which design and development of Digital Homecare services has taken place over the years has resulted in the current situation whereby solutions have been developed in silos that close reflect how healthcare is delivered. Telemedicine has focused on replicating some of the services provided by community General Practitioners and community nurses, monitoring physiological parameters. Telecare has focus on monitoring activities of daily living once patients are at home which to some extent replicates some of the services provided by domiciliary and informal carers.

New suppliers seeking to enter this market have tended to focus on either one of these further exacerbating the siloed approach. Monitoring COPD or Diabetes are examples of this. Although these are broad definitions, a common problem has up until now has limited the rate at which physicians or social services, that is care services provide to patients in the community, will adopt the solutions. Given the number of installations that are being considered, patients and their immediate network of carers need to be able to deal with much of the data and information that is generated. If they do not, the growth in Digital Homecare will lead to a data and communication explosion as data that is generated by installed devices is transferred to remote applications and becomes the responsibility of professional healthcare personal.

In many developed economies, consumerised Digital Healthcare products are already available at some level. In the UK for example, blood pressure, heart monitors and other devices can be purchased in high-street supermarkets, pharmacy chains or on the internet. Consumers are sign-posted to these suppliers through magazine, TV or internet advertising and access to information on the internet informs their decision making.

The reality however is that only the simplest of solutions tend to be purchased by consumers directly and where they are purchased there is typically no connectivity to remote services. The question also remains as to whether any General Practitioner would use the data if it were made available to them by their patients as the source and accuracy would be unknown.

Consumers in this sector include the "worried well" as well as those with know health problems.

Digital Homecare for future consumers

From a product development perspective it is necessary to determine, and be clear about the scope and level of technology that can be realistically provided in the home, who it is provided to and under what circumstances it is provided. It is also important to ensure that consideration is give to how solutions would need to change over time as the patient's condition and attitude to the technology changes or as better more cost effective technology comes available. All of these issues will have an impact on product and service development so an assessment of the type of patients or potential segments is required to determine the nature of the products that should be developed.

Typically, a clinical view is taken when assessing a patients' state of well-being in order to determine what level and kind of care is required. The outcome of such an assessment can be indicated on a continuum of care such as that show in Fig 1.

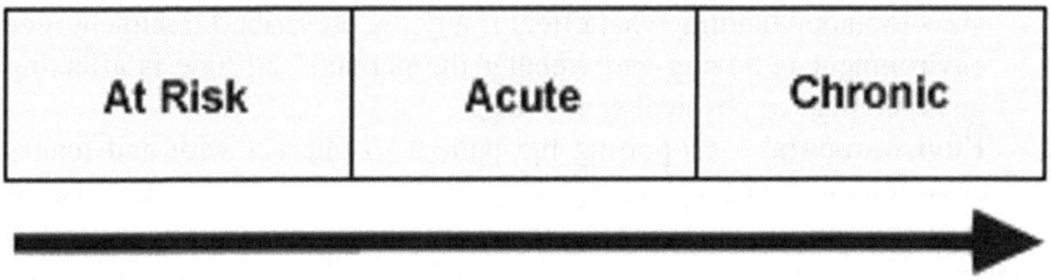

Figure.1 Basic Continuum of Care

This groups patients into silos based on a measure of risk to their well-being, how much care they require and how much it will cost. It does not indicate what type of technology solutions would be appropriate. Irrespective of a patients' condition or prognosis, taking a holistic view of Digital Homecare implies that that technology should aim at providing support across four areas as shown in Fig 2.

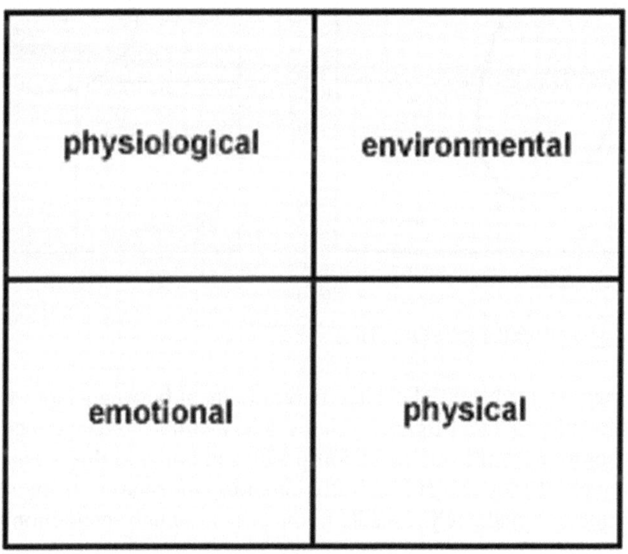

Figure.2 Four Aspects of Care

- **Physiological** - monitoring parameters such as blood oxygen, heart rate, blood pressure and weight. Solutions that focus on these areas, generally known as Telemedicine have been ongoing for several years. Typically users will use one or more medical devices to measure and transmit data via a dedicated Home Gateway to a remote monitoring station.
- **Physical** - monitoring parameters such as movements of joints, sight, hearing and level of pain
- **Emotional -** monitoring the state of mind that the patient is in either with a view to understanding what effect if any the prescribed treatment regime or environment is having and whether the patients' attitude is affecting their physiological or physical well being.
- **Environmental -** supporting the patient to interact with and manage the environment that they are in where their condition may otherwise make it difficult.

Clearly, a patients care and support requirements do not fit neatly into just one of these areas. At any given moment the focus could be spread across all four areas especially where the prognosis is multiple chronic illnesses. On an ongoing basis and over the longer term, the focus of support required will change, usually in an unpredictable way. The example in Fig 3 shows, for a particular patient, where the focus of their care needs are at different moments in time.

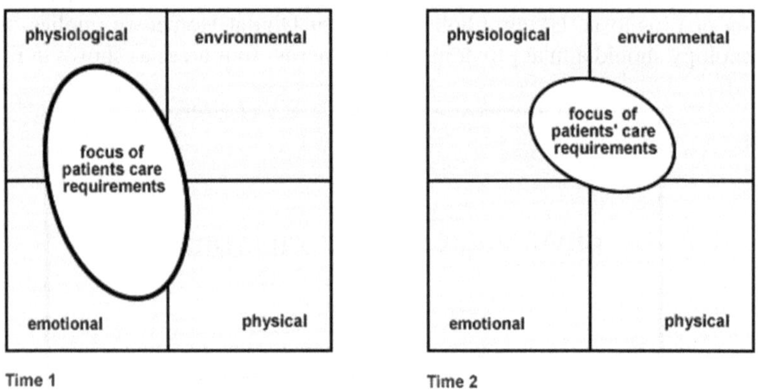

Figure.3 Change in Focus of Care Over Time

Whilst there is a substantial change in requirement between Time 1 and Time 2 it is not feasible to reconfigure systems every time a change occurs. Digital Homecare solutions deployed to support patients at home in this scenario will only work effectively if they can successfully integrate information from all four of the aspects of care and make adjustments to the way in which interaction with the patient is managed. One key ambition of the next generation of Digital Homecare products is that they enable this. Additionally, solutions that can be easily upgraded, downgraded or changed as the patient, their circumstances or environment change without requiring the consumers to relearn technology or make major changes to their regime are what a consumer market requires. In this context, upgrading or downgrading systems can be achieved by deactivating or activating application software that is installed on the devices and on the overall system rather than by changing the devices.

Referring to the Fig 3, each aspect of care has its' own specialists and even within a group of specialists there could be a range of views as to what technology package should be provided to a particular patient. Even in the simplest of cases when a patients' requirements fall into just one of these areas it can be necessary to hold case conferences involving multi-disciplinary teams in order to determine the best cause of action. The situation becomes more complex when patients requirements are distributed across two or more of these areas because more cross group collaboration will be required. When dealing with these situations a great amount of Collective Intelligence and experience informs decision making. It is essential that this is built into future Digital Homecare solutions.

The Importance of Collective Intelligence

Collective Intelligence across all aspects of care is ultimately responsible for determining whether patients could live independently at home or in the community without increased risk to their well-being and if so the tools and services that enable them to do this. Applying Collective Intelligence is a time consuming process and acts as a bottleneck where demand for service is high. Specifically:

- there is a vast amount of data to process and the data can be of variable quality
- key decision makers could be in conflict
- there are complex rules governing the process of combining viewpoints from different actors
- actors in this process are able to count or discount elements of data as well give higher or lower weight to other data elements based on experience

It is difficult to build technology that can deal with all of these points but in centre based clinical facilities where these observations also apply, initiatives such as Care Pathways and Practice Guidelines have been developed and deployed to capture this Collective Intelligence and improve efficiency and consistency of its application.

- **Care Pathways -** since the early 1990s investments in the design, development and application of care pathways as defined by Hill[1] have contributed to consistent, auditable application of clinical knowledge and best practice. The result has been better co-ordination across multi-disciplinary teams and generally better outcomes for patients.
- **Practice Guidelines** – are also relevant in this context although the emphasis is directed towards quality and co-ordination of care

These beneficial and much used initiatives represent an encoding of Collective Intelligence, experience and best practice in a form that can be easily understood shared and distributed. The concept should be developed for Digital Homecare in the broadest possible sense. This would require a general acceptance by the healthcare professionals that whilst traditional Telecare and Telemedicine initiatives are beginning to be considered in long tem care planning, much more can and should be done to achieve a full integration of Digital Homecare in care pathways and ensure that the widest range of solutions are made available as part of the process. One example of how innovative thinking can drive the implementation of consumer oriented solutions is the use of Nintendo's Wii in a number of professionally prescribed solutions to difficult healthcare cases. In this example, Dementia patients in the UK are using the Wii to help the elderly stay mentally and physically active. The local council who fund the program see this as "an excellent example of the use of new technology to improve the lives of the most vulnerable"[2]. Apart this and a few other exceptions it is unlikely at this time that many clinicians would recommend a Wii as part of a home care plan.

Creating a set of pathways to help define, deploy and manage Digital Homecare is a much harder process than defining pathways in a clinical setting for a number of reasons:

- Actors in the decision making process span many groups including professional groups, patient groups, community workers, friends and family. Some of these groups would not be involved in defining clinical care pathways but do need to be consulted in the development of a similar concept for Digital Homecare.
- There are many more device classes that must be considered since solutions as described earlier need to support physical, physiological, emotional and environmental care. The way in which devices communicate across each area needs to be formulated as does the situation interpretation when devices are in a certain state.
- Solutions need to be highly personalised and many of the parameters required to do this such as the patients state of mind and their environment are often those in which the health care service provider has no control and limited ability to determine.

However difficulty this might be, it should not be avoided and the focus should be directed towards developing an intelligent gateway that does incorporate Collective Intelligence, device intelligence and system intelligence as shown in Fig 4.

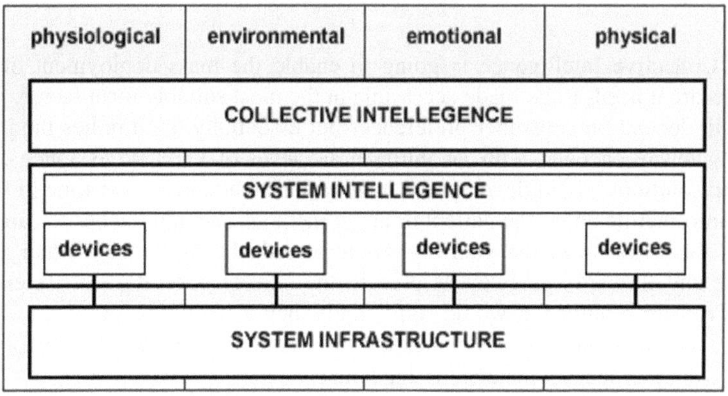

Figure.4 Combining Collective Intelligence with Device and System Intelligence

It will use pathways as templates for on-going home care but take into account changing contexts and deal with vague or fuzzy information and data. Dealing with vague or fuzzy information might mean for example obtaining a required piece of information indirectly or from alternative sources before making a diagnosis or recommendation. An example would be in using utility bills to assess the aspects of patients' daily activity that relate to the consumption of energy and water where appropriate sensors where not available in the home. This increases the degree of "intelligence that" system can exhibit and makes it more useful and applicable to a wider range of scenarios.

Finally to keep solutions both adaptable and practical, they should be able to deal with changing contexts without the constant need for reconfiguration. The ability to "understand" whether a patient alarm was triggered as a result of genuine problem rather than a change in behaviour that is actually perfectly normal in a given context will be one of the critical factors for mass adoption. The inability to deal with situations like this will render the majority of deployments useless quite quickly. Every time the context changed a potential system reconfiguration would be required. At the very least, this would require someone from the patient's care team to carry out an assessment. For members of the patients' care network, having to reconfigure the system every time the context changed would mean that the system would become too onerous to use. For sceptical professionals the continual manual intervention gives credence to the notion that rather than provide a benefit, these systems merely transfer workload and costs to other departments.

The home security industry provides an example of what happens when there little or confidence in installed systems. In this case enforcement agents and neighbourhood watch schemes do not necessarily respond to the activation of burglar alarms because the chance of it being a false alarm is high.

Making Collective Intelligence Accessible

If Collective Intelligence is going to enable the mass deployment of Digital Homecare it needs to be made accessible in the most suitable form factor. Suitability will depend on consumer preferences but essentially this implies the inclusion of a gateway encoded with an initial basic level of knowledge. Once commissioned solutions would develop and modify their "thinking" over time in line with new information about the patient or about methods and approaches to care.

At this basic level the gateway would already be more useful than a typical "store and forward" gateway as used in the current generation of Telemedicine and Telecare solutions. It would additionally include facilities to:

- assemble and process contextual information from a wide range of sources not just sensors installed in the home
- allow it to be interrogated remotely and in an ad-hoc manner, by care professionals or members of the patient's extended care network
- perform local configuration, trouble shooting and maintenance using its' own system intelligence

In total and as a key component of future Digital Homecare solutions, an Intelligent Gateway should therefore be capable of:

- executing encoded Collective Intelligence, pathways and protocols in a way that enables multi-disciplinary care teams, patients, friends and family to deliver provide appropriate and manageable support to patients at home
- providing high levels of assurance that actions are based on the accurate application of knowledge
- learning both in the context of their local in-home implementation and by receiving updated data or knowledge from relevant centres of excellence either on regular basis or on as "as need" basis
- understanding the context that they are attached to at a given time
- transferring only *relevant* data and information to and from remote processing centres or trusted individuals
- creating and delivering outputs for different types of users and ensuring that these are clear and auditable
- "understand" when a situation is beyond its' comprehension and handover processing to more knowledgeable sources

The overwhelming evidence is that this level of sophistication is not being engineered into current Digital Homecare solutions. Whilst there are an abundance of new products, enhancements have focused on providing better more user friendly designs, miniaturisation, increased networking capabilities and faster processing. The technology enhancements are positive developments as they create solutions that enable more complex decision making, however decision trees are generally pre-programmed and mainly static which limits the ability to deal with uncertain situations and is therefore still far removed from the ideal consumer oriented Digital Homecare solutions.

Factors That Limit Future Digital Homecare

Most of the technology components that are required to develop the kind of solutions capable of sustaining large scale consumer adoption of Digital Homecare solutions are readily available and at reasonable cost.

At the infrastructure level broadband and mobile communications ensure that users can remain constantly connected to everyone in their network of carers. Communications also enables frequent and rapid updates of knowledge in the form of data or improved decision making algorithms from remote centres anywhere in the world. The number and type of connected devices that can be used in monitoring the patient and their environment is increasing and industry initiatives such as those led by Continua will ensure the device interoperability required to create choice in the market.

The electronic manufacturing industries' ability to embed complex software applications on single chips and integrate these with diagnostic products is well understood and already widely used process.

The Collective Intelligence that has been discussed earlier and which is a key element of future systems can be encoded using techniques such as those found in the implementation of Artificial Intelligence, Expert Systems and Fuzzy logic. Research shows that the application of these methods can add significant value by way of implementing complex decision making that can generate appropriate outputs even when the inputs are vague and uncertain. Some of the most recent research in this area continues to focus on application of the methods to the provision of care to the elderly at home[3].

Since from a technical perspective the future generations of Digital Homecare solutions can be developed, with clear information about the worsening state of healthcare, the knowledge that a step change is required to improve the situation and the technical know-how to do this why is it not being done? Possible explanations include:

- The fact that at the present interest and motivation to do the research in this area rests largely with academic led institutions rather than commercial companies
- because of the long term of focus on monitoring - Telecare/Telemedicine and efficient transmission of data between patient and remote monitoring centre, existing industry collaborations and alliances that are working to drive the industry forward are, for now, more focused on technology standards and interoperability issues
- there exists even amongst the keenest of supporters a view that these kind of products would not get approval from authorities or gain acceptance in the market

With increasing number of new entrants to the Digital Healthcare space and specific industry initiatives such as those led by the Continua Health Alliance there is huge potential to drive towards Digital Homecare solutions that are holistic, intelligent, can be widely deployed and deliver the benefits that healthcare solution providers need to enjoy in order to continue to deliver quality care for all that require it.

Creating the Step Change

There are several ways in which such step changes could be stimulated and initiatives are already underway to increase product and service development

- Governments / Large Healthcare institutions who have the most to gain as well as the most to loose if they do not act, could invest the huge sums of money required, lay down the standards and drive the industry.
- Outside investors could back existing innovative companies unencumbered by existing customers and aging products or services in an effort to take a lead in this market.
- Outside of the healthcare sector other well established industries could continue to enter the market bringing assets and expertise in some of the areas that would be required to help generate a consumerised market. This approach leverages their huge momentum with millions of potential users right across the target demographics for Digital Homecare.

Government Sponsorship is increasing across the world but moving from Research and Development to trial status has been, and continues to be slow primarily because the focus continues to remain on establishing proof of value both in terms of healthcare benefits and commercial return on investment. Start-ups tend to focus on is niche areas. Outside industries are getting involved at an increasing rate. The next section briefly reviews who these new entrants are and shows how they can assist in the development of the market.

New Entrants

The increased focus on the global healthcare issue that has been raised by several think tanks, government bodies and healthcare authorities has attracted the attention of many industries not normally associated with the delivery of healthcare services. These "outsiders" are carrying out extensive research and development, sponsoring many studies with the aim of determining when and how to attack a market that is seen by all as lucrative and long term. Generally it is regarded as a strategic decision to create organic business growth by leveraging their trusted and respected brands to provide existing customers with additional services. These outsiders include business from the Telecommunications, Home Security, Home Automation, Consumer Electronics and Software Publishers and are summarised below.

Telecoms

Telcos, both fixed and mobile continue to improve the quality and range of services. Their existing markets are flat and in some instances declining. Consumers' ability to communicate via the phone or over the internet has become essential and this has created a captive market. Telcos are global companies with the manufacturing capability to create, deliver and manage product in volumes. They have huge operational capacity that covers sales support, help desk, field support, customer relationship management and billing. They have strong brand identities that register well with the target demographics and have long established relationships with them.

Although for Mobile operators the last 10 years has seen explosive growth across nearly all sectors of society, the target demographics are not as well served, at least not directly. Elderly patients with advanced stages of chronic illnesses for example are unlikely to adopt mobile phones as a tool for managing their care but their relatives and carers probably would. None the less mobile operators like their fixed line counter parts have robust operational infrastructures, very strong bands and global manufacturing.

Home Security

Well established security companies like ADT and Securicor have been supplying home security systems for years. Successful companies in this industry supply security devices as well as 24 * 7 monitoring and support with links to emergency services. These are the types of capability that will be a required if Digital Homecare is deployed widely. Whether or not they reach out to the target demographic is debatable. In contrast to fixed line telecoms companies which have a product considered to be essential, home security products are expensive and often seen as a luxury.

Home Automation

The home automation industry is very much a hobbyist industry. Whilst the majority of people would like increased automation around the home, the lack of standards and lack of products have kept this industry focused in niche markets. Products that are available tend to enable control of doors, taps, windows and lights. Whilst products are industrial in nature they are absolutely indispensable to patients who have physical disabilities and who could cope only if a dedicated carer were constantly available.

Software Publishers

In the software industry the term Health 2.0 is used to describe a concept in which Rich Internet Applications provide healthcare consumers with easy access to healthcare related applications, services and relevant communities. This together with the rise in deployment and speed of broadband and mobile data services has seen a number of initiatives from the software publishers whose technologies enable the creation of these applications and services. Microsoft and Google for example have both been active. Microsoft's Health Vault is an information based system aimed at putting the patient in control of their healthcare. Google Health is a health information storage program really focused on putting Electronic Patient Records in the hands of the owners.

Social Networks

Some aspects of care at home may be purely informational in that either the patient or an informal carer such as a relative would like more information on a condition of symptoms. In these scenarios, there is no requirement for a set of sensors or dedicated patient gateway, a PC or TV/Set-top box combination connected to the internet will suffice. Connectivity in this situation enables consumers to access:

- the internet to search for relevant information
- dedicated healthcare social networks which are growing in number and popularity

How the consumer chooses to act once they have received this information is a matter for them but in the context of Digital Homecare, access to healthcare social networks such as PatientsLikeMe[4] and wego[5] health are more interesting. These satisfy consumers' thirst for knowledge in a specific way and provide direct links to other people in the same position. Patients and there carers can compare their care plans and approach to care with others who have similar conditions. The information gathered from portals like these is not currently subject to any standards and may not be accurate but there is a sufficient body of knowledge to influence the thinking and actions of those who are being cared for and those who are providing the care. One possible response having found relevant information will be to consult a professional carer who is part of the patients care team, discuss the information and determine whether any of is relevant to their condition. If so changes can be made in consultation with the care team. At the other extreme, the patient or their informal carer may choose to adopt another method of care without consulting the care team. Both scenarios could generate long term problems in healthcare provision by causing healthcare professionals to spend more time discussing information and options presented by lay people or by having to "undo" unprescribed modifications to treatment.

Consumer Electronics

Ultimately Digital Homecare will require large numbers of devices to be designed, manufactured and delivered. Whereas this market was previously the preserve of the medical device industry, consumer electronics manufacturers are now extremely interested. In recent times Nintendo with its' Wii and Intel have both made highly publicised announcements regarding their commercial intensions in the healthcare sector. Nintendo's Wii product has already revolutionised gaming and its application in treating elderly people with Alzheimer's is starting to revolutionise thinking in the provision of technology driven healthcare solutions to this and other physical and cognitive rehabilitation applications. Intel's recently (July 2008) announced Personalised Health Guide[6] leverages Intel's position as a global manufacturer of high tech products, offers a more standardised approach to using medical devices for home monitoring but is focused only on the Telemedicine silo.

The table below summarises in general terms the contribution that each group of participants can make in the development of this industry.

Table.2 New Industry Participants

Industry Sector	**Potential Contribution to Digital Homecare Solutions and Services**
Telecoms (Fixed)	❑ Fixed line and Broadband infrastructure ❑ Central home unit (modem) with the connectivity to wider infrastructure and services
Telecoms (Mobile)	❑ Mobile and Broadband infrastructure ❑ Personalised unit (mobile or GSM modem) providing with connectivity to wider infrastructure and services and which can be used at home or on the move
Home Automation	❑ Controllers able to monitor and mechanically control appliances ❑ Expertise in remote monitoring and control of equipment and devices
Home Security	❑ Home security systems ability to offer round the clock monitoring ❑ Expertise in connecting and liaising with emergency services ❑ Service, support and logistics experience
Software Publishers	❑ Web based software applications and web services enabling easier access to applications and data from many different platforms
Social Networks	❑ User driven networks directly relevant to patients condition providing a global source of self help, support and encouragement
Consumer Electronics	❑ Expertise in developing low cost networked devices for the consumer industry

Amongst the strength of these organisations is that they have:

- large installed bases of long term customers which means that they understand how to do product development, provide continuity of service and ongoing support to a wide range of customer types in large markets
- service and support infrastructures that have been built and managed over several years thus ensuring that they could implement and manage the operational infrastructure that would be required to support the new services that would be generated
- global manufacturing capability that is critical to the delivery of products for widespread consumer adoption and their involvement will help drive costs down even further
- the ability to create the online presence that will enable consumers to get involved with providing large scale input to product and service development and to get connected with others in similar position which will help to drive the consumer market
- have a business led focus and are not interest in purely academic exercises and would therefore focus on products that would succeed in the market place

The weakness of these organisations is they typically have

- limited or no experience of delivering healthcare services
- limited relationships with patients' extended care network which is critical in delivering future digital home care

So given the number and type of new entrants into this market place, is it likely that with all of the new input, products based on new thinking and fit for a widespread consumer market will emerge. Certainly, all of the new players can make a significant contribution to this growing market either directly or indirectly but they tend to be really focused on leveraging skills and assets to generate new revenues from new markets. The Vice President of Mobile Operators' health program stated in November 2007, *"We are aiming to be the driving force of eHealth. This is a huge market because of trends, and because patients are unaware of its possibilities. We want to be able to provide services to both the medical services and services to the elderly and disabled markets. In an industry worth €450 billion for eHealth, we believe that our technology will allow health to adapt to the changing world around us"*[7]. In most consumer markets this is a perfectly acceptable business goal. It seems that is less acceptable in healthcare although the emergence of a new product that was truly consumerised with low costs might mitigate against this. Whilst these participants do have attributes that lend credibility to their ambitions, there is much that is missing so it is not obvious from the summary of entrants that this will be the case.

Consumers are familiar with a wide range of technology enabled devices around the home. These include Internet ready televisions and set top boxes, modern security alarms and of course broadband enabled personal computers. This is an appropriate setting for future home care in which case the focus should be directed to installing additional devices and linked services that deliver the health care functionality. This approach speaks partly to the rise of the smart home a concept which is not new but also not widely employed and also the deployment of Collective Intelligence. Smart homes have not been widely deployed as typically the focus is on new builds rather than retrofits. The decline in costs of technology components means that once again the high tech industry is pushing a SMART homes agenda where homes are designed with so much embedded technology that the whole house can be considered a Digital Platform. The embedded technology will typically include network infrastructure capable of supporting voice, data and video communications within the home as well as into and out of the home.

Within this sort of architecture, the environment would have a main controller - any device able to present application interfaces - through which all components are managed and integrated. The controller could be a computer, internet enable TV or dedicated platform. Visitors either from within the home or from a remote location could use a smart phone to access services that were relevant and they were authorised to access. In this context, Digital Homecare becomes just another service layer alongside entertainment or house hold management. There is however work to be done in order to ensure that components installed in SMART homes can operate in an intelligent was rather than just work within the limits of their programming[8].

Other Industry Initiatives

Industry initiatives are designed to enable leading players and those with vision to come together, share ideas and deploy resources at level and rate guaranteed to create the step change required. The initiative led by the Continua Health Alliance with its focus on technical consistency between devices from different vendors is improving openness and interoperability at the device level. This removes the debate about which vendor's device to use in a particular application but in any Digital Homecare solution however simple, the device technology is still only a component of the overall solution. There is an expected configuration of devices, application software, communications and services so whilst Continua's work will provide a stable platform for later development of Digital Homecare solutions which enjoy device interoperability and are adaptable, work is still required in order to incorporate Collective Intelligence.

Conclusion

There is no doubt that the burden of providing long-term care to all patients that require it is straining healthcare systems everywhere. There is also no doubt that where patients supported by a knowledgeable network of carers are able to manage their conditions when they are at home, there are considerable benefits to the patient, to their healthcare provider and to their friends and family. In much the same way that the personal use Glucometer revolutionised the management and treatment of Diabetes, more widely distributed Digital Homecare solutions will revolutionise the management of care for people at home.

Globally, the requirement for advanced solutions to be developed and widely deployed is almost universally acknowledged. This is a process that will change the way in which patients and their healthcare providers will interact. It will also have a profound affect on the way in which the patients' informal care network interacts and assists the patient. Technology will be at the heart of this change and it must be capable of supporting users at all levels of confidence and ability. Certainly, all of the technology components required to create appropriate solutions are available and collectively, the combined skills and assets of new entrants to this sector provide a platform on which the technology and supporting operations can be delivered to mass markets. The demand is there, the know-how is there, industry participants need to formulate the right partnerships to deliver.

References

1. Hill: Clinical Pathways: multidisciplinary plans of best clinical practice. OpenClinical (1998), http://www.openclinical.org/clinicalpathways.html (retrieved September 04, 2008)
2. The British Journal of Healthcare Computing & Information Management. Wii keeps elderly active in care homes, February 7 (2008), http://www.bjhcim.co.uk/news/2008/n802012.htm (retrieved August 12, 2008)
3. The British Journal of Healthcare Computing & Information Management. Fuzzy logic could aid monitoring and decision support in care for the elderly, December 18 (2007), http://www.bjhcim.co.uk/news/2007/n712020.htm (retrieved August 18, 2008)
4. patientslikeme, http://www.patientslikeme.com (accessed September 11, 2008)
5. wego health, http://www.wegohealth.com (accessed September 11, 2008)
6. Moody, R.: Intel launches first medical device. Portland Business Journal, August 22 (2008), http://Portland.bizjournals.com/portland/stories/2008/08/25/story4.html (retrieved September 2, 2008)
7. Bihan, E.: Orange Healthcare launched in France. eHealthEurope, November 14 (2007), http://www.ehealtheurope.net/news/3217/orange_healthcare_launched_in_france (retrieved August 3, 2008)
8. Valero, M., Pau, I., Vadillo, L., et al.: An Implementation Framework for Smart Home Telecare Services. Future generation communication and networking (2008) doi:10.1109/FGCN.2007.63

Privacy and Digital Homecare

Allies not Enemies

Kirsten Van Gossum and Griet Verhenneman

Abstract When developing new digital homecare applications, including services that enable the exchange of health data between the homecare professionals and the hospital (like an electronic health record), the legal requirements are often considered as a serious bottleneck. However, only a few principles have to be taken into account for the development of a privacy-friendly eHomecare application and they come with a bonus: an easier acceptance and uptake of the application by the public. This chapter therefore wants to set forth a minimum set of legal requirements for the use of eHealth tools in Europe. The project development of an EHR in the homecare sector will function as an example.
When developing an eHomecare application, such as an EHR, mainly Medical Law and Privacy regulations need to be taken into account. The European healthcare sector is regulated by different national regulations, including Medical Law and Patients' Rights. Although on international level the same basic principles apply in most countries, there is no European harmonization or coordination. With regard to Privacy regulations, the opposite is true. Within Europe the Data Protection Directive harmonizes the protection of personal data being processed. In sequence, the applicability, the basic legal concepts, the health data protection regime and the roles taken up by the different actors in an eHomecare project are being discussed. Next to Medical Law and Privacy it is also important to check - on a case-by-case basis - whether other legislation (such as the eCommerce and ePrivacy Directive, or sector specific laws) is relevant.
Secondly the chapter sets up a manual for the development of an eHomecare project. Points of particular interest are the question whether the project is dealing with primary or secondary use of personal data, the filing of a notification, the drafting of an informed consent for the patient and the healthcare professional and the need for an appropriate level of security.
Finally the chapter formulates ten practical recommendations, crucial to a successful privacy-friendly eHomecare project and / or application, in coherence with the timeline of a project. Going from the creation of awareness, over compliance with the law, to the protection of the patient and the healthcare professional and keeping evidence.
Related ICMCC chapter: Ann Ackaert et al., "A multi-disciplinary approach towards the design and development of value+ eHomeCare services".

K. Yogesan et al. (Eds.): Handbook of Digital Homecare, BIOMED, pp. 117–149.
springerlink.com

Table of contents

Introduction

e-Health tools or solutions often include products, systems and services that enable the exchange of health data between the different healthcare professionals. The best example of such an eHealth tool is an electronic health record [19].

The Article 29 Data Protection Working Party[1] defines an electronic health record (hereinafter: "EHR") as "*a comprehensive medical record or similar documentation of the past and present physical and mental state of health of an individual in electronic form and providing for ready availability of these data for medical treatment and other closely related purposes*"[18]. This means that – by using an electronic health record - the health data of a patient will be accessible anytime and anywhere by all the healthcare providers involved in his treatment, including his homecare professionals. Through close collaboration with the general practitioner (hereinafter: "GP") and the hospital via the EHR, they will be able to offer a more personalized and adequate homecare[2]. In other words, an EHR brings about better quality of treatment because of better information about the patient [18].

In this sense, an EHR differs from a personal health record (hereinafter: "PHR"[3]), which is initiated and maintained not by a healthcare professional but by an individual in order to enable him to understand and to manage his own medical information. A PHR will however not be the subject of this chapter and will only focus on the healthcare professional.

However, both the healthcare professional as the patient have an increasing concern about the legal consequences of exchanging patients' health data through

[1] The Article 29 Data Protection Working Party is an advisory and independent body constituted by the 95/46/EC Directive. It is compound by a representative of the supervisory authority or authorities designated by each Member State and of a representative of the authority or authorities established for the Community institutions and bodies, and of a representative of the Commission.
See: http://ec.europa.eu/justice_home/fsj/privacy/workinggroup/index_en.htm.
[2] For more information see IBBT project websites of the E-hip and TranseCare projects, http://www.ibbt.be/en/projecten.
[3] Such as Google Health and Microsoft Health Vault.

an EHR (Kuner 2007): where the healthcare professionals mainly have questions about their professional secrecy and liability, the patients worry about their personal privacy.

The purpose of this chapter is to set forth a minimum set of legal requirements for the use of eHealth tools in Europe. The project development of an EHR in the homecare sector will function as an example. This chapter starts off with an overview of the legal framework (see Sect. 1), addresses secondly a manual for developing an eHealth project (see Sect. 2) and ends with some practical recommendations to implement such a project (see Sect. 3).

1 Legal framework

When developing an EHR for the homecare sector, both medical regulations (see Sect. 1.1) and data protection laws (see Sect. 1.2) should be taken into account.

1.1 Medical regulations

In Europe, the healthcare sector is regulated by different national regulations, including Medical Law (or "Health Law") and Patients' Rights. Apart from some fundamental Patients' Rights articulated in European Conventions, these regulations are not further harmonized at a European level [1 and 2].

In addition tot these European conventions, there are no intercontinental nor international Conventions, Acts or Policies about Medical Law or Patients' Rights. Nevertheless, most countries apply the same basic principles. For example both Europe as the USA and Australia use the principle of negligence[4] to assess the liability of physicians. There are however large differences in the implementation of these medical regulations. While in Europe most countries regulate patients' rights

[4] Negligence can generally be defined as conduct that is culpable because it falls short of what a reasonable person would do to protect another individual from a foreseeable risks of harm.

in national laws, the USA consider health law still as common law[5] rather than statutory law[6] (Furrow et al. 2005 and Chalmers 1998).

Since there is no harmonization or coordination of the Patients' Rights or Medical Laws in Europe, medical regulations can be considered as a bottleneck in the project development of an EHR. For each European country involved in the project, different rules will apply, therefore the focus of this chapter will be on national and not on European legislation.

1.2 Data protection legislation

1.2.1 Introduction: the EU Data Protection Directive

In contrast with the medical regulations, the national data protection laws in Europe are harmonized by the EU Data Protection Directive of 24 October 1995 (hereinafter DPD) [3]. The main purposes of this Directive are (1) to safeguard an equivalent data protection in all European member states (recital 9 DPD), (2) to remove the obstacles to flows of personal data in the internal market and (3) to ensure that the transfer of personal data outside the EU (e.g. cross-border flow) is regulated in a consistent manner (recital 8 DPD).

In an eHealth context, the latter will be important when - for example - setting up a tele-expertise, e.g. consulting a specialist outside the EU by means of electronic multimedia communications via the general practitioner[7]. In principle, such a data transfer is prohibited, but exceptions are provided by the Directive (article 25 and 26 DPD). As a general rule, data transfers outside the EU are only allowed when the third country ensures an adequate level of protection (Article 25.1.

---

[5] Common law is created and refined by judges: a decision in the case currently pending depends on decisions in previous cases and affects the law to be applied in future cases. When there is no authoritative statement of the law, judges have the authority and duty to make law by creating precedent. The body of precedent is called "common law" and it binds future decisions.

[6] Statutory law or statute law is written law (as opposed to oral or customary law) set down by a legislature or other governing authority such as the executive branch of government in response to a perceived need to clarify the functioning of government, improve civil order, to codify existing law, or for an individual or company to obtain special treatment.

[7] The term "tele-expertise" is defined in article 2, 11° of the old "Government bill concerning the processing and computerization of the health data and the applications for tele-medicine", http://www.svh.be/behealth.htm and http://www.absym.be/behealth.html, 45 (*in Dutch*).

DPD). In this chapter, we will however only deal with data transfers inside the EU.

1.2.2 Applicability of the EU Data Protection Directive

The applicability of the EU Data Protection Directive depends on the location of the "controller" (article 4 DPD). The controller is "*the natural or legal person, public authority, agency or any other body which alone or jointly with others determines the purposes and means of the processing of personal data*" (article 2.d) DPD). In an eHealth project the purposes and means of the data processing are often jointly determined by all the members of the project consortium, acting as "joint controllers".

EU member states shall apply their national data protection provisions (harmonized by the DPD) to the processing of personal data where:

(a) the data processing is carried out in the context of the activities of an establishment of the controller on the territory of an EU member state[8];
(b) or he controller is not established on an EU member state's territory, but in a place where its national law applies by virtue of international public law;
(c) or the controller is not established on Community territory and, for purposes of processing personal data makes use of equipment, automated or otherwise, situated on the territory of the said Member State, unless such equipment is used only for purposes of transit through the territory of the Community (article 4.1. DPD). In this case, the controller has to designate a representative established in the territory of that member state (article 4.2. DPD).

1.2.3 Basic legal concepts of the EU Data Protection Directive

The DPD applies to the *"processing"* of *"personal data"*.

"Processing" is defined in article 2 (b) of the DPD as "*any operation or set of operations which is performed on personal data whether or not by automatic means such as collection, recording, organization, storage, adaptation or alterna-*

[8] When the same controller is established on the territory of several member states, he must take the necessary measures to ensure that each of these establishments complies with the obligations laid down by the national law applicable, see article 4.1.a) DPD.

tion[9]*, retrieval, consultation, use, disclosure by transmission, dissemination or otherwise making available, alignment or combination, blocking, erasure or destruction*" (article 2.b) DPD). This definition is very broad and includes both *"the processing of personal data wholly or partly by automatic means"*, as [...] *"the processing otherwise than by automatic means of personal data which form part of a filing system or are intended to form part of a filing system*" (article 3.1. DPD). This means that any processing of personal data in a health record – electronically or not - must comply with the rules set out in the DPD [17].

Furthermore, "personal data" is described in the DPD as "*any information relating to an identified or identifiable natural person*". This person is the so-called *"data subject"* (article 2.a) DPD). In a healthcare setting, the data subject will often be the patient involved. As a patient, the data subject will have additional rights with regard to his data processing. This will be discussed later (see Sect. 2.4. and 3.2.3.).

As the definition of "processing", the term "personal data" too, needs to be interpreted very extensively. It can comprise not only texts, but also images, sounds and even radiofrequencies (such as used in RFID-applications) [16 and 21].

The DPD will however only apply when the personal data are related to an *identified* or -at least *identifiable* - natural person. This implies that the personal data can be used to identify a particular person (Kuner 2007) [16]. To determine whether a particular person is identifiable, account should be taken of all the means likely reasonably to be used to identify the data subject (recital 24 DPD). According to the DPD an identifiable person is "*one who can be identified, directly or indirectly, in particular by reference to an identification number or one or more factors specific to his physical, physiological, psychological, economical, cultural or social identity*" (article 2.a) DPD).

Nevertheless, when the data are rendered anonymous in such a way that the data subject is no longer identifiable, the DPD will not be applicable (recital 24 DPD).

1.2.4 The different actors in an eHealth project

Before the start-up of an EHR development, it is most important to identify the different actors in the project. In accordance with the DPD, the three most central

---

[9] From a data protection perspective, "adaptation" and "alternation" have a different meaning: adaptation, refers to an adjustment of the data in order to keep these data accurate and up-to-date, whereas "alternation" implies a complete data interchange introducing new data in the data processing.

actors are the data subject (e.g. the patient), the controller and the processor. Both the data subject and the controller have already been discussed above (see respectively Sect. 1.2.3. and 1.2.2.). The latter is defined in article 2 (e) of the DPD as "*the natural or legal person, public authority, agency or any other body which processes personal data on behalf of the controller*" (article 1.e) DPD). This processor will be an external person or organization, e.g. a third service provider (De Bot 2001).

The processor, who is acting only on instructions from the controller (article 17.3. DPD), will naturally have less responsibilities than the controller himself. The controller stays liable for most of the data protections obligations that have to be met under the DPD. If the data processing of a controller is carried out by a processor, all liability issues have to be governed by a contract or legal act binding the processor to the controller (article 17.3. DPD).

In consequence, classifying the different actors in a project, implies the identification of all liability issues related to the project[10].

1.2.5 The processing of health data

In an eHomecare project, the processed personal data often relates to a person's health. In this case, the processing is considered to be more particularly sensitive then the processing of "normal" personal data and therefore requires a more strict protection [17].

In principle, the DPD prohibits the processing of any "data *concerning* health" (hereinafter: "health data")(article 8.1. DPD). This prohibition applies to all personal data which have "a strong and clear link" with the description of the health status of a person [5]. Therefore, all data contained in an EHR (including the patient's contact details) should be considered as "health data" [17].

However, this does not imply that all medico-related data are to be considered "health data". A holiday picture of a disabled person in a wheelchair in a traveling brochure e.g., is not to be qualified as health data, if the picture does not have a direct connection or link with the person's health [16].

[10] Please note that it will be difficult as a healthcare professional to escape certain liabilities: most national regulations require that healthcare professionals keep a medical record of their patients. Since they are legally required to determine the purposes and the means of the data processing in this medical record, they are (always) to be considered as "controllers". (De Bot, D. 2001. *Processing of personal data.* Antwerp: Kluwer: 46-47, (*in Dutch*)).

On the other hand, data, like e.g. "genetic data" should -on the contrary- in some contexts always be considered as health data. Not only paves the decoding of the DNA blueprint "the way to new discoveries and uses in the field of genetic testing, but it also can identify individuals, link them to others, and *reveal* complex data about the future health and development of those individuals and other people to whom they are genetically related" [15].

From this perspective, the data processing of genetic data is "more" privacy intrusive, since it concerns not only the data subject, but also his family. In this case, additional rules will apply. This will however not be dealt with in this chapter.

1.2.6 Health data protection regime

As already explained above, the DPD prohibits on the one hand the processing of health data in general (article 8.1. DPD), but provides at the same time several exemptions to this general prohibition (article 8.2., 3. and 4. DPD). On the other hand, personal data "only *revealing* health[11]" do not fall under the scope of this special protection and are subject to the "normal" data protection regime (see also Sect. 1.2.4).

Nevertheless, both regimes are based on the same four data protection principles: the transparency principle, the proportionality principle, the finality principle (or purpose / use limitation principle), and the lawfulness principle (article 6.1. DPD). All these principles are related to the quality of the personal data being processed and have to be complied with by the controller (article 6.2. DPD).

1.2.6.1 The four Data Quality Principles

The transparency principle

The transparency principle relates to the obligation of every controller to give a minimum of information about the data processing and its purposes, to the data subject prior to the collection of the data (article 10 DPD). This obligation will be explained further when dealing with the informed consent (see Sect. 2.3.1.). The transparency principle thus implies that all personal data must be processed fairly (article 6.1.a) DPD). This means e.g. a transparency level must be guaranteed to

[11] "Personal data *revealing* health" must be opposed to "personal data *concerning* health". As illustrated above (see Sect. 2.2.4.) this means a direct, strong and clear connection or link with the health of the person is required in order for data relating to the health of a person to be qualified as health data in the way defined in the DPD.

the data subject at every stage and every moment of the data processing, especially when collecting the data (De Bot 2001).

In particular for a project developing an EHR, this means the controller(s) within the project, will have to inform the patients participating in the project about the implications and possible risks of the data processing in an EHR. This will allow the patient to make a risk analysis of his data being processed and to choose whether or not he wants to participate in the project. Since the homecare professionals are, as key players between the different healthcare providers, most closely related to the patient's home environment, they are the best in place to perform this task (Leonard and Poullet 1999).

"Fairly" also means that the personal data cannot be stored any longer than necessary for the purposes for which the data were collected (Vandendriessche 2004 and De Bot 2001). This implies that restricted retention periods for the data storage have to be taken into account when setting up an EHR. Please note however that national medical regulations sometimes also require a minimum retention period for the data collected in a health record, as is the case in Belgium[12].

Proportionality principle

Secondly, the processing of personal data must always be adequate, relevant and not excessive in relation to the purposes for which the data are collected and/or further processed (article 6.1.c) DPD). As a consequence, it is not allowed to process personal data "en bloc", but a selection will have to be made based on the relevance of the data for the purposes for which the data are processed (De Bot 2001). In practice, this implies that the healthcare professional will have to balance the patient's interests between the patient's wish for privacy and his need for medical care.

The patient's wish for privacy is often related to the degree of data sensitivity. Depending on the that degree, the collected data can be divided into three main data categories: (1) the administrative data, (2) the data accessible for all healthcare providers (like vaccinations and allergies) and (3) the data only accessible to the attending GP or specialist. This data distinction is also a possible approach on how to organize the access to an EHR in a proportionate manner (Dhont and Poullet 1999-2000).

Additionally, the data need to be processed in an accurate way (article 6.1.d) DPD). This obliges the healthcare professional to permanently manage the quality of the collected data including taking every reasonable step to keep these data up-to-date and to ensure that data which are inaccurate or incomplete, with regard to

---

[12] In a Belgian hospital health records must be stored for at least 30 years [8 and 10].

the purposes for which they were collected or for which they are being further processed, are erased or rectified (article 1.d) DPD).

Due to the particularity of a homecare setting, data accuracy is one of the most important issues when exchanging health data in an EHR. Therefore, also the appropriate technical and organizational measures have to be taken to protect the data against accidental or unlawful destruction or accidental loss, alteration, unauthorized disclosure or access, in particular where the processing involves the data transmission over a network (article 17.1. DPD). A common used measure to secure data in a network connection is the public-private key encryption.

Finality principle

Thirdly, personal data can only be collected for "specified, explicit and legitimate purposes". These purposes have to be set out before initiating the data processing. When data are further processed in a way incompatible with the initial purposes, this will be considered illegitimate (article 6.b) DPD).

In order to determine whether or not further data processing is compatible with the initial purposes, the healthcare professional will have to take into account both the patient's reasonable expectations regarding the initial purposes and the legal or other regulations restricting these purposes[13].

However, further processing of data for historical, statistical or scientific purposes shall never be considered as incompatible, provided that the member state involved cares for appropriate safeguards (article 6.b) DPD) (see Sect. 2.1.). In Belgium, these safeguards are provided by a Royal Decree [13].

Lawfulness principle

Finally, the personal data need to be processed in a "lawful" manner (article 6.1.a) DPD). Personal data are "lawfully" processed when it complies with the legal framework applicable in the context of the data processing, in this case a homecare setting. As a consequence, the processing will be considered "unlawful" whenever a legal provision is not complied with. In that case, a patient will be able to take his healthcare professional, as a controller to court (De Bot 2001).

Furthermore, the purposes of the data processing have to be "legitimate" (article 6.1.b) DPD). The data processing is in other words, not permitted without a le-

---

[13] Please note that since the assessment of the patient's reasonable expectations, is –in most cases- entirely based on "facts", it seems to be more sensible to set out each of the purposes separately and explicitly, even though they might be compatible with one another.

gitimate basis. The legitimate bases to process health data (in an EHR) can be found in article 8 of the DPD and will be discussed in the next section.

1.2.6.2 The legitimate bases to process health data

Health data can only be processed when permitted by article 8 of the DPD. The following exceptions are provided:

- the data subject has given his explicit consent to the processing of his health data; or
- the data processing is necessary for the purposes of carrying out the obligations and specific rights of the controller in the field of employment law in so far as it is authorized by national law providing for adequate safeguards; or
- the data processing is necessary to protect the vital interests of the data subject or of another person where the data subject is physically or legally incapable of giving his consent; or
- the data processing is carried out in the course of its legitimate activities with appropriate guarantees by a foundation, association or any other non-profit-seeking body with a political, philosophical, religious or trade-union aim and on condition that the processing relates solely to the members of the body or to persons who have regular contact with it in connection with its purposes and that the data are not disclosed to a third party without the consent of the data subjects; or
- the data processing relates to data which are manifestly made public by the data subject or is necessary for the establishment, exercise or defense of legal claims (article 8.2. DPD); or
- the data processing is required for the purposes of preventive medicine, medical diagnosis, the provision of care or treatment or the management of health-care services, and where those data are processed by a health professional subject under national law or rules established by national competent bodies to the obligation of professional secrecy or by another person also subject to an equivalent obligation of secrecy (article 8.3. DPD).

Please note that for reasons of substantial public interest, an EU member state may lay down additional exceptions (either by national law or by decision of the supervisory authority), as long as these exemptions are subject to the provision of suitable safeguards (article 8.4 DPD). As will be discussed later, the explicit consent is however the most frequently used legal basis to process health data in a project phase (see Sect. 2.4.).

1.3 Other relevant legislation

In some cases, and depending on the business model chosen by the project management, additional regulations may interfere with the data protection legislation. As these regulations do not always apply in an eHealth context, they will only be briefly explained.

1.3.1 The e-Commerce Directive

Since an EHR is meant to be accessible anytime and anywhere by all the healthcare professionals involved in the patient's treatment, the e-Commerce Directive [5] will often be applicable. The e-Commerce Directive applies to "*any service normally provided for remuneration, at a distance, by electronic means and at the individual request of a recipient of services*" (article 2.a) eCommerce Directive and article 1.2.a) Directive 98/48 EC), this is e.g. an "information society service". As a consequence, every provider of an information society service established in the EU is subject to this Directive (article 3 eCommerce Directive). Examples of an information society service in the homecare sector are: tele-expertise, telemedicine and tele-monitoring.

Crucial to the applicability of the e-Commerce Directive, is the condition of the service provided from a distance. If the patient and the health provider are both present in the same space, the Directive is not applicable.

The e-Commerce Directive has two main goals. First, it obliges the service provider to render a minimum level of information to the user or recipient of the service. This information has to be easily, directly and permanently accessible and should enable the user to identify the service provider in the "physical" world and to understand the different technical steps in the application [10]. Additionally, the e-Commerce Directive provides a specific liability regime for internet service providers acting as "intermediaries" with regard to mere conduit, cashing and hosting[14]. Nevertheless, this liability regime covers only cases where the activity of the

[14] "Mere conduit" can be defined as information society service that consists of "the transmission in a communication network of information provided by a recipient of the service, or the provision of access to a communication network", "cashing" can be defined as "the automatic, intermediate and temporary storage of the transmitted information in a communication network provided by a recipient of the service performed for the sole purpose of making more efficient the information's onward transmission to other recipients of the service upon their request" and "hosting" can be defined as "the disposal of a server containing stored information". See Article 13-15 eCommerce Directive; Van Eecke, P. 2001. Electronic Health Care Services and the e-Commerce Directive. In *A decade of research ad the crossroads of law and ICT*, ed. Jos Dumortier. Brussels: Larcier.

information society service provider is limited to the technical process of operating and giving access to a communication network over which information made available by third parties is transmitted or temporarily stored, for the sole purpose of making the transmission more efficient (recital 42 eCommerce Directive).

When the information society service provider is not only involved in the technical process but as well in the data processing as a third service provider, he acts as a processor and therefore, all liability issues have to be governed by a contract (article 17.3. DPD).

1.3.2 The e-Privacy Directive

In some cases, the use of new advanced digital technologies (and in particular the Internet) in the development of an EHR, requires specific data protection. In this case, the e-Privacy Directive [6] is applicable which translates the data protection principles set out in the DPD into specific requirements for the telecommunications sector (recital 4 ePrivacy Directive). This Directive applies to "*the processing of personal data in connection with the provision of publicly available communications services in public communications networks in the Community*" (article 3 ePrivacy Directive).

An "electronic communications service" is defined in the Framework Directive as: "*a service, normally provided for remuneration, which consists wholly or mainly in the conveyance of signals on electronic communications networks, including telecommunications services and transmission services in networks used for broadcasting, but excludes services providing, or exercising editorial control over, content transmitted using electronic communications networks and services; it does not include information society services,* [...] *which do not consist wholly or mainly in the conveyance of signals on electronic communications networks*" (article 2.c) Directive 98/48 EC).

When the service of a digital homecare application thus merely exist in the transmission of data via e.g. the Internet (without offering any additional services) the e-Privacy Directive will be applicable.

An example is e.g. the automated transmission of results of blood pressure measurements or testing glucose to an hospital via an Internet-connected application at the patient's home[15]. If the service of this application only exist in transmitting the data from the patient's home to the hospital, the e-Privacy Directive ap-

[15] For a more detailed description of such a service we refer to the Flemish IM3 project of IBBT (http://www.ibbt.be/en/project/im3).

plies. However, as soon as the service includes additional services, like a first assessment of the data by a nurse or is linked to an emergency call centre, the e-Privacy directive will not be applicable anymore. In this case the rendered services then exists of more than merely the transmission of information. Since the automated collection and transmission of health data will in most of the eHomecarecases only be useful in case these data are also the subject of a sort of assessment, the e-Privacy Directive will hardly ever be applicable.

2 Set-up manual for eHomecare projects

In an integrated approach to an eHealth project[16], it is most important to take some basic data protection principles into account.

2.1 Primary and secondary data processing

As already explained, the DPD will be applicable when processing health data in an eHomecare project. If these data are directly collected from the patient, the specific data protection regime for health data will be applicable. In most of the projects, this requires the explicit consent of the patient. By giving his consent, the patient will agree his data to be processed for the scientific and statistical purposes set out by the project.

When processing data for historical, statistical or scientific purposes, it is however also possible to re-use data which were initially collected for other purposes (by the project consortium or another "external" controller). In principle, personal data are not allowed to be further processed in a way incompatible with the initial purposes. Further processing of data for historical, statistical or scientific purposes is however not to be considered as incompatible when the member state, in which the controller is located, provides appropriate safeguards (article 6.1.b) DPD). These safeguards are in the Belgian jurisprudence referred to as the data protection regime for "secondary" data processing, which is elaborated in the Royal Decree of February 13, 2001 [13], attached to the Belgian Data Protection Act [8]. Basically, this regime consists of a three-layered classification with the use of anonymous data as a starting point (Article 3 Belgian Royal Decree of 13 February 2001).

---

[16] See chapter Ackaert, A. et al. A multi-disciplinary approach towards the design and development of value+ eHomeCare services.

"Anonymous data" in the sense of the DPD can be defined as “any information relating to a natural person where the person cannot be identified, whether by the data controller or by any other person, taking account of all the means likely reasonably to be used either by the controller or by any other person to identify that individual”.

When re-using data for historical, statistical or scientific purposes, this means that these data should be in principle rendered anonymous (or so called: “anonymised”) in such a way that the data subject is no longer identifiable and identification will not be possible anymore” [16].

If however the use of anonymous data proves to be impossible, considering the purposes of the data processing, the use of pseudonymous or key-coded data will be allowed (article 4 Belgian Royal Decree of 13 February 2001). In this case, “information relates to individuals that are earmarked by a code, while the key making the correspondence between the code and the common identifiers of the individuals (like name, date of birth, address) is kept separately" [16].

Only if also the use of pseudonyms seems to be impossible, the controller can use non-coded personal data (article 5 Belgian Royal Decree of 13 February 2001). Logically to each of these three levels apply different conditions, which become stricter as the data become “less anonimized”. Therefore, before processing health data “secondary”, the appropriate level of protection within the scope of the project will need to be identified.

2.2 Notification

Prior to the data processing, the controller needs to notify the national supervising data protection authority (hereinafter: “data protection authority”)(article 18.1. DPD). This notification has to include a minimum of information and at least:

- the name and address of the controller and of his representative (if any) and;
- the purpose or purposes of the processing;
- a description of the category or categories of data subject and of the data or categories of data relating to them;
- the recipients or categories of recipients to whom the data might be disclosed;
- proposed transfer of data to third countries;
- a general description allowing a preliminary assessment to be made of the appropriateness of the measures taken to ensure security of processing (article 19 DPD).

Each member is required to publicize all notifications in a public register (article 21 DPD) to ensure transparency of the data processing to the general public.

In some cases, a notification is however not considered adequate to guarantee the fair processing of the data. If certain processing operations are likely to present specific risks to the rights and freedoms of data subjects, member states have the possibility to introduce a prior checking of these operations by the data protection authorities (article 20.1. DPD).

On the opposite, there are cases in which it is not deemed necessary to notify the data protection authority. Therefore, member states may also provide for the simplification of or exemption from notification under strictly defined circumstances and conditions (article 18.2., 18.3. and 18.4. DPD). Please note that such an exemption does however not release the controller of his other data protection obligations.

2.3 Privacy notice for the patient

2.3.1 Need for an informed consent

As already explained above (see Sect. 1.2.6.2), the explicit and informed consent of the patient will in many eHealth projects be the only legitimate ground to process health data (article 8 DPD). Especially regarding projects, consent will often be the safest solution to hold the health data processed in a "lawful" way.

However, consent is not always required. In a medical context, the processing of health data is allowed without the patient's consent whenever the data processing is necessary for the purposes of preventive medicine, medical diagnosis, the provision of care or treatment or the management of health-care services. It must be noted that in this case, it is additionally required that those data are processed by a health care professional subject under national law or rules established by national competent bodies to the obligation of professional (medical) secrecy (or by another person also subject to an equivalent obligation of secrecy) (article 8.3. DPD). Since the scope of a project is often encloses more than only those mentioned above, this derogation will however not cover all data processing with regards to the research purposes of a project, such as the technical development of an EHR (De Bot 2001) [17].

Secondly, an informed consent is not required in case of an emergency (article 8.2.c) DPD). As for the previous exemption, this exemption too has to be interpreted very restrictive[17]. It can only be applied if the data processing is absolutely necessary to protect the vital interests of the patient, e.g. when a coma patient is in need for urgent surgery[18]. In this case, the data subject is physically incapable of giving his consent. Also, the legal incapability of giving consent will be considered as a legitimate ground to process health data when the person involved is in risk of one's life.

Finally, national laws or other regulations too might provide for a legitimate ground to process health data without the consent of the patient, if those data are not disclosed to a third party (article 8.2.d) DPD). In Belgium, e.g. national regulations oblige each GP to keep a General Health Record (hereinafter: "GHR") of his current patients [12]. In principle, the GP is not required to ask the patient's consent to store his data in this GHR. Only if the GP wants to exchange the data of the GHR with other colleagues who are involved in the patient's treatment, the patient's consent needs to be obtained before sharing the data (Article 4 Belgian Royal Decree of 3 May 1999 on the General Health Record).

In any case, an informed consent will always be a way out to ensure the legitimacy of the data processing in eHealth projects. By integrating a well-considered patient consent management in the project or application, the data processing will be more transparent and people will be less reluctant to participate.

2.3.1.1 Requirements on the informed consent

The informed consent of the data subject (e.g. the patient) is defined in the DPD as: "*any* (1) *freely given* (2) *specific and* (3) *informed indication of his wishes by which the data subject signifies his agreement to personal data relating to him being processed*" (article 2.h) DPD). This definition contains the three basic conditions for "consent".

First of all, the consent must be given *freely*. This means it is not allowed to put any pressure on the patient when asking for his consent. Sometimes pressure can arise just from the inferior position of the patients towards his healthcare provider.

---

[17] This is because the derogations provided in article 8 of the DPD are limited and exhaustive and need to be construed in a narrow fashion. See Article 29 Data Protection Working party, Working document of 15 February 2007 on the processing of personal data relating to health in electronic health records (EHR): 8.

[18] This in contrast with article 5.d) DPA. In this case the controller must not proof the data subject was unable to consent. Important to notice is that in this case too only a vital interest of the data subject can allow the processing. The exemption is not applicable when the processing of the health data is necessary for protection of vital interests of another person. See De Bot, D. 2001. *Processing of personal data*. Antwerp: Kluwer: 132-133 (*in Dutch*).

In a project, it is most important to avoid such situations: e.g. no discrimination with regard to quality of the homecare provided to the patient will be allowed between patients consenting and not consenting with the processing of their health data in an EHR. Please also note that unless the patient's consent is given to receive a certain advantage, the Royal Decree attached to the Belgian Data Protection Act explicitly prohibits to process health data with as a sole legal basis the informed consent in cases there might be an inferior position of the patient towards the healthcare professional (article 27 Belgian Royal Decree of 13 February 2001). Since eHomecare projects have as main goal the improvement of the patient's homecare, this prohibition will however not be considered as a bottleneck for the project.

Secondly, the consent must be *specific*, e.g. the data processing and its purposes must be adequately described in a clear and transparent manner. For the controller, this is not always an easy task. Special attention will have to be paid (1) to the description of the purposes which may not be too vague, but also not too detailed so the information becomes too intricate to understand for the patient and (2) to the identification of the different data streams in the application (like an EHR).

Finally, the consent must also be *informed*, e.g. the controller has to give the patients participating in the project, all the necessary information to assess the implications and possible risks of their data being processed (De Bot 2001). As a consequence, consent based on false or wrongly provided information, has no legal value.

Like indicated before, the controller has to provide the data subject with a minimum of information. One way to provide this information is by including it in a written privacy notice.

In particular, the data subject has to be informed about the identity of the controller and (if any) of his representative (article 10.a) DPD) and about the purposes of the processing for which the data are intended (article 10.b) DPD). Additionally and in so far as necessary with regard to the specific circumstances in which the data are collected, the controller will have to provide the patient with any information necessary to guarantee fair processing in respect of the data subject. This can include the recipients or categories of recipients of the data, whether replies to the questions are obligatory or voluntary, as well as the possible consequences of failure to reply, and the existence of the right of access to and the right to rectify his own data (article 10.c) DPD).

2.3.1.2 Vulnerable patients unable to consent

As already indicated, some patients are unable to give their consent due to a physical or legal incapability. In cases where there is no emergency, the DPD does however not give a clear answer on how to process health data of people without a will (e.g. demented elderly or Alzheimer patients). In this case, the general principles of civil law concerning legal representatives and national regulations on patients' rights will provide for a solution [18].

2.3.1.3 The informed consent in practice

Although for the processing of health data, a written consent is usually not required in most of the EU member states, it will be most preferable to have it for all data subjects involved in the project. From the perspective of the burden of proof, a written consent has several advantages (Vandedriessche 2004). It is for example not always easy for a healthcare professional (acting as a controller) to proof he has made enough efforts to inform the patient about his data processing and it is even more difficult to verify whether the patient involved has understood this information or not. Research demonstrates that patients generally do not remember much of the oral information given by their healthcare professional during consultation. A written consent, in the form of a privacy notice, will allow the patients to reread the information whenever they want (Dijkhofz 2003-2004).

2.4 Privacy and security policies

2.4.1 Additional data protection documents

Equally important as the privacy notice, are the privacy and security policies. These policies consist of a set of different documents reflecting the controller's obligation to take all appropriate technical and organizational measures to protect the collected, or in any other way processed, personal data against accidental or unlawful destruction, accidental loss, alternation, unauthorized disclosure or access and against all other unlawful forms of processing (article 17.1. DPD). Examples are guidelines for the employees, a data protection manual or an incident plan.

These technical and organizational measures have to ensure an appropriate level of data security, taking into account the state of the art, the implementation costs, the nature (sensitivity) of the data and the potential risks for a security breach (article 17.1. DPD).

Since the processing of health data in an EHR over the Internet encounters a lot of security threats, the project partners will need to implement a very strict privacy and security policy.

2.4.2 The processor contract

The obligation to maintain an appropriate level of security does not only include the controller, but, if any, also the processor.

When the data processing action is carried out by a processor on the controller's behalf, the controller must choose a processor who provides sufficient guarantees in respect of the technical security measures and organizational measures. Naturally, the controller also has to ensure compliance with those measures (article 17.2. DPD).

Therefore, the carrying out of processing by way of a processor must always be governed by a contract or legal act binding the processor to the controller. This contract has to stipulate that (1) the processor shall act only on instructions from the controller and that (2) he too has to implement an appropriate level of protection (article 17.3. DPD).

Unlike the privacy notice to the data subject, this contract has to be in writing, or equivalent form, for the purposes of keeping evidence (article 17.4. DPD).

3 Practical recommendations for the start-up of an eHomecare project

From the very first start of an eHomecare project, it is important to include legal research as one of the basic steps in determining the bottlenecks. In most cases, these bottlenecks can be derived from the general principles of the legal framework applicable to the project. When identifying the "legal" bottlenecks in advance, a lot of integration problems can be avoided with regards to the implementation in "real-life".

In the second stage of the project, legal research needs to be focused on drafting and implementing adequate privacy notices and policies (see Sect. 2.4.). These policies have to ensure that the deployment of the application will be both functional as legally acceptable. This is the most difficult part of the project since the legal requirements need to be translated into technical terms, which then have to be implemented in the architecture of the application. At this stage multidisciplinary teamwork becomes a key issue.

In the last stage of a project, the legal research activities have to focus on the legal validation. This validation implies a permanent "legal" follow-up to ensure the continuous compliance of the technical aspects of the project with the existing legal framework.

Within each of these project stages, different legal issues occur. Based on our experiences in the TranseCare[19] and eHip[20] project, we tried to translate these issues into ten main principles. These principles can be used to develop a privacy-friendly application.

3.1 First stage: before the project kick-off

3.1.1 Principle one: identify all actors and the purposes of the data processing in the project and determine the legal basis to process these data

When starting a project involving the processing of data, it is most important to know whether you will act as a processor or as a controller. Depending on your role in the project, different liabilities and obligations will be evoked (see Sect. 3.1.2).

In order to delimit your role in the project, you will first have to identify the different data streams and related data processing actions, not only within the project, but also within in the application you want to develop, bearing in mind all potential data flow scenarios and schemes.

These data flow scenarios and schemes are related to the purposes of the data processing in your project. When drafting these scenarios, it is prudent to make already a first distinction between the primary and secondary use of personal data, since both regimes ask for a different approach (as explained in Sect. 2.1.).

Please note that - depending on the scenario you have in mind - the different data processing actions can have different purposes, e.g. the purposes of the data processing in a "proof of concept" are different to those of a "real life" implementation.

As will be explained below, these purposes have to be described as accurately as possible because (1) you will have to verify if there is any legal basis to process health data for these purposes and this will be easier to assess if the purposes are distinctively described and because (2) you will have to inform the data subject (e.g. patient) of these purposes before the actual data processing and this information has to be as accurate as possible. When the data processing is based on the informed consent of the patient, this will allow him to make a risk analysis of his data being processed and to choose whether or not he wants to participate in the

[19] See: http://www.ibbt.be/en/project/e-hip.

[20] See: http://www.ibbt.be/en/project/transecare.

project. As a consequence, it is prudent to describe the different scenarios in which the data processing is envisaged, by referring to well-defined, concrete situations.

Please also note that a general agreement of the data subject to collect his data for generally defined purposes, can be considered as void. Defining the purposes of the data processing in your project has thus a lot of legal implications and is equal to already half of the legal work.

3.1.2 Principle two: all project partners should be aware of their liabilities

As already explained, different liabilities and obligations will be evoked depending on your role as a processor or as a controller in the project (see Sect. 3.1.2.).

After having identified the role of each actor in the project, the different obligations and liabilities have to be set out and appointed to the different project partners. In this sense, a well-drafted contract between the controller(s) and the processor(s) in the project will provide a solution to divide the liability concerning data protection issues.

Liabilities can however also occur in other contexts apart from the data protection framework, like e.g. product liability (with regard to the offered products or services) or medical liability. Depending on the relation between the actors involved, a basic distinction needs to be made between contractual liability and extra-contractual liability.

As a consequence, assessing liability includes more than only verifying the liability regime set out in the DPD. Other specific regulations have to be considered as well, including e.g. the e-Commerce Directive and its liability regime for hosting, cashing and mere conduit.

3.2 Middle stage: during the project

3.2.1 Principle three: well-built identification systems

During the first steps in a project developing an EHR system, identification of both the patient and the healthcare professional is often recognized as one of the crucial bottlenecks in the project.

"Identification" refers to the description of an individual by identifiers like his name, date of birth and address[21].

In order to ensure the identified person is the person he claims to be, this description will have to be officially certified by e.g. a birth certificate, an electronic ID or a health card. This is the so-called "authorization" of the person.

3.2.1.1 A patient identification system

In view of the fact that an incorrect identification of a patient can have detrimental (medical) consequences, the implementation of a well-built patient identification system (hereinafter: "PIS") based on unique patient identifiers is absolutely necessary when developing an EHR.

One example of a unique identifier is the national (identification) number. Since the DPD allows member states to determine the conditions under which a national number may be processed (article 8.7. DPD), it seemed a logical step to introduce this number in the health sector.

Some member states, like Belgium and the Netherlands, did however not want to use the national number for healthcare purposes in order to avoid any interconnectivity with other related sectors as for example the Social Security (article 8.7. DPD). In Belgium, this discussion has now come to an end by the new Act on the implementation and organization of an eHealth platform [9] introducing the national number as patient identifier.

3.2.1.2 An identification system for the healthcare professional

In order to prevent the unauthorized access of users to an EHR, it will be also essential to develop an identification system for the healthcare professionals, allowing the authentication and authorization of each healthcare professional who wants to access the EHR. Such an identification system should be based on a role-based access policy which ensures for each healthcare professional the access to the health data to be strictly limited to what is necessary for the exercise of his profession and his role in the treatment of the patient (by analogy article 16, §2, 2° DPA).

This is the so-called "*need to know*" principle: only health care professionals or authorized personnel of healthcare institutions who are presently involved in the patient's treatment, have the right of access to this patient's EHR[22].

---

[21] Article 29 Data Protection Working Party, Opinion 4/2007 on the concept of Personal Data, 12-13.

3.2.2 Principle four: patient consent management

As already explained above (see Sect. 2.4.1.), the patient's consent is for eHomecare projects often the only possible legal basis to process health data and therefore frequently considered a bottleneck. If the patient does not consent, the whole project can be delayed or, even worse, cancelled.

In practice, this means it is most important to be as transparent as possible about the data processing in the EHR. This will result in an easier acceptance and uptake of the application by the public. As already explained, writing a clear privacy notice is however not always an easy task. On the one hand, a privacy notice has to contain some legally required information (see Sect. 2.4.1.1.) taking into account the patients' rights and on the other hand a privacy notice also needs to be compact and easily comprehensible for the patient.

In addition, the privacy notice is linked with the written informed consent of the patient (see Sect. 2.4.1.3.) (Vandendriessche 2004 and De Bot 2001). Since this consent must be specific, it must relate to a well-defined, concrete situation in which the processing of health data is envisaged [17]. This implies that the patient should have the possibility (1) to give his consent for a limited or unlimited period of time, (2) to decide whether he consents in the processing of a specific category of health data or all his health data and (3) to regulate which (categories of) healthcare professionals at which level are granted access to the health data[23] [17].

From this point of view, it will be necessary to document the EHR with electronic proof of the patient's specific consent for each data processing action in the EHR [17].

---

[22] Please note that access should never be allowed on a "nice to know" basis. This means that it should not be possible for a healthcare professional to have access to the EHR of a patient if he is not involved in the treatment of this patient. In order to prevent that healthcare professionals would take access to an EHR on a nice to know basis logging and tracing mechanisms should be installed.

[23] Please note that this includes his right to block the access to certain health data for a particular healthcare professional and to withdraw his consent. This choice is derived from the patient's free choice of practitioner and hospital or clinic. See article 6 of the Belgian Act on Patients' Rights of 22 August 2002, *Belgisch Staatsblad* 26 September 2002 (*in Dutch*).

3.2.3 Principle five: implement a correct procedure for the right of access

Not only the DPD, but also a lot of national Laws on Patients' Rights allows every patient a right of access to or information about his health data which are being processed[24] (article 12 DPD).

3.2.3.1 The right of access according to the DPD

In accordance with the DPD, the health care professional will have to give the (identified) patient, upon request, access to the personal information in his EHR. This implies the right of access to be an active right, meaning the information will only be given after the patient has asked for it. This action distinguishes the right of access from the right to be informed (see Sect. 2.4.1.1.), which is a passive right. The controller has to give a minimum of information in advance, with or without request, in order to give the patient the possibility to assess the risks of his data being processed and to consent to it or not.

In the case of right of access, the DPD requires the controller (often a health-care professional) to inform the data subject (often a patient) on whether or not data relating to him are being processed and about the purposes of the processing, the categories of data concerned, and the recipients or categories of recipients to whom the data are disclosed. The controller is also obliged (1) to communicate to the data subject in an intelligible form about the data undergoing processing and about any available information as to their source and has (2) to inform the patient about the logic involved in any automatic processing and about the opportunity to file an appeal and get access to the public register (article 12 DPD).

3.2.3.2 The right of access according to medical law and patients' rights

In addition to the DPD, national medical laws often explicitly allow the patient a direct right of access to his health record. This right is related to the human right to physical and human integrity [9].

In some cases, the patient must however be protected against himself. Therefore, most national laws provide some exceptions to the right of access to a health record as will be illustrated by the Belgian Act on Patients' Rights (hereinafter: "APR").

---

[24] This is at least the case in the Belgian Act on Patients' Rights of 22 August 2002.

First of all, the APR does not allow the patient to have a right of access at all times. He can only re-exercise his right after a reasonable amount of time he checked his health record the previous time (Nys and Vinck 2003).

Secondly, the healthcare professional will also refuse access when he considers that the permission to access information would obviously harm the patient's health. This is the so-called "therapeutic exception". However, before taking this decision, the healthcare professional needs to consult a colleague and add a written statement to the patient's health record on his refusal. Additionally, the healthcare professional has to inform the trusted party if appointed by the patient (article 7§4 DPA) (Trouet and Dreezen 2003).

Finally, please note that the right to be informed does not only imply "a right to know", but also "a right not to know" [9]. On the one hand, the "right to know" clearly gives the patient the right to be informed about his health condition. This is e.g. information about the diagnosis and the use of medication. It is most important that this information is communicated in a clear and understandable way taking into account the situation and capabilities of each individual patient (see Sect. 2.4.1.2.)[25]. On the other hand, the right of information contains also a "right not to know", meaning that a patient has the right not to be informed about his health condition. In this case, the health professional shall not give information to the patient unless this obviously causes serious harm to the patient himself or any other person [9].

3.2.3.3 In practice

In practice, the right of access has an enormous impact on the technical requirements of an EHR. First of all, both the patient and his healthcare professional (involved in his treatment) have the possibility to block each other's access to parts of the EHR, which complicates the writing of the access policies from a technical point of view. In any case, it will be necessary to equip the EHR with a feature to block the access of certain information and to provide the healthcare professional with a feature to indicate when he uses the therapeutic exception to prevent the patient being harmed by the information in his EHR[26].

---

[25] It is important to note that the "right to know" in this sense has nothing to do with the right to be informed before preceding the treatment; Dijkhofz, W. 2003-2004 'The Law on Patientrights. Part III. The right to information and informed consent.': *Tijdschrift Gezondheidsrecht.* 104 (*in Dutch*).

[26] Please note that this is also relevant for other healthcare professional accessing the EHR.

Secondly, the right of access of the healthcare professional needs to be based on the “need to know” principle and a role-based access policy. This can be technically translated to the installation of “modular access rights”. To implement modular access rights, the medical information in the EHR must be divided in different categories of health data, (like e.g. a category for allergies and data required during an emergency case) to which the access is limited to specific categories of healthcare professionals [17].

3.2.4 Principle six: comply with all applicable laws

The legal requirements of an eHomecare project often do not only relate to data protection and medical legislation. Depending on the different scenarios developed in an eHomecare project, also sector specific (national) regulations need to be taken into account.

For instance, one of the scenarios in the TranseCare project included a video monitoring system with the installation of cameras at the patients’ homes. In the project, two different kinds of systems were discussed: (1) a system which can be switched on in alarming situations and (2) a system which monitors continuously. Based on the higher privacy risk to process data under the second system, the partners of the TranseCare project decided only to work with the first system. This assessment did however not merely include data protection issues, but also involved a study on the right of personal portrayal and specific regulations on the use of cameras.

This example illustrates that for each project scenario, the scope of the legal framework applicable to the project (1) practically always needs to be extended to more specific (sector) regulations (than only data protection and medical legislation) and (2) has to be assessed on a case-by-case basis.

3.2.5 Principle seven: implement the necessary security measures

As already explained, the controller of an EHR needs to take all appropriate technical and organizational measures to protect the personal data collected in the EHR. However, not all national data protection laws contain specific provisions for implementing such security measures. In this case, the controller has to decide which measures are to be implemented or not.

According to Belgian legislation, at least the following security measures have to be implemented when processing health data in an EHR:

- first of all, the controller must ensure that all data are up-to-date and will be erased or corrected if inaccurate, incomplete and irrelevant or if the data processing is illegitimate;
- as already explained above, he also has to limit the access to the data for all persons acting under his authority to what is strictly necessary for the fulfillment of their profession;
- furthermore, he has to make sure that all persons acting under his authority are informed about all relevant legislation pertaining to the protection of health data in an EHR;
- Finally, he has to ensure that the application of the EHR is -from a technical point of view- in accordance with the information provided in the notification (see Sect. 2.2.) (article 16 §2 of the Belgian DPA).

Other possible security measures are for example: the drafting of a security policy, the appointment of a security officer and the use of logging and tracing mechanisms.

3.2.6 Principle eight: the privacy of the healthcare professional

When applying logging and tracing mechanisms, certain personal data of the healthcare professionals accessing the EHR will be processed. Especially when the healthcare professional is not the controller, but an employee of the controller or the processor (e.g. a specialist working for a hospital), the same rules apply to him as to the patient. In this case, he has to be considered as a data subject. However, since the data processed from the healthcare professional are normally no health data, the "normal" data protection regime will be applicable.

Please also note that in a professional relationship most probably additional regulations on labor law will apply. Especially when the log data are not only used for security reasons, but are also intended for monitoring purposes (e.g. to control the health care professional), additional protection needs to be provided to the healthcare professional.

3.3 Final stage

3.3.1 Principle nine: validate the project from a legal point of view

During the previous stages of the project, legal research focused on translating the legal requirements into technical terms which needed to be implemented in the architecture of the EHR. In the last stage of the project, it is most important to evaluate and validate this translation from a legal point of view. By using a check list which can be easily derived from the research done in the previous stages, the functioning of the application (e.g. HER) and its architecture need to be "legally double-checked" to ensure that the EHR is both functional as legally acceptable.

3.3.2 Principle ten: implement the application in real-life and keep up-to-date

When deploying the application, the nine principles as set out above can be used as a checklist to see whether all data protection requirements are also met in "real-life".

In addition, the controller of the EHR must however also ascertain that all technical and organizational measures are regularly checked. After all, the technologies on information systems are constantly evolving which means that the controller has to keep technically up-to-date to react on possible security breaches. On a regular basis, he will need to verify whether his security policy is still up-to-date and meeting an appropriate level of security.

Ensuring the continuous compliance of the technical aspects of the application with the existing legal framework, implies as well a permanent "legal" follow-up. In an innovative and emerging sector as eHealth, it is most important to monitor any relevant changes in the legal framework which may occur during the implementation of an EHR, since new legislative initiatives in such a sector are very likely to arise.

4 Conclusion

When developing an eHomecare application mainly national medical regulations and data protection laws need to be taken into account. Unfortunately, most of the medical regulations in Europe are not harmonized, which makes it very difficult to develop one legally acceptable application that can be implemented in whole Europe.

With regard to data protection laws, the opposite is however true. Within Europe the Data Protection Directive harmonizes the protection of personal data being processed all over Europe. Before starting an eHomecare project it is most important to understand the basic principles and concepts of this Directive which make it possible to identify the different actors in the project. In accordance with the DPD, the three central actors are the data subject (e.g. the patient), the controller (mostly a healthcare professional) and the processor (acting as a third service provider). Where the controller is liable for most of the data protection obligations, the processor will only held liable for the obligations governed by his contract with the controller.

After having identified all actors in the project, some basic legal steps need to be taken to be compliant with all data protection requirements. Points of particular interest are (1) the question whether the project is dealing with primary or secondary use of personal data, (2) the notification to the Data Protection Authority, (3) the drafting of an informed consent (for the patient and the healthcare professional) and (4) the need for an appropriate level of security.

At this point, legal research does however not come to an end. In order to avoid a lot of integration problems when implementing the application in "real-life", it is most important to include legal research from the very first beginning of an eHomecare project.

Therefore, legal research should also be focused on drafting and implementing adequate privacy notices and policies ensuring that the deployment of the application will be both functional as legally acceptable. In practice, this means that all legal requirements need to be translated into technical terms and need to be implemented in the architecture of the application. At this stage of the project, the two main issues at stake are the implementation of (1) a patient consent management and (2) a correct procedure for the right of access to the EHR: since both the patient and his healthcare professional(s) (involved in his treatment) have the possibility to block each other's access to parts of the EHR, it will be necessary to equip the EHR with technical features to indicate when a data processing action is allowed or not.

This translation of legal requirements into technical terms can only be achieved by multidisciplinary teamwork and ensures that the developed technologies can be deployed in real-life without violating any legal requirements or harming patients' rights.

Reference list

Regulations and soft-law:

[1] Article 8 Convention for the protection of Human Rights and Fundamental Freedoms (November 4, 1950)
[2] Article 4 Convention for the Protection of Human Rights and Dignity of the Human Being with regard to the Application of Biology and Medicine: Convention on Human Rights and Biomedicine (April 4, 1997)
[3] Directive 95/46/EC of the European Parliament and of the Council of 24 October 1995 on the protection of individuals with regard to the processing of personal data and on the free movement of such data
[4] Directive 98/48 EC amending Directive 98/34/EC laying down a procedure for the provision of information in the field of technical standards and regulations

[5] Directive 2000/31 of the European Parliament and the Council of 8 June 2000 on certain legal aspects of information society services, in particular electronic commerce, in the Internal Market (Directive on electronic commerce)
[6] Directive 2002/58 EC of the European Parliament and the Council of 12 June 2002 concerning the processing of personal data and the protection of privacy in the electronic Communications sector (Directive on privacy and electronic communications)
[7] R (97) 5 on the Protection of Medical data, European Council, 2 (February 13, 1997)
[8] Act of 8 December 1992 protecting private life with regards to the processing of personal data, Belgisch Staatsblad (March 18, 1993) (in Dutch)
[9] Belgian Act on Patients' Rights of 22 August 2002, Belgisch Staatsblad (September 26, 2002) (in Dutch)
[10] Art. 7 § 1 Belgian Act of 11 March 2003 concerning certain aspects legal of information society services, Belgisch Staatsblad (March 17, 2003) (in Dutch)
[11] Act on the implementation and organization of the eHealth platform, Parl. St. House of Representatives 2007-2008, nr. 52-1257/006; Parl. St. Senate 2007-2008, nr. 4-863/3
[12] Article 2 Belgian Royal Decree of 3 May 1999 on the General Health Record, Belgisch Staatsblad (July 17, 1999) (in Dutch)
[13] Articles 2 – 24 Belgian Royal Decree of 13 February 2001 to implement the Law of 8 December 1992 protecting the private life with regard to the processing of personal data (in Dutch)
[14] Article 46 Belgian Medical Code of Conduct, `http://www.ordomedic.be/web-Ned/deonton.htm` (in Dutch)
[15] Article 29 Data Protection Working Party, Opinion 6/2000 of 13 July 2000 on the Human Genome and Privacy, 2
[16] Article 29 Data Protection Working Party, Opinion 4/2007 on the concept of Personal Data, 7-17
[17] Article 29 Data Protection Working party, Working document of 15 February 2007 on the processing of personal data relating to health in electronic health records (EHR), 6–8
[18] Article 29 Data Protection Working party, Working document 132/2007 on the processing of personal data relating to health in electronic health records (EHR), 4
[19] Communication from the Commission to the Council, the European Parliament, The European Economic and Social Committee and the Committee of the Regions of 30 April 2004 on eHealth - making healthcare better for European citizens: An action plan for a European e-Health Area, 7
[20] The European Standards on Confidentiality and Privacy among Vulnerable Patient Populations (July 8, 2005), `http://www.eurosocap.org`
[21] Belgian Data Protection Commission, Advice 34/1999 on the processing of images in particular in relation to the use of video-surveillance, 5 (in Dutch)

Doctrine and literature

Chalmers, D.: Australia. In Medical Law. In: Nys, H., Blanpain, R. (eds.) International Encyclopedia of Laws, pp. 28–29. Kluwer Inernational, The Hague (1998)
De Bot, D.: Law on the protection of personal data' in X., Persons and Family Law. In: Comments on the articles and survey of jurisdiction and doctrine, Kluwer Rechtswetenschappen, Antwerp (2001)

De Bot, D.: Processing of personal data. Kluwer, Antwerp (2001) (in Dutch)
Dhont, J., Poullet, Y.: The General Medical Record: a correct assessment between efficiency of the state, independancy of the health care professional and the privacy of the patient. Tijdschrift Gezondheidsrecht, 251–252 (1999-2000) (in Dutch)
Dijkhofz, W.: The Law on Patientrights. Part III. The right to information and informed consent. Tijdschrift Gezondheidsrecht, 104–115 (2003-2004)
Furrow, B., et al.: United States of America. In Medical Law. In: Nys, H., Blanpain, R. (eds.) International Encyclopedia of Laws, p. 29. Kluwer Inernational, The Hague (2005)
Kuner, C.: European Data Protection law, Corporate Complinace and regulation, vol. 92, p. 552. Oxford University Press, Oxford (2007)
Leonard, T., Poullet, Y.: The protection of personal data in full (r)evolution. The Act of 11 December 1998 implements the Directive 95/46/EC' Journal des Tribunaux: 380 (1999) (in French)
Nys, H., Vinck, I.: New regulations on patient rights, pp. 112–113. Kluwer, Mechelen (2003)
Trouet, C., Dreezen, I.: Legal protection of the patient: Nieuw Juridisch Weekblad, 6 (15 January 2003) (in Dutch)
Van Eecke, P.: Electronic Health Care Services and the e-Commerce Directive. In: Dumortier, J. (ed.) A decade of research ad the crossroads of law and ICT. Larcier, Brussels (2001)
Vandendriessche, J.: Protection of private life. In: De Corte, R. (ed.) Practical Guide for law and the Internet, pp. 16–17. Vanden Broele, Brugge (2004) (in Dutch)

List of abbreviations

- **EHR**: Electronic Health Record
- **GP**: General Practionner
- **DPD**: Directive 95/46/EC of the European Parliament and of the Council of 24 October 1995 on the protection of individuals with regard to the processing of personal data and on the free movement of such data
- **DPA**: (Belgian) Data Protection Act 8 December 1992
- **e-Privacy Directive**: Directive 2002/58 EC of the European Parliament and the Counsil of 12 June 2002 concerning the processing of personal data and the protection of privacy in the electronic Communications sector (Directive on privacy and electronic communications)
- **e-Commerce Directive**: Directive 2000/31 of the European Parliament and the Counsil of 8 June 2000 on certain legal aspects of information society services, in particular electronic commerce, in the Internal Market (Directive on electronic commerce)
- **Data protection authority**: National supervising data protection authority
- **GHR**: General Health Record
- **PIS**: Patient Identification System
- **APR**: (Belgian) Act on Patient Rights of 22 August 2002

VirtualECare: Group Support in Collaborative Networks Organizations for Digital Homecare

Ricardo Costa[1], Paulo Novais[2], Luís Lima[1], José Bulas Cruz[3] and José Neves[2]

[1]College of Management and Technology - Polytechnic of Porto, Felgueiras, Portugal

[2]DI-CCTC, Universidade do Minho, Braga, Portugal

[3]University of Trás-os-Montes e Alto Douro, Vila Real, Portugal

Abstract Collaborative Work plays an important role in today's organizations, especially in areas where decisions must be made. However, any decision that involves a collective or group of decision makers is, by itself complex, but is becoming recurrent in recent years. In this work we present the *VirtualECare* project, an intelligent multi-agent system able to monitor, interact and serve its customers, which are, normally, in need of care services. In last year's there has been a substantially increase on the number of people needed of intensive care, especially among the elderly, a phenomenon that is related to population ageing. However, this is becoming not exclusive of the elderly, as diseases like obesity, diabetes and blood pressure have been increasing among young adults. This is a new reality that needs to be dealt by the health sector, particularly by the public one. Given this scenarios, the importance of finding new and cost effective ways for health care delivery are of particular importance, especially when we believe they should not to be removed from their natural "habitat". Following this line of thinking, the *VirtualECare* project will be presented, like similar ones that preceded it. Recently we have also assisted to a growing interest in combining the advances in information society - computing, telecommunications and presentation – in order to create Group Decision Support Systems (GDSS). Indeed, the new economy, along with increased competition in today's complex business environments, takes the companies to seek complementarities in order to increase competitiveness and reduce risks. Under these scenarios, planning takes a major role in a company life. However, effective planning depends on the generation and analysis of ideas (innovative or not) and, as a result, the idea generation and management processes are crucial. Our objective is to apply the above presented GDSS to a new area. We believe that the use of GDSS in the healthcare arena will allow professionals to achieve better results in the analysis of one's Electronically Clinical Profile (ECP). This achievement is vital, regarding the explosion of knowledge and skills, together with the need to use limited resources and get better results.

K. Yogesan et al. (Eds.): Handbook of Digital Homecare, BIOMED, pp. 151–178.
springerlink.com

Table of Contents

Introduction

As the human population is ageing, it is a matter of fact that the elderly in need of special attention is also growing. Old age brings new problems (e.g., health, loneliness), aggravated with the lack of specialized human resources to assist their needs. However, this is not exclusive of the elderly, as diseases like obesity, diabetes, and blood pressure have been increasing among young adults [1]. As a new reality, it has to be dealt by the health sector, and especially by the public one. Thus, the importance of finding new and cost effective ways for health care delivery are of particular importance, especially when one wants them not to be removed from their “habitat” [2]. Besides that fact, pressures exist in government and society (e.g., budgetary restraints, cost of medical technologies and cost of internment) that will force readjustments of actual health care practice, which may also affect other co-related public systems [3, 4].

Motivation

In the last years we have assisted to a proliferation of various research projects in order to increase the quality of care services and reduce the associated costs, especially the ones that require the patient to be delocalized from his natural habitat (Home). Normally these tend to be simple and basic reactive alarm systems without many requirements from the support platform point of view [5]. In our opinion these systems were very useful to delineate a path for others to follow. Taking this path we have presented the VirtualECare project [6, 7] which we believe will be the next generation of remote proactive healthcare system with, in our case, Group Decision techniques for problem solving through the use of today's available, low cost, technology making this way a very promising approach to a possible solution for some of the health sector problems.

Collaborative Networks in Digital Homecare

The use of collaborative networks in the care of the elderly may be an important part of a social development process, yet it has not been studied in depth. This work looks at the role that collaborative networks and learning plays within the innovative processes of a smart home for care of the elderly, and suggests a framework that will allow an organization to strategically model a collaborative environment that may be conducive to innovation. Such a framework will identify key areas of the Inter-Virtual Organizations Co-operation for Care of the Elderly, which should be discussed in line with the collaborative tool requirements of the care providers. A theoretical ontology based tool is also briefly discussed to capture and identify how the services of the elderly project team are innovating and provide care providers with collaborative tools, which will reflect their collaborative and knowledge needs.

Some work on the above problem has been made, namely using alarm systems that can be triggered by the monitored people in case of necessity, to more modern ones, using almost any artifacts that the new technologies have to offer [4, 8].

The major goal in our work is to take the work already done to a next level, enhancing elderly quality of life [3]. The path to pursue relies on a mix of different contributions from Artificial Intelligence, such as Collaborative Networks, Ambient Intelligence and Knowledge Representation tools coupled whit different computational paradigms and methodologies for problem solving, such as Agent Based Systems and Group Decision Support Systems. To achieve such a result, we will enrich any space (e.g., houses, buildings, critical areas in hospitals) with smart artifacts so that through the use of automated or semi-automated Group Decision Support Systems we may diagnose healthcare problems (and more) and present solutions on time [9].

The challenges faced by both business and academy in recent years, in association with the advances in information and communication technology, lead to the creation of a large variety of Networks, namely Collaborative Networks (CN). Basically, CN let professionals and organizations to seek complementary and joint activities, allowing them to participate in new and more competitive businesses opportunities, reaching new markets and/or fostering scientific excellence, either in forms of services or products. This can be done, namely, through highly integrated supply chains, virtual enterprises/organizations, professional virtual communities, value constellations and/or virtual laboratories [10].

Group Decision Support Systems

Group Support Systems

By definition, any Collaborative Network Organizations (CNO) has to support collaborative work, that presupposes the existence of a group of people that has as mission the completion of a specific task [11]. The number of elements involved in the group may be variable, as well as the persistency of the group. The group members may be at different places, meet in an asynchronous way or may belong to different organizations. Collaborative work has not only inherent advantages (e.g., greater pool of knowledge, different world perspectives, increased acceptance), but also assertive goals (e.g., social pressure, domination, goal displacement, group thinking) [12].

Meeting phases

Group Support Systems (GSS) intend, as we shall see, to support collaborative work. In this work we will call "meeting" to all the processes necessary to the completion of a specific collaborative task. A meeting is a consequence or an objective of the interaction between two or more persons [13]. Physically, a meeting can be realized in one of the four scenarios: same time / same place, same time / different places, different times / same place and different times / different places. Each one of these scenarios will require from the GSS a different kind of support.

Until now we discussed collaborative work and present group members as the only persons involved in the process. However, it is very common to see a third element taking part in the course of action, the facilitator. The meeting facilitator is a person welcomed by all the members of the group, neutral and without authority to make decisions, which intervenes in the process in order to support the group in the identification of a problem and in the finding of a solution, in order to increase group efficiency [14].

According to Dubs and Hayne [15] a meeting has three distinct phases, as it is depicted in Figure 1.

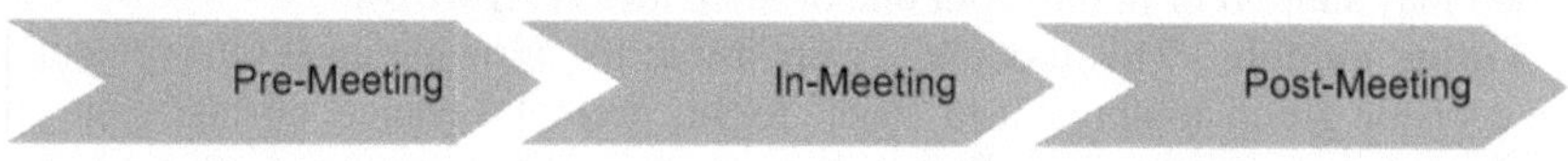

Figure 1. Meeting Phases

In the Pre-Meeting phase the facilitator prepares the meeting, i.e., establishes the meeting goals, proceeds with the group formation (making sure that all the participants have the necessary background), selects the best supporting tools, informs the meeting members about the goals and distributes among them the meeting materials.

In the In-Meeting phase the participants will be working in order to accomplish the meeting goals, and the facilitator has the task of monitoring the meeting interactions (e.g., to observe the relationship between the group members) and to intervene if necessary.

In the Post-Meeting phase, it is important to evaluate the results achieved by the group, as well as by how much each group member is acquit with the achieved results (satisfied/unsatisfied). Still, in this phase it is very important to identify and store information that can be useful in future meetings (e.g., how to actualize the participant's profile for future selection).

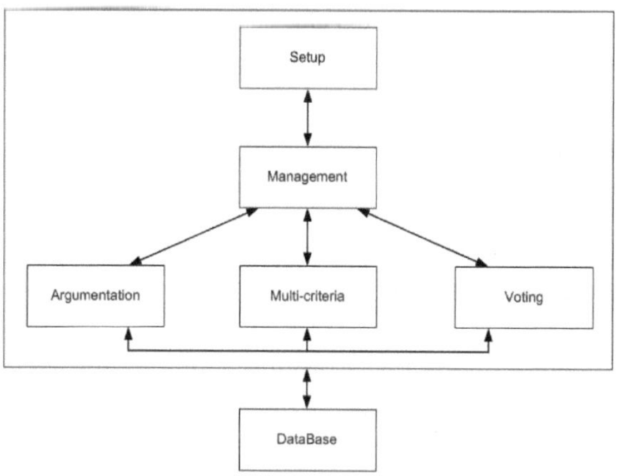

Figure 2. VirtualECare Group Decision Architecture

Setup module – will be operated by a *facilitator* during the pre-meeting phase that will do several configuration and parameterization activities;

Multi-criteria module – will be operated by a *facilitator* during the pre-meeting phase, being in charge of the definition of the evaluation criteria and scales and, eventually, in deleting dominated alternatives.

Argumentation module - This module is based on the IBIS (Issue Based Information System) argumentation model developed by [16] and his colleagues in the early 70's. According to this model, an argument is a statement or an opinion which may support or pointed out one or more ideas (Figure 3).

Voting module - This module is responsible for allowing each intervenient of the decision group component to "vote" for his preferred choice, normally the one most similar to his "opinion" (Figure 3).

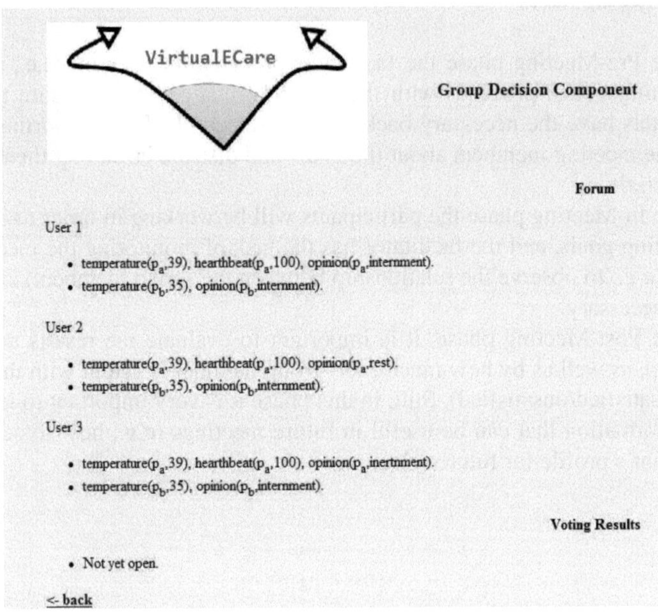

Figure 3. VirtualECare Forum

Recommendation System

Idea Generation

The ***Group Decision*** module, as it was said before, is a major module of our system. This fact, associated with the importance of decision-making in today business activity and with the needed celerity in obtaining a decision in the majority of the cases that this key module will be defied to resolve, requires a real effectiveness of the decision making process. Thus, the need for an Idea Generation tool that will support the meetings, being those face to face, asynchronous or distributed, becomes crucial.

The flow of new ideas is central in an environment as the one presented above. Several idea generation techniques were popularized during the early 1950's in order to assist organizations to be fully innovative. These techniques, although primarily born and used in the advertising world, can be applied to an infinite number of emerging areas. Many idea techniques emerged from that time and continue to current days, such as Brainstorming, Nominal Group Technique (NGT), Mind-mapping and SCAMPLER, among others.

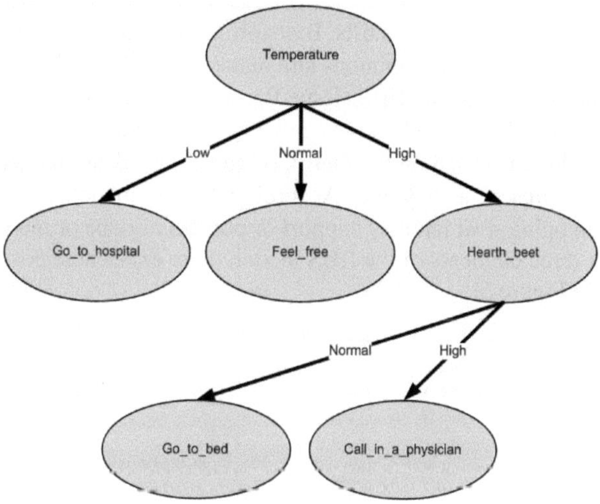

Figure 4. A decision tree of a specific problem

In order to face the real challenges that this module have to deal with, we selected two idea generation techniques for different situations:

Brainstorming – it is probably the best-known creative tool. It can be used in most groups, although in most cases the rules that oversee it must be perceived by the group elements. It comes with all its potential when and independent facilitator manages the process (so the group can focus on the creative tasks). Normally, a brainstorming has duration somewhere between 30 minutes to 1 hour, depending on the difficulty of the problem and the motivation of the decision group. Due to this fact it cannot be used in situations of life or death, but it can and is going to be used in assessing patient's quality of life;

Mind-mapping – it is best used when one needs to explore and/or develop ideas for a specific problem, or when we need to take notes and/or summarize meetings. It can be used to obtain immediate answers in critical situations.

In Mind-mapping the specific problem is presented in the form of a decision tree, being the vital data obtained, for instance, from the sensors attached to the **Supported User** (Figure 4).

Argumentation

After establishing individual ideas (through the above presented tools, or simply by intuition) the participants are expected to "defend" those ideas in order to reach consensus or majority. Each participant will, therefore, and in a natural way, argue for the most interesting alternatives or against the worst alternatives, according to his/her preferences and/or skills. By expressing their arguments, participants expect to influence the others' opinions and make them change their own [17].

This module is based on the IBIS (Issue Based Information System) argumentation model developed by Rittel and his colleagues in the early 70's [18]. The core of this methodology is based on the matrix of questions, ideas and arguments that, all combined, represent a dialogue. According to this model, an argument is a statement or an opinion which may support or pointed out one or more ideas.

Among the three elements of the IBIS model, there exists nine possible links, as it is depicted in Figure 5.

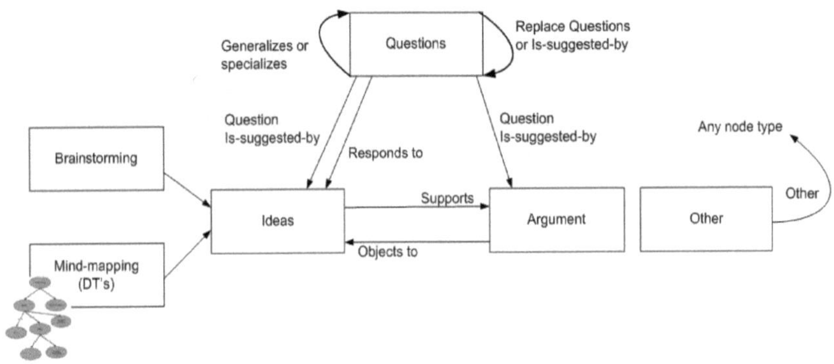

Figure 5. IBIS model adapted from Conklin and Begeman

In the implementation process of the Group Decision apparatus, and the respective support software, some modifications to the model have been made.

The **question** in the IBIS model is, in the Group Decision apparatus, the **goal** of the meeting.

Ideas are the alternatives of the multi-criteria decision problem and arise from the idea generation tool throughout brainstorming or through mind mapping.

Arguments in IBIS can be pros or cons vis-à-vis a given idea. In the Group Decision module they are based in two types of information: Patient Electronic

Clinical Profile and a set of Decision Trees. Additionally, the possibility for one participant to argue using an argument from another member is real.

This module is paramount on the in-meeting phase. It is used by the participants to defend their positions, but can also be used in the post-meeting phase by the facilitator (e.g. if the group does not reach a solution, the facilitator may use this module to check which is the most consensual alternative).

The IBIS model has been often used in the development of GDSSs, the first implementation being gIBIS [19]. By adopting this model, the Group Decision module should enable a better organization of the arguments exchanged by the participants. This may facilitate opinion convergence, and at the same time to reduce the meetings "noise".

Once a decision has been made, it is (automatically) sent to the monitored person (***Supported User*** in Figure 10) by a mobile device (Figure 6), in order to keep him/her informed.

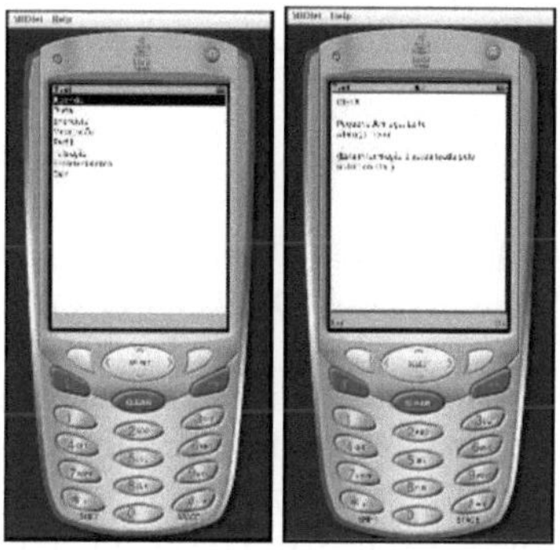

Figure 6. A Group Decision assessment reported on a person mobile device

Quality of Information

VirtualECare Group Decision Support System deals with information and knowledge in an environment of uncertainty. The information available must always be considered incomplete and imperfect.

How does a decision maker is confident about the reliability of the information at hand? In group decisions each person that participates in the final decision must be confident on: The reliability of the computer support system; The other decision makers; The information rolling in and out of the system and the information exchanged between participants. The Group Decision of the VirtualECare system operates in such environment. We leave the first issue to others and concentrate in the last two, proposing a model for computing the quality of information.

A suitable representation of incomplete information and uncertainty is needed, one that supports non-monotonic reasoning. In a classical logical theory, the proof of a theorem results in a *true* or *false* truth value, or is made in terms of representing something, with respect to one may not be conclusive. In opposition, in a logic program, the answer to a question is only of two types: *true* or *false*. This is a consequence of the limitations of the knowledge representation in a logic program, because it is not allowed explicit representation of negative information. Additionally, the operational semantics applies the Closed-World Assumption (CWA) [20, 21] to all the predicates. The generality of logic programs represents implicitly negative information, assuming the application of reasoning according to the CWA.

An extended logic program, on the other hand, is a finite collection of rules of the form [22, 23]:

$q \leftarrow p_1 \wedge \ldots \wedge p_m \wedge not\ p_{m+1} \wedge \ldots \wedge not\ p_{m+n}$	(1)
$?\, p_1 \wedge \ldots \wedge p_m \wedge not\ p_{m+1} \wedge \ldots \wedge not\ p_{m+n}$	(2)

where ? is a domain atom denoting falsity, the pi, qj, and p are classical ground literals, i.e. either positive atoms or atoms preceded by the classical negation sign ¬. Every program is associated with a set of abducibles. Abducibles can be seen as hypotheses that provide possible solutions or explanations of given queries, being given here in the form of exceptions to the extensions of the predicates that make the program.

The objective is to provide expressive power for representing explicitly negative information, as well as directly describe the CWA for some predicates, also known as *predicate circumscription* [24]. Three types of answers to a given question are then possible: *true*, *false* and *unknown* [21]. The representation of null values will be scoped by the ELP. In this work, we will consider two types of null values: the first will allow for the representation of unknown values, not necessarily from a given set of values, and the second will represent unknown values from a given set of possible values. We will show now how null values can be used to represent unknown information. In the following, we consider the extensions of the predicates that represent some of the properties of the participants, as a measure of their skills for the decision making process:

```
area_of_expertise: Entities x StrValue
role: Entities x StrValue
credible: Entities x Value
reputed: Entities x Value
```

The first argument denotes the participant and the second represents the value of the property (e.g., `credible(luis, 100)` means that the credibility of the participant `luis` has the value `100`).

```
credible(luis,100)
¬credible(E,V)←
            not credible(E,V)
```

Program 1. Extension of the predicate that states the credibility of a participant

In Program 1, the symbol ¬ represents the strong negation, denoting what should be interpreted as false, and the term *not* designates negation-by-failure.

Let us now admit that the credibility of another possible participant *ricardo* has not, yet, been established. This will be denoted by a null value, of the type unknown, and represents the situation in Program 2: the participant is credible but it is not possible to be certain (affirmative) about its value. In the second clause of Program 2, the symbol ⊥ represents a null value of an undefined type. It is a representation that assumes any value as a viable solution, but without being given a clue to conclude about which value one is speaking about. It is not possible to compute, from the positive information, the value of the credibility of the participant *ricardo*. The fourth clause of Program 2 (the closure of predicate credibility) discards the possibility of being assumed as false any question on the specific value of credibility for participant *ricardo*.

```
credible(luis,100)
credible(ricardo,⊥)
¬credible(E,V)←
            not credible(E,V),
            not exception(credible(E,V))
exception(credible(E,V))←
            credible(E,⊥)
```

Program 2. Credibility about participant ricardo, with an unknown value

Let's now consider the case in which the value of the credibility of a participant is foreseen to be 60, with a margin of mistake of 15. It is not possible to be positive, concerning the credibility value. However, it is false that the participant has a credibility value of 80 or 100. This example suggests that the lack of knowledge may only be associated to a enumerated set of possible known values. As a different case, let's consider the credibility of the participant *paulo*, that is unknown, but one knows that it is specifically 30 or 50.

```
credible(luis,100)
credible(ricardo,⊥)
¬credible(E,V)←
            not credible(E,V),
            not exception(credible(E,V))
exception(credible(E,V))← credible(E,⊥)
exception(credible(carlos,V))← V ≥ 45 ∧ V ≤ 75
exception(credible(paulo,30))
exception(credible(paulo,50))
```

Program 3. Representation of the credibility of the participants carlos and paulo

Using Extended Logic Programming, as the logic programming language, a procedure given in terms of the extension of a predicate called *demo* is presented here. This predicate allows one to reason about the body of knowledge presented in a particular domain, set on the formalism previously referred to. Given a question, it returns a solution based on a set of assumptions. This meta predicate is defined as: `Demo: Question x Answer`

Where Question indicates a theorem to be proved and Answer denotes a truth value (see Program 4): true (T), false (F) or unknown (U).

```
demo(Q,T)← Q
demo(Q,F)← ¬Q
demo(Q,U)← not Q ∧ not ¬Q
```

Program 4. Extension of meta-predicate demo

Let i ($i \in 1,\ldots, m$) represent the predicates whose extensions make an extended logic program that models the universe of discourse and j ($j \in 1,\ldots, n$) the attributes of those predicates. Let $x_j \in [min_j, max_j]$ be a value for attribute j. To each predicate is also associated a scoring function $V_{ij}[min_j, max_j] \rightarrow 0 \ldots 1$, that gives the score predicate i assigns to a value of attribute j in the range of its acceptable values, i.e., its domain (for simplicity, scores are kept in the interval $[0 \ldots 1]$), here given in the form: `all(attribute_exception_list, sub_expression, invariants)`

This denotes that *sub_expression* should hold for each combination of the exceptions of the extensions of the predicates that represent the attributes in the *attribute_exception_list* and the *invariants*.

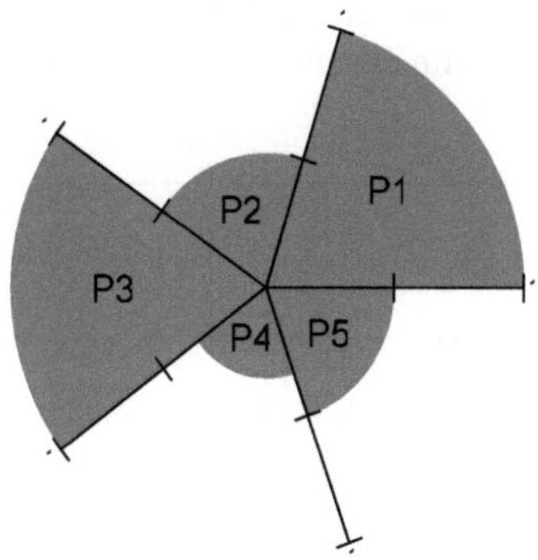

Figure 7. A measure of the quality of information for a logic program or theory P

This is further translated by introducing three new predicates. The first predicate creates a list of all possible exception combinations (pairs, triples, ..., n-tuples) as a list of sets determined by the domain size (and the invariants). The second predicate recurses through this list and makes a call to the third predicate for each exception combination. The third predicate denotes sub_expression, giving for each predicate, as a result, the respective score function. The Quality of Information (QI) with respect to a generic predicate P is therefore given by $QI_P = 1/Card$, where Card denotes the cardinality of the exception set for P, if the exception set is not disjoint. If the exception set is disjoint, the quality of information is given by:

$$QI_P = \frac{1}{C_1^{Card} + \cdots + C_{Card}^{Card}} \quad (3)$$

where C_{Card}^{Card} is a card-combination subset, with *Card* elements.

The next element of the model to be considered is the relative importance that a predicate assigns to each of its attributes under observation: w_{ij} stands for the relevance of attribute j for predicate i (it is also assumed that the weights of all predicates are normalized, i.e.:

$$\forall i \sum_{j=1}^{n} w_{ij} = 1 \quad (4)$$

It is now possible to define a predicate's scoring function, i.e., for a value $x = (x_1, ..., n)$ in the multi dimensional space defined by the attributes domains, which is given in the form:

$V_i(x) = \sum_{j=1}^{n} w_{ij} * V_{ij}(x_j)$	(5)

It is now possible to measure the QI that occurs as a result of a logic program, by posting the $V_i(x)$ values into a multi-dimensional space and projecting it onto a two dimensional one.

Using this procedure, it is defined a circle, as the one given in Figure 3. Here, the dashed n-slices of the circle (in this example built on the extensions of five predicates, named as $p_1 \ldots p_5$) denote de QI that is associated with each of the predicate extensions that make the logic program. It is now possible to return to our case above and evaluate the global credibility of the system. Let us consider the logic program (Program 5).

```
¬credible(E,V)← not credible(E,V),
             not exception(credible(E,V))
exception(credible(E,V))← credible(E,⊥)
credible(luis,100)
credible(ricardo,⊥)
exception(credible(carlos,V))← V ≥ 45 ∧ V ≤ 75
exception(credible(paulo,30))
exception(credible(paulo,50))
role(luis,⊥)
role(ricardo,doctor)
exception(role(carlos,doctor))
exception(reputed(luis,80))
exception(reputed(luis,50))
exception(reputed(ricardo,40))
exception(reputed(ricardo,60))
reputed(carlos,100)
```

Program 5. Example of universe of discourse

As an example we represent the QI associated with participants *luis* and *ricardo*, depicted in Figures 4 and 5.

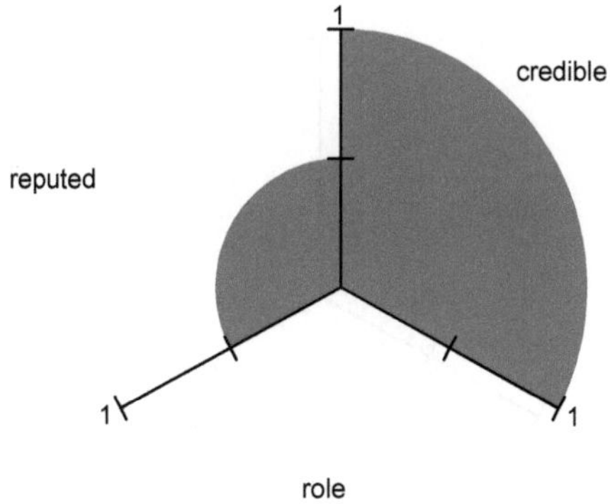

Figure 8. A measure of quality of information about participant luis

In order to find the relationships among the extensions of these predicates, we evaluate the relevance of the QI, given in the form $V_{credible}(luis) = 1$; $V_{reputed}(luis) = 0.785$; $V_{role}(luis) = 0$. It is now possible to measure the QI associated to a logic program referred to above: the shaded n-slices (here n is equal to three) of the circle denote the QI for predicates *credible*, *reputed* and *role*. However, in order to accomplish the main goal of this work, we need to further extend the purpose of Figures 4 and 5, i.e., we may define a new predicate, *trustworthiness*; whose extension may be given in the form of the example (Program 6).

```
¬trustworthiness (X,Y)←
            not trustworthiness (X,Y),
            not exception(trustworthiness (X,Y))
trustworthi-
ness(luis,((credible,1),(reputed,0.785)(role,0)))
trustworthi-
ness(ricardo,((credible,0),(reputed,0.785),(role,1)))
```

Program 6. Measuring the global quality

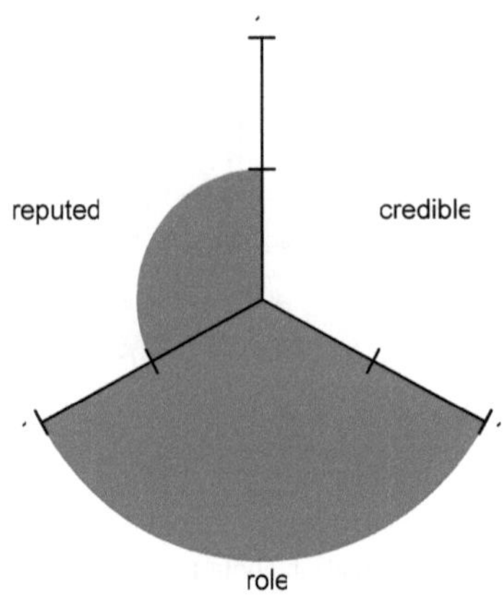

Figure 9. A measure of quality of information about participant ricardo

Besides being able to evaluate the quality of individual actors and individual pieces of information that flows in a group decision system, we aim to have an overall mechanism that allows one to measure the global quality of the system itself and, consequently, the outcomes from it. There is too much in stake when we deal with healthcare, and one must raise the confidence on decisions, especially in an environment of uncertainty, incomplete and imperfect information. The same mechanism used to evaluate individual parts of the system is consistently used to evaluate all the system, through an extension process.

Applications Scenarios

The main goal of VirtualECare is to improve end user's quality of life allowing them to enjoy the so-called active ageing. To achieve this purpose we will take advantage of the enormous evolution new technologies have assisted in past years.

To better understand the amplitude of VirtualECare, let's consider the following scenario [25]:

"John has a heart condition and wears a smart watch that takes his blood pressure three times a day. His watch also reminds him to take his medications and the proper dosage for each medicine. If anything is unusual, his watch alerts both him and the Group Decision Support System (GDSS). John also has a PDA that contains an interactive health control table where he can monitor his medications, schedule his exercises, manage his diet and log his vital statistics. The GDSS has access to this table so they can keep up to date on his condition. Currently, John's watch detects that his blood pressure is unusually high. The GDSS receives a grade B and calls him to check what might be causing his high blood pressure (diagnose). At the same time John receives a checklist of possible causes to re-

view. John compares this list to his own health control table in his PDA to see what might be wrong. Meanwhile, the GDSS decides John should come to an appointment."

The presented scenario requires an infrastructure to support all the several intervenient and provide basic interaction mechanisms. On top of this infrastructure an extensive number of services can be deployed and/or be developed.

VirtualECare Project

Our objective is to present an intelligent multi-agent system not only to monitor and to interact with its costumers (being those elderly people or their relatives), but also to be interconnected to other computing systems running in different healthcare institutions, leisure centres, training facilities or shops. The VirtualE-Care [9] architecture is a distributed one, being their components unified through a network (e.g., LAN, MAN, WAN), and each one with a different role (Figure 1):

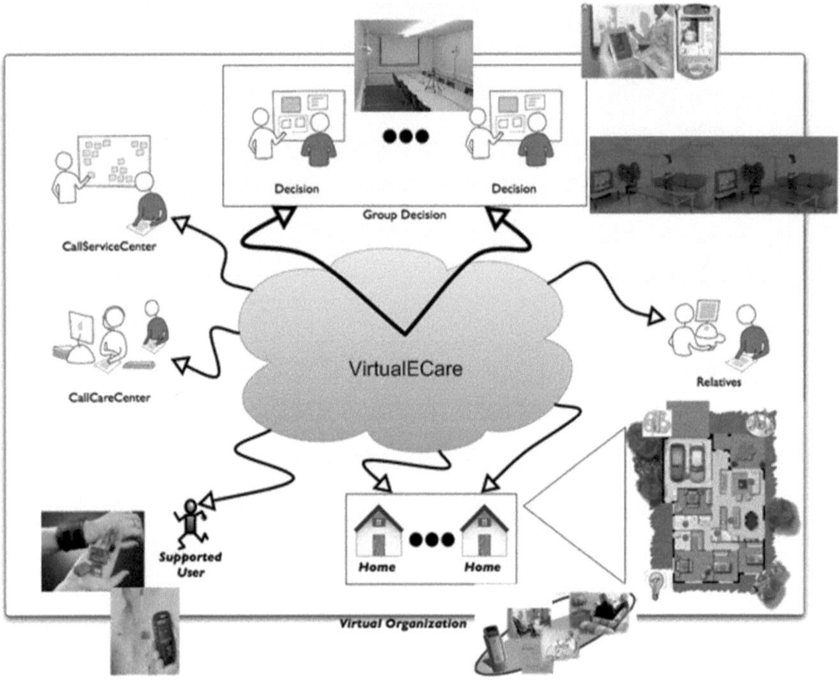

Figure 10. VirtualECare

SupportedUser – Elderly people with special healthcare needs, whose critical data is sent to the ***CallCareCenter*** and forwarded to the ***Group Decision Supported System***;

Home – ***SupportedUser*** natural premises. The data collected here is sent to the ***Group Decision Supported System*** through the ***CallCareCenter,*** or to the ***Call-ServiceCenter*** (which speak for themselves);

Group Decision – It is in charge of all the decisions taken at the VirtualECare platform. Our work will be centred on this key module;

CallServiceCenter – Entity with all the necessary computational and qualified personal resources, capable of receiving and analyze the miscellaneous data and take the necessary actions according to it;

CallCareCenter – Entity in charge of the computational and qualified personal resources (i.e., healthcare professionals and auxiliary personnel), capable of receiving and analyze the clinical data, and to take the necessary actions.

Relatives SupportedUser - Relatives which may and should have an active role in the supervising task of their love ones, providing precious complementary information (e.g., loneliness).

In order to the Group Decision Support System take their decisions, one needs of a digital profile of the SupportedUser, which may provide a better understanding of his/her special needs. In this profile we may have different types of data, ranging from the patient Electronic Health Record to their own personal experiences and preferences (e.g., musical, gastronomic). It will provide tools and methodologies for creating an information-on-demand environment that can improve quality-of-living, safety, and quality-of-patient care.

Technology Overview

Infrastructure

Considering the above scenario, and the needs it implies, we have designed a first proposal of a generic, configurable, flexible and scalable infrastructure as presented in Figure 11. It is expectable that on top of it an extensive number of services will progressively arise. These services must, and will be, developed as Web Services, thus allowing the coexistence of several, different, software languages interacting with each other through the use of common messages.

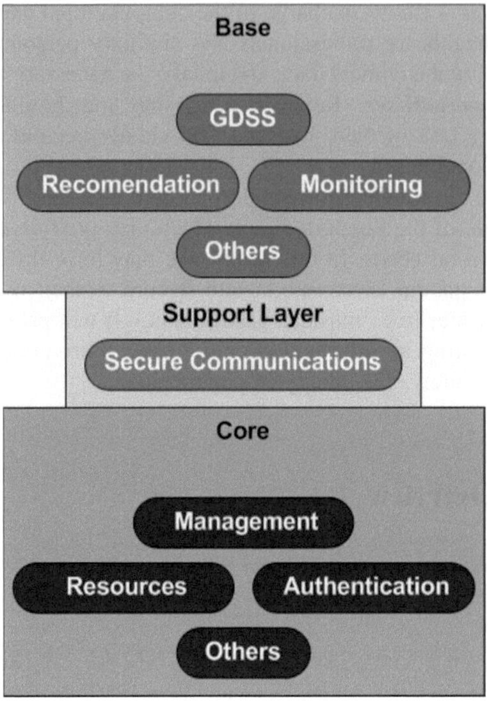

Figure 11. VirtualECare Infrastructure

The fundamental components of the proposed infrastructure are:

- *Secure Communications* – in order to all the components interact, a secure communication infrastructure is mandatory;
- *Management* – responsible for configure and monitor the involved components;
- *Resources* – responsible for every component registration and manage the resources catalog;
- *Authentication* – every component must authenticate itself in order to be able to interact with others;
- *Recommendation* – responsible to make problem solving recommendations;
- *Monitoring* – responsible for interacting with all the sensors and report its results to the GDSS;
- *GDSS* – responsible for Decision Making.

Architecture

The VirtualECare architecture is a distributed one, composed of a series of different elements eventually geographically separated (Figure 12). It is also a dynamic one since elements can enter and leave at any time, logically or geographically, or the services they provide may vary. The main components of the architecture are the End User and its House, a Monitoring module, the Recommendation System, the Group Decision, the Database, an HL7 module, among others. Each element of the architecture may be very different in its functionalities or software language, calling for an heterogeneous architecture. These are the main issues that were addressed and are detailed in this section: how we make our architecture distributed, modular, dynamic, extensible, flexible, scalable and compatible. To achieve this, we adopted open and widely used technologies and standards, such as OSGi, R-OSGi, FIPA or Web Services.

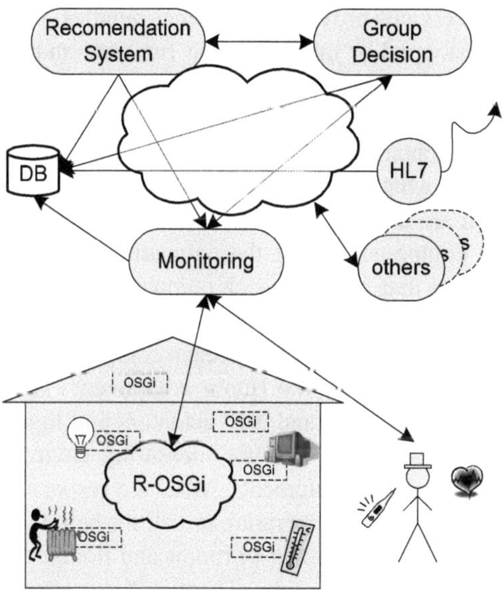

Figure 12. VirtualECare Architecture

To ensure the communication and compatibility between the different components, the Web Services paradigm was used. Web Services can be seen simplistically as a way of sharing information over a network and they are platform independent, being ideal for this kind of systems. Each of the components which provide information declares Web Services that are then requested by the other components which need to access that information. A component can, however, be at the same time a server and a client. The Recommendation System, for example, uses Web Services provided by both the House and the Database and provides, as a service, the Recommendation that is used by the Group Decision. The communication protocol and examples of communication sequences and messages needed for all this components to work together are detailed further ahead.

In Figure 12 we can look at a simplified view of our architecture. The arrows represent Web Services which allow the several components to exchange information. The arrows can be seen as "uses service from" pointing from the client to the server. The House is a little more detailed, showing OSGi and R-OSGi subcomponents responsible for interconnecting different kinds of elements

Let us now detail the technologies used in the components by moving to a more close view of the architecture. At this level, two well known standards where used: OSGi and R-OSGi. OSGi is an initiative that intends to establish standards in Java programming, highly specific, catering for the sharing of Java classes, that may be achieved in terms of a services platform paradigm [26, 27]. The use of this technology will let developers build Java applications on a modular basis. The resulting modules are called bundles, which are not only competent to provide services, but also to use services provided from other bundles. In OSGi, a bundle can be installed, started, stopped or un-installed at run-time and without any kind of system reboot, which makes OSGi-based technologies very modular and dynamic.

R-OSGi is an extension to OSGi which allows the access of services provided in remote OSGi implementations, in a completely transparent way, much like they were local services. But what are this technologies good for in our case?

OSGi and R-OSGi are used in our architecture to achieve two main objectives at the level of each component: grant the compatibility and communication between the different parts that make up each component (much like we need to do at a higher level) and establish a logical organization inside the component. These issues come from the multitude of parts that each component can be made of.

Let us look, as an example, to the House component. The House is made of physical parts like 1-Wire sensors and X10 actuators and logical ones like Multi-agent Systems (MAS). 1-Wire is used for measuring environmental values and X10 to control appliances and equipments. MAS are responsible for taking basic reactive actions like control the temperature or call for help in case of need. Moreover, the house may have a big number of rooms and floors which, like the rest of the components, can vary along the time. There is, firstly, the need to organize all these components logically. In order to achieve this we create several OSGi implementations. For each group of similar sensors in each room, a bundle is created. This means that for each room, there will be a bundle reading values from the temperature sensors, another one reading the values from the luminosity sensors and so on. These bundles provide, as a service, the mean value of the last values obtained from the respective sensors. As for the actuators, there is one bundle controlling each equipment or appliance, which is able of sending X10 commands to the equipment it controls. The services these bundle provide are the X10 commands that can be issued to each equipment.

The bundles of the same type in each floor run in the same OSGi implementation, i.e., in each floor there is an OSGi implementation for the temperature bundles, another one for the luminosity bundles, and so on. Likewise, there is an OSGi implementation for the appliances of each type on each floor, i.e., an OSGi for lights, another for air conditioning, etc. In addition, there can also be OSGi implementations inside the House that are just software, like the Multi-agent System that is responsible for taking the basic actions. How we adapted our MAS to be fully integrated with OSGi is described further ahead. Each of these OSGi implementations has at least one additional bundle: a R-OSGi bundle which provides remote access to the implementation. This bundle acts as the bridge between the exterior and the sensors or actuators controlled by the implementation. Its services are the operations that can be performed on the components controlled by the implementation it is in. In the case of the sensors, this bundle is remotely requested to provide the values of sensors and, in the case of the actuators, is through this bundle that the X10 commands arrive to the correct appliance. In this case, the bundle also guarantees that the command is valid and that the consequences of it being executed don't go against pre-established security policies (e.g. establishing the temperature of the air conditioning in some room to a dangerous value). R-OSGi is therefore the way of integrating each piece inside an OSGi-based component of the architecture, granting the communication between OSGi implementations.

Finally, let's describe how a MAS is merged inside this system. The MAS is responsible for regularly checking the values of sensors, acting on the actuators accordingly (e.g. the temperature suddenly dropped, turn the heat on) and calling for help in case of need, as well as registering all the events and decisions taken into the Database. Let's now see how we integrate our MAS with the rest of the architecture. The aim is to make accessible the functionalities of an agent (e.g., its methods) as services to other bundles. It would not be advisable to convert each agent into an OSGi bundle, since it would increase the development time and throw away the advantages of MAS based methodologies for problem solving. Therefore, the decision was to create an OSGI bundle that could make the bridge between regular bundles and Jade: the MAS bundle. This bundle can deal with one Agent Container (AC) and implement the methods declared in the interface of the agents in that AC as its own services. Moreover, this bundle must be able to start and stop agents, which in practice, corresponds to the start and stop of the services provided by them. The bundle, upon the reception of an invocation for an offered service from any other bundle, sends the invocation to the correspondent agent and delivers the respective result to the calling bundle. It must be noted that an agent, when trying to satisfy an invocation, may require the services provided by other bundles currently available. This is possible through the MAS bundle.

As for the interface between the MAS bundle and the Jade system, a Jade-Gateway agent (JGa) is being used. The task of this agent is to act as a bridge between Jade and non-Jade code. This agent is created when the MAS bundle is started, along with the other agents. The JGa has the knowledge of which services are provided by each agent running so, whenever a request from a service arrives to the MAS bundle, it knows to which agent the request should be forwarded.

Likewise, if an agent needs to use a service from another bundle, it contacts the MAS bundle, which is responsible for contacting the correct bundle, invoking the service and forwarding the result back to the agent. This way, we create a bundle which allows for Jade instances to run behind OSGi implementations in a completely transparent way.

We have hereby detailed our architecture. At a high level, it is composed of components which share information based on Web Services. Each one of these components can then be detailed and looked closer in means of the pieces they are made of: sensors, actuators, MAS, software, etc. The communication inside the components is based on OSGi and R-OSGi open standards, granting extensibility, modularity, dynamics and a logical hierarchical organization of the pieces that make part of each component.

Communications

Let us take a closer look to the challenge of making such different components to work together. This challenge comes not only from the fact of the architecture being distributed but also from the fact that components may be programmed in different languages and even be running in different platforms. There is therefore the need to establish a mean of communication that is possible to use on all the platforms or all the languages that the components can use. More than just choosing the mean of communication, the language used must be specified so that interoperation between components is possible.

As we have stated before, we have chosen the Web Services to implement the communication between components since they are platform independent and work over networks. The information that is shared through Web Services is in XML format and what our Web Services share is FIPA-ACL messages represented in XML [6]. This FIPA standard allows a description of the main content of the message without having to read the content by using concepts like ontology, language or speech-acts. This way, messages can be forwarded and sent to the final agents without the need to check the content.

However, we have defined a way of structuring the actual content of the message in XML. Examples of content are the temperatures in a room or in an entire house (a list of rooms), an aspect of the Electronic Health Record (EHR), the whole EHR or a recommendation coming from the Recommendation System. As an example we have below a simple message from the Recommendation System, asking the house about the values of the temperature and movement on all the rooms of the house:

```
<?xml version="1.0"?>
<fipa-message>
 <act> request </act>
 <msg-param>
  <sender>
   <agent-identifier>
    <name> groupdecision </name>
    <addresses>
     <url> http://abc.com/groupdecisionwebservice
</url>
    </addresses>
   </agent-identifier>
  </sender>
 </msg-param>
 <msg-param>
  <receiver>
   <agent-identifier>
    <name> house </name>
    <addresses>
     <url> http://def.com/housewebservice </url>
    </addresses>
   </agent-identifier>
  </receiver>
 </msg-param>
 <msg-param>
  <content>
   <sensors room="all"> temperature </sensors>
   <sensors room="all"> movement </sensors>
  </content>
 </msg-param>
 <msg-param>
  <conversation-id> 88273847728729 </conversation-
id>
 </msg-param>
</fipa-message>
```


As an example of a sequence of communication, we can look at Figure 13. All the process is triggered by the bundle responsible for monitoring the vital signs of the Supported User. This bundle detects an irregular heart beat and warns the House central OSGi, where the MAS is running using R-OSGi. The MAS requests information from the movement sensors in another OSGi and asks again about the cardiac rhythm to the bundle that started the process to ensure that there was no reading error. Having gathered the information, the MAS decides that it cannot do anything to correct the situation and informs the Group Decision sending the anomalous values. This one contacts the Recommendation System which reads all the values of the sensors of the House and generates a recommendation which is then issued back to the Group Decision. After communicating with some more elements (like specialized doctors) and having in consideration the answer from the Recommendation System, two actions are taken: an ambulance is sent to the Home and Lights in the room of the user are turned on.

Dashed arrows represent R-OSGi services being invoked, regular arrows stand for FIPA ACL messages being exchanged through Web Services and circles represent some major processing or communication with local bundles using OSGi. Due to lack of space, this picture is simplified. For example, in the last two lines, a request from the GD to turn on the lights would arrive to the Home central, from there to the OSGi lights implementation bridge bundle and from there to the bundle that control the lights of the room the user is in, which would issue the respective X10 command. The Sensors box also represents all the sensors in general and what really happens is that there is a group of OSGi implementations, each one of them controlling a type of sensors, grouped by room and by floor.

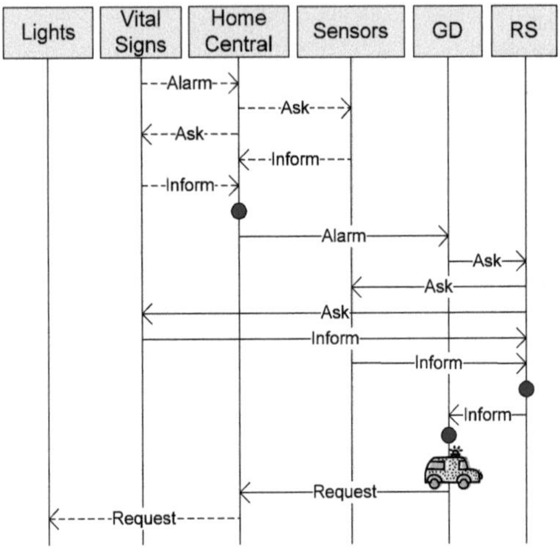

Figure 13. Sample Communication Sequence Diagram

The complete architecture has, therefore, much more components and is much more complex. However, using this approach we can, despite the complexity, create a logical and hierarchical organization that works well as long as each bundle knows the bundles it should directly communicate to. By doing so and defining the messages content structure, we implement the communication methodology needed to give life to the architecture.

Conclusion and Future Work

The new reality in the healthcare sector to allow a dignified care provisioning to all the population in general, and the elderly in particular imposes new approaches to provide specialized services, without delocalizing or messing up with their routines, in a more effective and intelligent way. This chapter describes the

VirtualECare project with special incidence on the Group Decision module that supports asynchronous and distributed meetings set up for solving multi-criteria decision problems. The system supports the meeting participants in constructing and sharing ideas and "defends" those ideas in order to reach consensus or majority. To defend his ideas, each participant, should argue for the most interesting alternatives or against the worst alternatives, according to his/her preferences and/or skills, expecting to influence the others' opinions and make them change their own. In future work the argumentation module will allow not only a simple way of justifying opinions, but also a persuasive argumentation in order to allow each element to try influence other through the confrontation of opinions.
Additionally, we are going to apply the presented Knowledge Representation with the respective Quality of its Information to the Group Decision module. Thus, the suggestions/decisions presented by this module, will consider the existence of incomplete information, and, even so, will present a possible way to try and, if possible, resolve the actual problem. Incomplete information may arise from several sources (e.g. unreachable sensors, incomplete Patient Electronic Clinical Profile), but what is important is to be able to measure the quality of the information we have access to and the quality of the ideas presented by the participants, based in factors like reputation, credibility, namely, in the discussion. However, we are certain, that some vital information, if incomplete, may even so, compromise any suggestion/decision but, in the majority of situations, we believe this will not be the case.

We have also presented, based on open standards, a framework to an early deployment of a prototype for the VirtualECare system. In future work, we expect to elaborate on real life scenarios and situations, in order to make the necessary's developments to set a working prototype, that could provide to the population in general, and the elderly, in particular, a certain amount of remote services (e.g., healthcare, entertainment), without delocalizing or messing up with their routines, in a more effective and intelligent way.
Attending to the presented scenarios and a possible ways to make it reality, we present how we may use collaborative networks as a support for different, but interconnected virtual organizations, that could provide to all the population in general, and the elderly, in particular way, a certain amount of remote services (e.g. healthcare, entertainment, learning), without delocalizing or messing up with their routine, in a more effective and intelligent way.

References

[1] Ford, E.S., Capewell, S.: JACC:2128-2132 (2007)
[2] WHO, Active ageing: towards age-friendly primary health care. World Health Organization (2004)
[3] Giráldez, M., Casal, C.: The Role of Ambient Intelligent in the Social Integration of the Elderly. IOS Press, Amsterdam (2005)
[4] Camarinha-Matos, L.M., Afsarmanesh, H.: Virtual Communities and Elderly Support. WSES (2001)
[5] Saranummi, N., Kivisaari, S., Sarkikoski, T., Graafmans, J.: Ageing & Technology - State of the art. Report for the European Commission, Institute for Prospective Studies, Seville, Spain (1996)

[6] Costa, R., Novais, P., Machado, J., Alberto, C., Neves, J.: Inter-organization Cooperation for Care of the Elderly. Springer, Wuhan (2007)
[7] Costa, R., Neves, J., Novais, P., Machado, J., Lima, L., Alberto, C.: Intelligent Mixed Reality for the Creation of Ambient Assisted Living. LNCS(LNAI). Springer, Heidelberg (2007)
[8] Sarela, A., Korhonen, I., Lotjonen, J., Sola, M., Myllymaki, M.: IST Vivago ® - an intelligent social and remote wellness monitoring system for the elderly. In: 4th International IEEE EMBS Special Topic Conference on Information Technology Applications in Biomedicine, Birmingham, UK, pp. 362–365 (2003)
[9] Augusto, J.C., McCullah, P., McClelland, V., Walden, J.-A.: Enhanced Healthcare Provision Through Assisted Decision-Making in a Smart Home Environment. In: 2nd Workshop on Artificial Inteligence Techniques for Ambient Inteligence (2007)
[10] Camarinha-Matos, L.M.: Virtual Enterprises and Collaborative Networks (IFIP International Federation for Information Processing). Kluwer Academic Publishers, Dordrecht (2004)
[11] Camarinha-Matos, L.: New collaborative organizations and their research needs. In: PRO-VE 2003. Kluwer Academic Publishers, Dordrecht (2003)
[12] Marreiros, G., Santos, R., Ramos, C., Neves, J., Novais, P., Machado, J., Bulas-Cruz, J.: Ambient Intelligence in Emotion Based Ubiquitous Decision Making. In: Proceedings of the International Joint Conference on Artificial Intelligence (IJCAI 2007) - 2nd Workshop on Artificial Intelligence Techniques for Ambient Intelligence, AITAmI 2007 (2007)
[13] Bostrom, R., Anson, R., Clawson, V. (eds.): Group facilitation and group support systems. Macmillan, NYC (2003)
[14] Schwarz, R.M.: The Skilled Facilitator: Practical Wisdom for Developing Effective Groups. Jossey Bass, San Francisco (1994)
[15] Dubs, S., Hayne, S.C.: Distributed facilitation: a concept whose time has come? Computer Supported Cooperative Work, 314–321 (1992)
[16] Rittel, H., Webber, M.: Policy Sciences 4, 155–169 (1973)
[17] Brito, L., Novais, P., Neves, J.: The logic behind negotiation: from pre-argument reasoning to argument-based negotiaion. In: Plekhanova, V. (ed.) Intelligent Agent Software Engineering, pp. 137–159. Idea Group Piblishing, USA (2003)
[18] Conklin, J.: The IBIS Manual: A short course in IBIS methodology. GDSS Inc
[19] Conklin, J., Begeman, M.: gIBIS: A Hypertext tool for exploratory policy discussion (1988)
[20] Hustadt, U.: Do we need the closed-world assumption in knowledge representation? In: Buchheit, N. (ed.) KI 1994 Workshop Baader, Saarbrüken, Germany (1994)
[21] Analide, C.: Antropopatia em Entidades Virtuais, Ph.D. Thesis. Engineering School University of Minho, Braga, Portugal (2004)
[22] Neves, J.: A Logic Interpreter to Handle Time and Negation in Logic Data Bases. In: Proceedings of the ACM 1984, The Fifth Generation Challenge, pp. 50–54 (1984)
[23] Gelfond, M., Lifschitz, V.: Logic Programs with Classical Negation. In: Proceedings of the International Conference on Logic Programming (1990)
[24] Parsons, S.: IEEE Trans. on Knowledge and Data Eng. 8 (1996)
[25] Holmlid, S., Björklind, A.: Ambient Intelligence to Go. In: AmIGo White Paper on mobile intelligent ambience (2003)
[26] Initiative OSG Osgi Service Platform, Release 3. IOS Press, Amsterdam (2003)
[27] Chen, K., Gong, L.: Programming Open Service Gateways with Java Embedded Server(TM) Technology. Prentice Hall PTR, Englewood Cliffs (2001)

Standard-Based Homecare Challenge

Advances of ISO/IEEE11073 for u-Health

M. Martínez-Espronceda[1], I. Martínez[2], J. Escayola[2], L. Serrano[1], J. Trigo[2], S. Led[1], and J. García[2]

[1] Electrical & Electronics Engineering Dep., Public Univ. Navarra (UPNA) - Campus de Arrosadía s/n. 31006 Pamplona, Spain.
{miguel.martinezdeespronceda, lserrano, santiago.led}@unavarra.es, phone: +34 948 169264, fax: +34 948 169 720

[2] Aragon Institute for Engineering Research (I3A/GTC), Univ. Zaragoza (UZ), c/ María de Luna, 3, 50018 Zaragoza, Spain.
{imr, jescayola, jtrigo, jogarmo}@unizar.es, phone: +34 976 761945, fax: +34 976 761945

Abstract Advances in Information and Communication Technologies, ICT, are bringing new opportunities in the field of interoperable and standard-based systems oriented to ubiquitous environments and wearable devices used for digital homecare patient telemonitoring. It is hoped that these advances are able to increase the quality and the efficiency of the care services provided. Likewise they should facilitate a home monitoring of chronic, elderly, under palliative care or have undergone surgery, leaving beds in the Hospital for patients in a more critical condition. In any case telemonitored patients could continue to live in their own homes with the subsequent advantages as more favorable environment, less need for trips to the hospital, etc.

At a time of such challenges, this chapter arises from the need to identify robust technical telemonitoring solutions that are both open and interoperable in homecare scenarios. These systems demand standardized solutions to be cost effective and to take advantage of middleware operation and interoperability. Thus, a key challenge is to design a plug-&-play and standard-based platform that, either as

Manuscript received April 15, 2008. This research work has been partially supported by projects TSI2007-65219-C02-01 and TSI2005-07068-C02-01 from *Comisión Interministerial de Ciencia y Tecnología* (CICYT) and European Regional Development Fund (ERDF), PET2006-0579 from *Programa de Estímulo de Transferencia de Resultados de Investigación* (PETRI), and FPI grant to M.Martínez-Espronceda (Res. 1342/2006 from Public University of Navarre).

M. Martínez-Espronceda, L. Serrano, and S. Led are with the Electrical and Electronics Engineering Dep., Public University of Navarra, Campus de Arrosadía s/n, 31006 Pamplona, Spain (e-mail: lserrano@unavarra.es). I. Martínez, J. Escayola, J. Trigo, and J. García are with the Communications Technologies Group (GTC), Aragon Institute for Engineering Research (I3A), University of Zaragoza (UZ), c/ María de Luna, 3, 50018 Zaragoza, Spain (e-mail: imr@unizar.es).

K. Yogesan et al. (Eds.): Handbook of Digital Homecare, BIOMED, pp. 179–202.
springerlink.com

individual elements or as components, can be incorporated in a simple way into different homecare environments, configuring Home and Personal Area Networks (HAN and PAN).

Nowadays, there is an increasing market pressure from companies not traditionally involved in medical markets, asking for a standard for Personal Health Devices (PHD), which foresee a vast demand for Ambient Assisted Living (AAL) and applications for ubiquitous-Health (u-Health). ISO/IEEE11073 (X73) standards is adapting from Intensive Unit Care (ICU) scope, focused on the Point-Of-Care (PoC), to Personal Health Devices (PHD), focused on ubiquitous environments, implementing high quality sensors, supporting wireless technologies (e.g. Bluetooth or Zigbee) and providing a faster and more reliable communication network resources. This X73-PHD version is adequate for the homecare challenge and might appear the best-positioned international standards to reach this goal.

In this chapter, a X73 compliant homecare platform, as a proof of concept, will be completely described explaining all steps implemented as well as tradeoffs needed for obtaining a working tool. Afterthat, both advances in PHD standardization and the evolution from PoC to PHD will be addressed. Finally, future trends and open points, according our knowhow, will be proposed.

Table of contents

Introduction

Homecare is one of the most common practices in telemedicine, and it is hoped that it can increase the quality of the care and the efficiency of services provided. In fact, it should facilitate a continuous or event-based monitoring of chronic, elderly, under palliative care patients or have undergone surgery, without having them occupying the beds that would be necessary for monitoring in-situ (leaving the beds for the use of patients in a more critical condition). In addition, telemonitored patients can continue to live in their own homes with the subsequent advantages: comfort, familiar environment, reduced amount of visits to the hospital, etc.

The communications and interfaces among components of patient monitoring systems and between these systems, become now very important in exploiting all the possibilities offered by the information gathered [1]-[3]. However, different manufacturers use their own software and communication protocols: building proprietary solutions that can only work alone or inside a single-vendor system. As each device *speaks* a different *language*, an interoperability problem emerges, leading to difficulties when a part of a system must be replaced as well as high costs [4]. Furthermore, the information acquired cannot be easily integrated into and exchanged with the Electronic Healthcare Record (EHR).

There is a need for developing open sensors and middleware components that allow transparent integration and plug-and-play interoperability of monitoring devices and systems (see Fig. 1). The use of communications standards seems to be an efficient way to solve these problems.

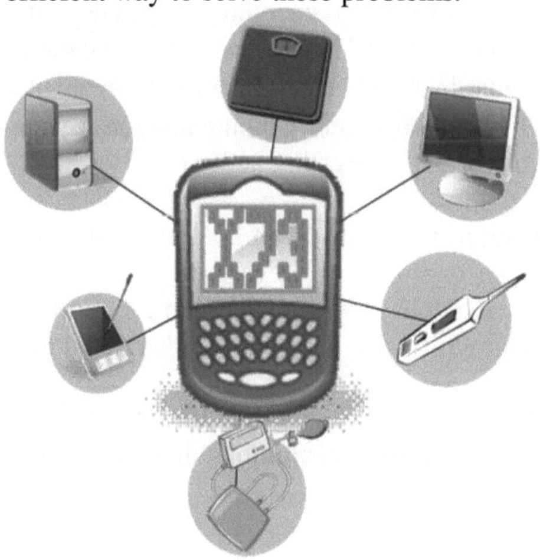

Fig. 1. Middleware need: medical devices interoperability

As it is shown in Fig. 1, the most used devices in telemedicine applications to measure parameters and biological signals are glucose meters, blood pressure and heart rate meters, pulse-oximeters, ECG monitors, digital scales, etc. Moreover, in last years, it is desirable that non-patient oriented devices that are part of a spectrum of use from fitness and wellness monitoring, through devices that support both independent and assisted living and self-managed informal monitoring, are also capable of playing a part in such an interoperable continuum of care. As the paradigms for health management change, in the face of societal and economic pressures, this continuity and flexibility will become increasingly important. Thus, it is common for medical devices to be wireless or wearable (with sensors incorporated into clothing, bracelets, etc.), that makes their use more comfortable. These collections of sensors around the patient make up what can be usually described as either a Body/Personal Area Network (BAN/PAN). Often, for monitoring elderly patients or those with limited mobility, these PAN or BAN networks are completed with presence detectors, movement sensors, or similar telecare devices, which are combined to form a Home Area Network (HAN).

The challenge of having telemonitoring systems that can interoperate and communicate with a middleware platform based on an open standard is complicated, somehow, because of the device features that are usually implied. Moreover, for these telemonitoring devices, the physical way of transmission is not always the same, being it either wired or wireless: (e.g. Bluetooth, Zigbee, Wibree, USB, etc.). Furthermore, they coexist with other medical and network devices such as PCs, routers, modems, mobile phones, etc. that use different technologies. Then, a modular layer design of the standard should have specializations for different low layer communications to be used.

To place the standard in context, we summarize other standards in the field of healthcare information systems oriented towards the encoding of signals and biomedical parameters, the standardization of the EHR, or the communication between medical applications using standardized messages. The main organizations focused on Medical Informatics and Information and Communication Technologies (ICTs) for e-Health that, including other interesting activities, coordinate the standards development are:

Committee European of Normalization (CEN) [5], with its Technical Committee CEN/TC251, is the main European organization in this field. In Spain, the Spanish Normalization Association (AENOR), with its Technical Committee AEN/CTN139 where our researching group works, is the standards-related institution, as a national CEN mirror.

International Standards Organization (ISO) and Institute of Electrical and Electronics Engineering (IEEE) [6], are the high level institutions that coordinate the previous national and international organizations.

And the main norms and standards for medical information interoperability that are being developed are:

Digital Imaging and Communications in Medicine (DICOM) [7], from the American College of Radiology (ACR) and National Electrical Manufacturers Association (NEMA). Its situation into the context of medical images is optimum due to its spreading over hospital and manufactures. It includes the main directives for biomedical signals intercommunication and it is ECG-oriented as SCP-ECG, from CEN/ENV1064, the specific standard for ECG.

Health Level 7 (HL7) [8], founded by American vendors of medical devices and recognized by American National Standards Institute (ANSI), is the international standard for medical messages exchange. It develops a specific syntax in the seven levels of the protocol stack, for information representation in a simple structure of segments, data types flags, and mapped fields.

EN13606 [9], from CEN and ISO/IEEE, specifies the information architecture for interoperable communications among services and systems that send, receive, store or exchange data with the EHR.

ISO/IEEE11073 (X73) [10], is a family of standards for medical devices interoperability developed by IEEE and adopted by ISO as standard, that groups the previous CEN norms that define the different levels of the communication model: MIB for lower levels, and INTERMED/VITAL for upper levels.

The integration in the use of standards and their huge scale implantation is a complex way. Thus, the role of external associations is even more important than standardization organizations. Integrating the Healthcare Enterprise (IHE) [11] is one of these associations: an organism with manufactures of all around the world (America, Europe and Asia) with the main objective not to develop new norms but adopt the most suitable available standards for each specific telemedicine application or service.

In this direction, an important hit occurs in June 2006, when 22 industry-leading technology and health companies joined forces and formed an open non-profit industry alliance named Continua Health Alliance [12]. According to its mission "*establish an ecosystem of interoperable personal health systems that empower people & organizations to better manage their health and wellness*", the alliance plans to select connectivity standards and set out guidelines for interoperability. Their main goal is not to develop new standards, but to leverage existing ones as much as possible, and to close recognized interoperability gaps by means of interoperability guidelines. Continua addresses the whole range from the medical device at the patient's home to the back-end services by defining interoperable interfaces. Besides technical aspects, an objective of the alliance is to establish a certification program with a consumer recognizable logo for the devices. Furthermore, the alliance plans to collaborate with government regulatory agencies regarding consistent policies for the use of hi-tech personal health devices at home, and to develop new ways for reimbursement of personal health systems.

X73 PoC implementation

One of the main challenges in the standard development is its real implementation in a telemedicine solution, transferable to the health system. There are some previous contributions developed. Firstly, the Dr. Warren's research group implementations [13]-[14], that studied the viability of applying standards in sanitary environments and implementing similar platforms to monitor patients in the PoC, and 2) PHD Working Group (PHDWG) [15] proof of concept implementations, whose aim was to test some aspect of their new standard. Nevertheless, till the creation of the PHDWG, presented later, there are not European antecedents in this field, nor proposals about global end to end solutions that introduce new patient telemonitoring use cases in ubiquitous environments and oriented to be X73 compatible, as it is being presented in this chapter.

The basic architecture of the ubiquitous telemonitoring platform (Fig. 2) is based in a logging element (Compute Engine, CE) that collects all the information acquired by different patient tracking Medical Devices (MDs) that define the PAN/BAN networks. This CE communicates, through the communication networks, with the remote hospital server that manages the different CEs and gathers all the information arriving from each patient monitoring scenario to update the EHR.

The implementation achieves that the proposed design does not depend either on the manufacturer proprietary MDs, or the connection interfaces, or the format of the different data bases, since all the communication chain follows standard protocols. Moreover this architecture includes:

- Customized interfaces for each use case (UC) and/or kind of patient/user allowing in some cases its active interaction.
- P&P methods for multiple MD management according to Ambient Intelligence (AmI) algorithms.
- Optimum wide band technologies selection mechanisms using advanced Quality of Service (QoS) estimation algorithms.

The characteristics of the different elements that form the system architecture, as well as the design specifications that have been followed in its implementation are described as follows:

MDs and X73 adapters. Currently it is an exception to find MDs conforming to the X73-PoC standard. Even though they include universal interfaces, their protocols are proprietary. Moreover, the standard only considers the use of RS-232 and IrDA. Therefore, in the development presented, proprietary medical devices without X73-PoC output are used including an adapter to the standard for both the physical interface and the transport. The devices used in the implementation are: a blood pressure (OMRON 705IT), and a pulse oximeter (DATEX-Ohmeda 3900).

CE X73. Gateway is designed as an X73 device or a manager, beneficiating from all those typical X73 functionalities: interoperability, service of alerts, supervision, and remote control. There are some risks because CE X73 is located in the patient's environment, where the conditions are out of the service provider's control. Consecuently, it has been necessary to consider some questions that have been, for example: intelligence of system (no dependence to external equipment to the home, so the CE needs a special intelligence module), or the confidence (the patient requires privacy for his/her personal medical information transmitted by using encryption methods).

X73/EN13606 Server. This communication hub is composed by two entities. The first one, the telemonitoring server, is in charge of receiving the data from the X73 CE through an experimental X73-PoC connection. It also manages the state of the network and CEs. The second one, EN13606 server, collects patient data through the telemonitoring server, verifies them and finally stores them in the patient EHR which is based on EN13606 standard.

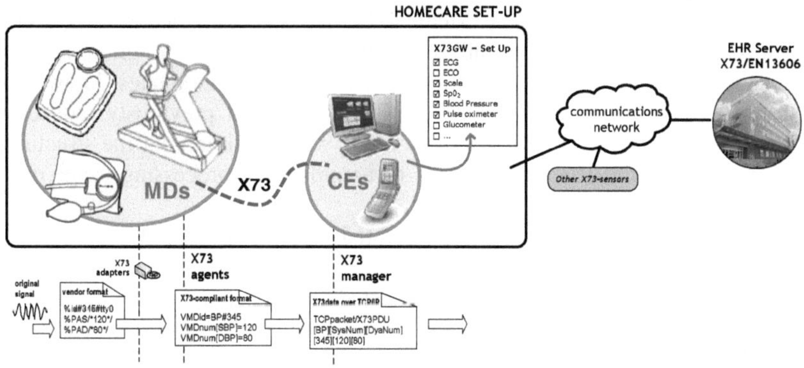

Fig. 2. Generic telemedicine integrating heterogeneous systems

When it comes to selecting the programming language, it has been taken into account the hardware capacities of the aimed devices. Hence, it is essential to make use of low level and/or native languages. Therefore the use of C/C++ is proposed. Moreover, the next features have been taken into account for its election.

- Use of pointers for the efficient management of objects trees, memory, and data frames.
- Development experience with C/C++ language.
- Low level hardware access.
- Possibility to develop in embedded systems.
- Integration with Application Development environments (RAD) for friendly window based applications in Windows platforms with Microsoft Foundation Classes (MFC).

The development environment for the solution has been basically Microsoft Visual Studio. While all the code belongs to the own protocol as the management of X73-PoC models (information, services and communications) is developed uniquely with the standard C/C++ libraries, the visual Graphic User Interfaces (GUI) have been implemented by using the MFC libraries. These libraries allow developing the protocol's code and required functionalities in simpler classes.

Moreover it provides the needed controls (buttons, information fields, lists, etc.) to allow for the creation of applications for terminal as well as applications based on windows in a simpler way not only for the Win32 platform but also for embedded systems based on Windows CE. The increment of libraries due to the use of MFC, despite reducing the code efficiency, does not reach the levels that would suppose the use of managed code (.Net, C#), and it is compensated with a reduction of development time.

All the elements, attributes, classes and messages in its abstract format are based on the Medical Device Data Language (MDDL) for their representation. Later they are defined as existing data types inside the C/C++ domain through the use of the Abstract Syntax Notation (ASN.1) descriptions. Finally, a marshalling process is issued following the Medical Device Encoding Rules (MDER) for transmission. This process determines mainly the design of the solution, if process efficiency is a key point in the solution. The use of frame templates (knowing the position of bytes in the transferred message) generated previously reduces the creation process to fill up the necessary fields while maintaining the structure of the remainder bytes. The requirements of memory and processing usage can be reduced.

The protocol stack layers were implemented keeping the next characteristics:

- The transport layer has been implemented as an adaptation to the transport stack to be used: The operating system's one in TCP/IP case (net socket), or a specifically designed one in the case of IrDA/RS-232.
- X73 session layer is minimized, disappearing all the synchronization services and control dialog.
- The X73 session layer is kept as a negotiation mechanism of the syntaxes to be used by the upper layers, defined in X73.
- Next, the association management Services Elements (SE) and data transfer are detailed:
- ACSE (Association Control SE). It manages the association state between the agent and the manager.
- CMDISE (Common Medical Device Information SE). This protocol implements the services of application level transmission of data between systems.
- ROSE/CMISE (Remote Operation SE/Common Management Information SE). It implements event or notification communication and the execution of operations remote systems.

The evolution of this implementation from X73-PoC in [16] to its next version based in X73-PHD requires the use of strategies that increment the efficiency of the process, given the limitations of PHD devices. The protocol stack modelling or X73-PHD models can be intelligently reorganized to reduce the complexity of the program. While in the previous solution all the OSI layers were implemented as well as functions and classes with their correspondent local variables and linking with other classes, now uniquely the message header is processed and then a ramified interpretation schema is followed according to the type of service of the header. In this way, it is possible to access to the information contained in the frame from the core application in certain cases.

The messages, object and data can be marshalled and added to the frame on-the-fly taking advantage of the MDER characteristics, as it has been mentioned previously. This strategy unloads the complexity in the execution stage far away to the compilation and development one. This is due to fact that the use of pointers in C/C++ and byte-array manipulation (transmission frames) have to be performed with extreme care in order to avoid execution time errors (buffer overrun, pointer to restricted zones, etc.). A comparison of the two models described previously is shown in Fig.3 .

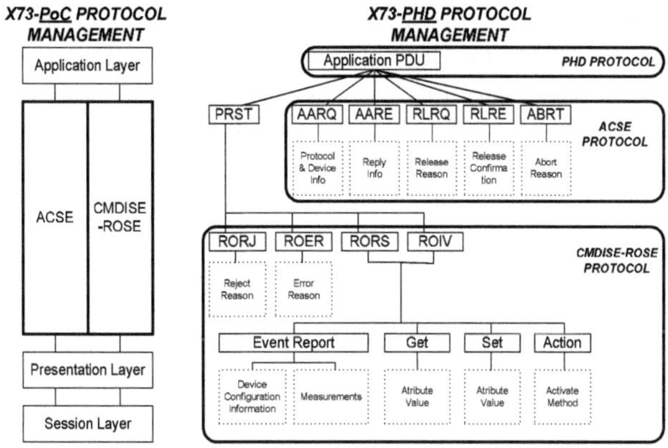

Fig. 3. Comparison of the X73-PoC and X73-PHD protocol stacks

ISO/IEEE 11073 challenges: evolution from X73-PoC to PHD

The family of standards X73 has undergone an evolutionary process from the beginning of its development to the present time, in which multitude of engineers have worked in colaboration with international universities, institutions and organizations. The first version, X73-PoC [17], as it has been seen in the previous section, dealt with the problematic of interoperability in the communication between different MDs around the patient (in the PoC) and the logger (denominated gateway) that centralizes the collected medical data of each one of them and standardizes the format of this information for its later transfer to the hospital or the telemonitoritoring server of the e-Health service.

The later development of new wearable MDs, with sensors of high quality and based on wireless technologies (like Bluetooth or ZigBee), and the increase of broadband accesses to multimedia networks has fueled the evolution of the X73 standard towards an optimized and adapted version to these new technologies and ubiquitous contexts: X73-PHD. With the previous technological background, the actual situation is met, with the standard being developed faster than before. This can be observed in the "Draft Standard for Health informatics IEEEP11073 - 20601 TM/D16" [18].With this evolution it changes the protocol architecture, the agent-manager communications model, Finite State Machine (FSM), and the transport stack that conform the X73-PHD protocol stack. Likewise, the design rules for the implementation of any system or e-Health solution based on X73 are modified, key objective of the X73-PHDWG work.

Basically, X73-PHD makes it possible the connection between MDs and CEs, acting as an extension of the so-called gateway in X73-PoC. This allows to evolve from common use cases which have been already used many times in e-Health solutions (home telemonitoring, patient follow-up, elderly patient care, etc.), towards a new ubiquitous solution context of u-Health (provided by X73-PHD) that spans the range of new use cases candidates for X73 as personal trainers, sports medicine, personal patient care, mobile scenario with wireless devices, etc.

There are two main reasons why it has been necessary to develop a new version of X73-PoC: its complexity and the e-Health evolution. The standard has a difficult structure, adopting contents from different standards. Its implementation requires of a long development processing time, some features are not still completed and, somehow the protocol itself seems to be obsolete. For the previous reasons and the new use cases, it is necessary the development of a new version. This way, X73 will not be just pushed into the background as a mere standardization attempt.

When designing the standard features, it is necessary to evaluate the UCs from the MDs to be implemented with X73-PHD so that the set of specifications supported by the standard is completely defined. In general the system features a typical star topology like Fig 1. in where the manager allocated in the center receives all the data coming from the agents. A preliminary list that contains the use cases considered for the development can be found in [18]. The main use cases are:

Healthy living / wellness & fitness
Imminent disease management
Assisted Ambient Living
Elderly patient care
Diabetes
Home monitoring of single cardiac patient

During the development, use cases have been arranged in three groups as it is showed in Fig.4. It is also included the associated medical devices to be standardized to X73-PHD. When the initial set of devices intended to work with X73-PHD was to be made, a survey was used to obtain data from the companies. In this survey, it was pointed out, for each device, the need to apply X73-PHD to its communications. Final classification was made based on the interest of experts in developing the standard or providing help for that during the process and the availability of a working group. Device specialization list which contains drafts under development are:

- 11073-10404 - Pulse oximeter
- 11073-10406 - Heart rate monitor
- 11073-10407 - Blood pressure monitor
- 11073-10408 - Thermometer
- 11073-10415 - Weighing scale
- 11073-10417 - Glucose meter
- 11073-10441 - Cardiovascular fitness and activity monitor
- 11073-10442 - Strength fitness equipment
- 11073-10471 - Independent living activity hub
- 11073-10472 - Medication Monitor

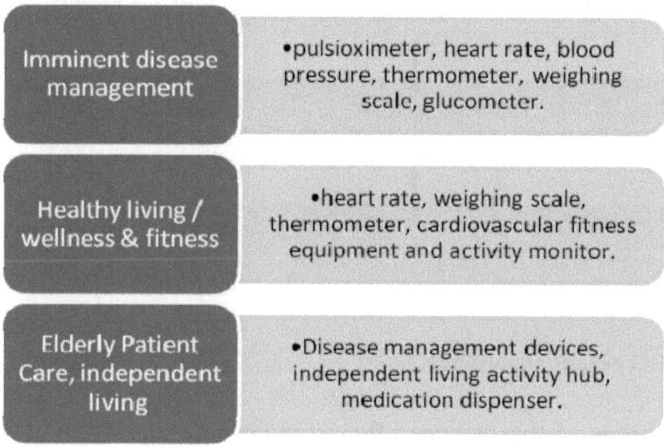

Fig. 4. Use Cases classification for X73-PHD.

X73-PHD model

A detailed description of the X73-PHD standard can be found in [18]. In the following lines, a basic description of its structure and the most interesting issues affecting the utilization of user's MDs are presented. PHD has thoroughly simplified the architecture of the protocol, defining perfectly the functionalities, now separated into three different models (see Fig. 5):

Domain Information Model (DIM) typifies the information inside an agent as a set of objects. Each object has one or more attributes. Attributes describe measurement data that are sent to the manager and elements that control the behavior of the device.

Service Model provides methods to access data that are sent between both systems (agent and manager) to establish the interchange of DIM's data. Within these methods, commands such as GET, SET, ACTION and Event Report extracted from the ROSE protocol can be found.

Communication Model describes the network architecture in which one or more agents communicate with a single manager via point-to-point connections. For each link, the FSM controls the system behavior. Another function of the communication model is to translate abstract syntaxes used in the DIM into transfer syntax. For instance, into binary messages using codification rules MDER. Other types of messages such as XML can be used.

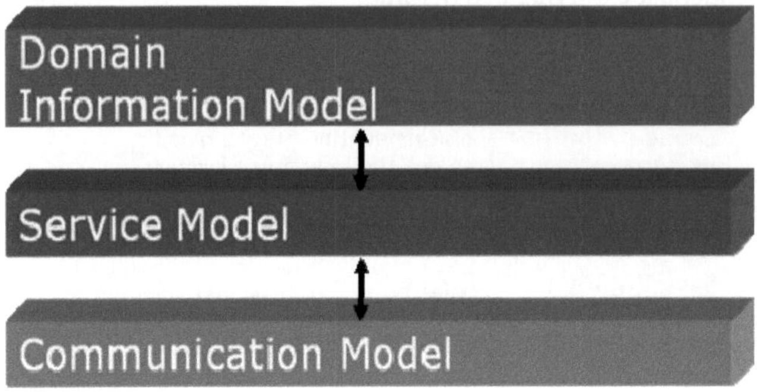

Fig. 5. X73-PHD generic architecture.

Specializations of the devices often contain new class definitions in the communication model in order to cover its particular functionalities. Besides, manufacturers can create their own specializations or extend the older ones, generating a modified scheme of objects and a list of defined attributes. It is manager's duty to identify these configurations in order to decide whether the association is accepted or not, based on the capabilities of the device.

X73-PHD protocol stack

X73-PHD includes a new architecture for the X73 protocol stack that makes possible the connection between MDs, or agents, and CEs or managers. This new X73-PHD stack is divided into three levels (see Fig. 6):

- **Device Specializations**. A set of model descriptions which collects the total of objects and attributes related to the device components, like an overall system's configuration (Medical Device System, MDS), Persistent Metric (PM-Store and Segments) or Metric Specifications. New MDs are continuously being added, by developing its MDS.
- **Optimized Exchange Protocol**. The main part of the standard consists of a medical and technical terminology framework (DIM) which will be encapsu-

lated inside the Protocol Data Unit (PDU). The first version of X73 defined this part as MDDL. Next, a Service Model defines a set of messages and instructions to retrieve data from the agent based on the DIM. In addition to this, it provides a data conversion from an ASN.1) to a Transfer Syntax, using optimized Encoding Rules (MDER), as well as standard Binary ER (BER) and even more effective Packet ER (PER) support. Service Elements taken from the previous X73 version for this purpose are: ROSE (optimized for MDER), ACSE, and CMISE. The communication model describes a point-to-point connection based on manager-agent architecture through a FSM.

- **Transport Layer**. Data transmission will be held over a transport technology due to X73 identifies assumptions that require direct support by this layer, allowing various transports to be implemented (X73-PoC established higher dependency between transport and upper and lower layers). Thus, transport specifications are out of the scope of X73-PHD, while other Special Interest Groups (SIG) are working towards profiles definition for Bluetooth, USB, ZigBee, etc.

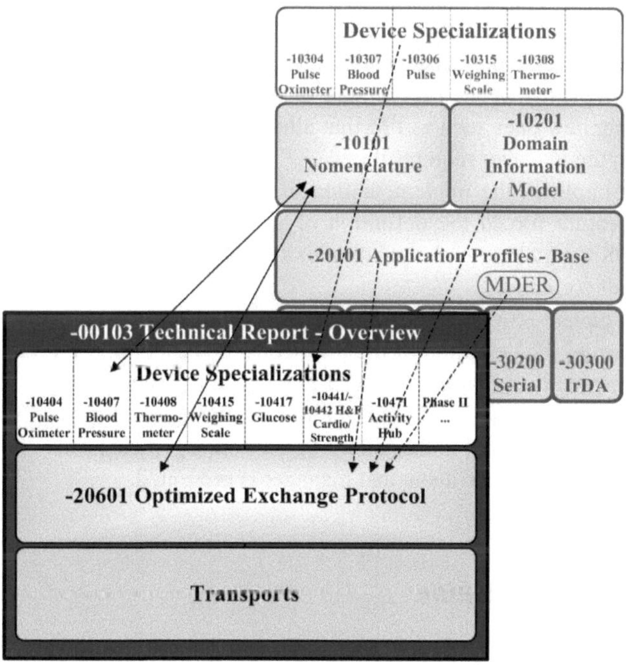

Fig. 6. Evolution of protocol stack from X73-PoC to X73-PHD

Going into the details of [18], something that enhances the previous protocol is that the three models are almost gathered in one single document. Its main characteristics are the following:

- Since the manager knows the standard specifications, the agent does not have to send its configuration unless it uses a different one. In that case, the manager will ask for that configuration in order to be able to work with that agent and to store this configuration for future occasions. This avoids the association procedure which can be a high time-consuming task in the case of multi-specialized devices (since they implement several devices at the same time, such as blood pressure and glucometer, for instance).

- It is independent of the transport layer. This significantly reduces the problems of the implementation. The protocol simply assumes a series of functionalities that the selected technology should fulfill. If that would not be possible, it admits the definition of functionalities through a shim layer.
- It defines different transport profiles, taking into account the conditions of the communication channel (application environment), and it classifies them according to these conditions:
  - Type 1: Transport profiles that contain both reliable and not reliable services. At least one or more virtual channels for reliable transport and zero or more channels for not reliable should exist.
  - Type 2: They contain only a unidirectional transport service.
  - Type 3: They only contain one not reliable transport service with one or more channels of this type.
- It reduces the complexity of the objects tree of the DIM, removing redundant classes and adding new ones such as PM that allows storing measurements that can be sent when the manager requires them.
- It considerably simplifies the implementation of multi-specialized devices. In X73-PoC, this feature forced the definition of a specific MDS type (Hydra-MDS). This MDS type, along with the complexity of the objects structure, was hard to implement correctly.
- A much more complete FSM is thoroughly described and tested to prevent any potential error during the operation of the protocol. The design of the FSM for PHD is more versatile than that used in X73-PoC since it has added new functionalities such as to have the agent configuration at manager's disposal. Since this is a key issue in X73-PHD, in the following section, a generic FSM scheme for the communication between agent and manager is presented.

X73-PHD Finite State Machine

The design of the FSM (see Fig. 7) is the key issue of any solution based on X73-PHD since it defines the fundamental procedure of behavior. In the design, the following states defined in X73-PHD must be taken into account: DISCONNECTED, CONNECTED, UNASSOCIATED, ASSOCIATED, CONFIGURING and OPERATING. The operating procedure would be as follows:

- When both devices are turned on, the local initialization procedure is executed (MDIB and other state parameters).

- From that initialization, a connection is established through the transport layer; if it has been successfully driven, then both devices enter into CONNECTED state (but UNASSOCIATED). In order to get associated, the agent sends an association request [AARQ] to the manager.
- If the manager already knows the agent's configuration, either because it is standard or because the manager has the configuration stored from previous operations, they enter into the ASSOCIATED state and they will be ready to operate. If not, then the manager will ask previously for the agent's configuration (CONFIGURING) and store it for future connections (this facilitates the plug-and-play functionalities).
- In the OPERATING state, the sending of measurements begins. They can be directly sent by the agent or on demand by the manager. Under this mode, the agent can perform either a single sending or successive, during a period of time which can be limited or not.

At any time both agent and manager can get disassociated because of error situations, end of measurements, or because of other circumstances. To do so, it exists a disassociation request [RLRQ] followed by a confirmation on the other side [RLQE], or a direct disassociation [ABRT].

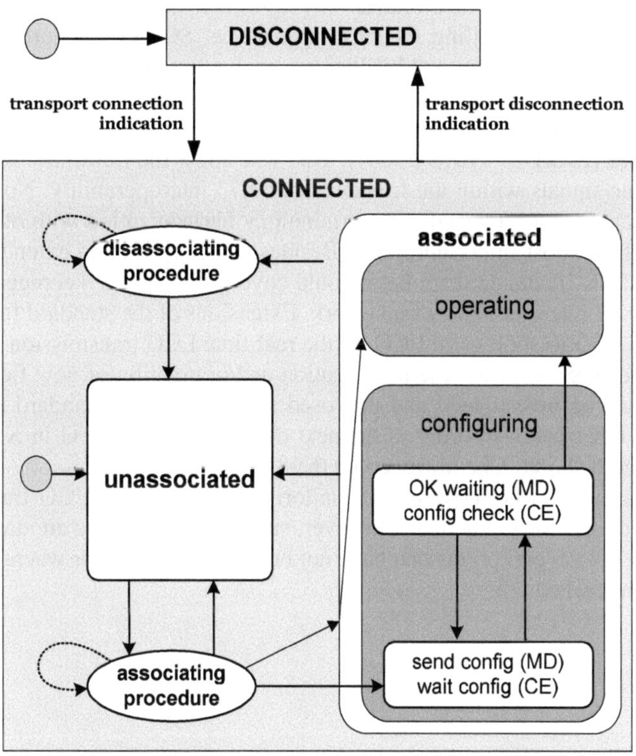

Fig. 7. Generic Finite State Machine (FSM)

Future trends and open points

Enhancements and harmonization of real-time signals, implementation into microcontrollers, integrated management for multiple devices, for homecare telemonitoring solutions are discussed below. Due to the protocol evolution and feature expansion towards a more efficient u-Health vital signs communication framework, new functionalities could now be incorporated allowing X73 to be used in a wider range of solutions:

Signal handling: harmonization and enhancements

The X73 standard can be easily adapted to MDs which register punctual values such as pulse, blood pressure, temperature, etc. However, it is highly desirable that the standard could also support some more complex biomedical data such as, for example, the ECG. Within the framework of X73-PoC standard, the ECG is already considered: there is a device specialization draft for the ECG (ISO/IEEE/CEN 11073-10306). Within X73-PHD, the ECG is not still defined but it is expected to be defined in the near future.

Other standards have been filling the ECG signals i.e. SCP-ECG (European Standard), HL7 aECG (American), or MFER (Japanese) among others. There is a close relationship between X73 and SCP-ECG. Recently, the latest version of the SCP-ECG standard (EN1064:2005+A1:2007) has been approved as part of the X73 family standard (ISO/DIS 11073-91064). This will allow the transmission of electrocardiographic signals within the framework of X73 interoperability. Nonetheless, several issues remain opened. The terminology harmonization with other standards is one of the most important items. Besides, it is expected to extend as much as possible the SCP standard so that it could cover new aspects, keeping always in mind the X73 interoperability framework. Extensions of the standard from diagnostic 12-lead ECG to short-term ECG, or the real-time ECG transmission are examples of that feature. Anyway, the modification and/or creation of new fields in the standard must be investigated and proposed so that the SCP standard can support it. On the other hand, in order to the next definition of the ECG in X73-PHD to be coherent, it should take into account the SCP-ECG standard.

In environments such as home care telemonitoring, the real-time ECG transmission is expected to be very practical. However, since these standards are under development, there are several points that have not been addressed yet or where no consensus has been reached.

Implementation into medical devices

Patient's data are usually collected via wearable MDs. A key point in these devices is ergonomics since it improves patient's quality of life. In order to improve the ergonomics, MD developers shall increase device's autonomy and decrease its weight which usually means that the board must use both batteries as small and soft as possible and low capacity embedded processing systems in order to minimize the power consumption. Typical components in a board are a microcontroller, a communication module and a sensor, but sometimes the unique component in the board is a System-on-Chip (SoC) module that integrates all these components in an only chip. Once the hardware has been selected, the required software solution has to be developed. The software framework for such a task is commonly determined by the hardware involved. For example in the Bluetooth or ZigBee case, the framework is determined by the communications stack that usually provides a proprietary Real Time Operating System (RTOS) and a proprietary Application Programming Interface (API) to access the RTOS functions. Typical features of medical device hardware used in medical applications are a few Kilobytes of Random Access Memory (RAM), a few tens of Kilobytes of non-volatile solid-state memory (typically flash or Read-Only Memory, ROM), and a few Megaflops processor. All these requirements are finally translated into software implementations that have in mind to reduce processor and memory as much as possible. As far as software is concerned, this type of devices do not require a high grade of intelligence and sources code are usually written in assembler, C, or embedded C++. Operating System (OS), in case it was used, is platform dependent and its API differs strongly from some devices to others.

This section proposes a general software architecture to implement MDs. It must be noticed that X73 defines completely a point to point communication between an agent and a manager and what that implies. That means that both syntaxes (the contents of each message, byte to byte) and semantics (the meaning of the message contents and its dynamics: what action to execute, how to respond, etc.) are defined for each transaction that usually entails any of this processes: a state change in the FSM, modifications in some of the DIM objects, and/or execution of some actions.

Based on our implementation experiences a guideline to incorporate X73 into MDs and how to proceed with a MD implementation is given below and it is based on the concept of pattern. A pattern is defined as a model that can be used to produce a copy exactly equal to a reference. The concept can be applied here to interchanged messages between a specific MD and its CE. Taking an X73 specific type of message it can be seen that there are some sections or blocks that keep constant and unchanged during all MD life.

These similarities appear because in each transaction one or more ASN1 structures are transmitted and its attributes are nearly always the same as they are needed only to enable interoperability and P&P and do not transmit information.

Blocks of bytes that do not differ can be extracted for a specific type of message, following the 11073 standard. We have coined each of them as pattern since they allow building X73 messages. All of the patterns needed to construct a message in a point to point communication between a MD and its CE are stored into what we call patterns library. Starting from the patterns library, each of the messages interchanged between MDs and its CE can be reproduced with a minimum of code lines. An example of the process is shown in Fig. 8 in which the message of interest is filled with patterns from patterns library, and a few program variables, such as Invoke-Id or an ObservedValue (obtained, for example, from the last blood pressure measurement). Messages generated in this way can be compared with incoming ones, or transmitted.

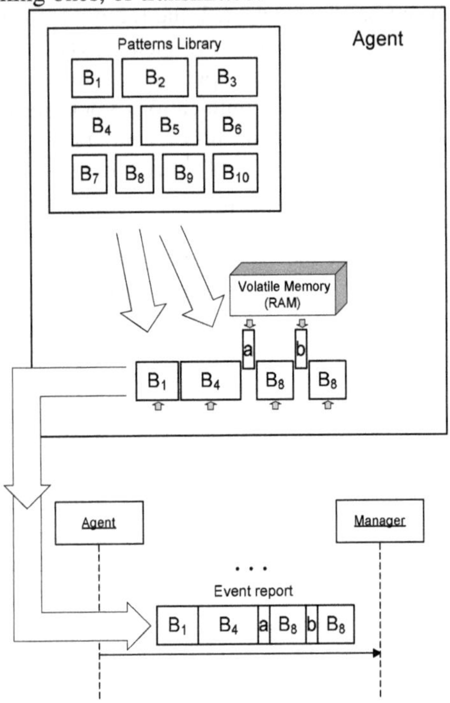

Fig. 8. X73 Messages synthesis from patterns

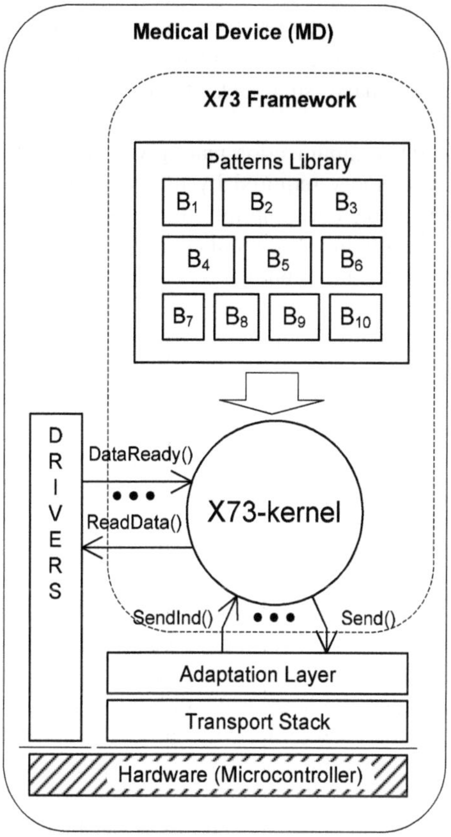

Fig. 9. Architecture proposed for X73 MDs implementation

The architecture of components for software development is proposed in Fig. 9 and it is composed by the patterns library [19], the X73-kernel, the drivers, the adaptation layer, and the transports. The X73-kernel is the task that copes with pattern assembling, processing, comparison and transmission. It also manages the state of the FSM, the state of objects in the DIM, and some system signals. The signals managed include data sent or data received signals, connection established, connection lost, timer signals for scanners (such as PeriCfgScanner), etc. Drivers provide basic functions that depend on the MD specialization that allow the X73-kernel manipulate the hardware. The adaptation layer provides services that allow the X73-kernel managing peer-to-peer communications through the transport.

The guidelines above can be used to produce MD implementations. Each of these implementations can be shared between more than one MDs but only when both devices share the same communication profile and specialization. For example it is possible to use the same implementation in a Bluetooth bathroom scale and a RS-232 laboratory weigh scale when both of them use polling profile (since both of them use the weigh scale specialization and the polling mode communication profile), but is not possible to use that implementation in a Bluetooth bathroom scale that use the baseline or PHD profile. These platforms usually use a common multiplatform programming language, such as C, to program the X73-kernel so it can be easily ported.

Untying these MD specialization-MD communication pairs gives great optimization in memory space. Most of the memory required by this solution is non-volatile type. Consequently, the low memory consumption makes possible to use the same X73-kernel and library of patterns in a big number of MDs that, at the same time, allows sharing it between different manufacturers improving interoperability.

An exhaustive analysis of the X73 standard is required to generate the patterns library and the X73-kernel. Our proposal is depicted in Fig. 10. Two-steps analysis is need: Firstly, to determine the set of messages that the device needs and the sequence they should follow, and, secondly, the analysis of this set of messages (typically a dozen) to obtain patterns. Once obtained, they are store in the patterns library. Duplicated ones are discharged in order to reduce memory consumption. Once the patterns library has been generated, the X73-kernel that provides all the functionalities is developed using object oriented analysis and design (OOA/D) principles following a stimulus-response schema.

Once developed, an implementation can be shared and it offers a RAD that will allow a novel X73 implementer to develop a MD with only a basic knowledge of X73 since the unique needed modules to be developed are the adaptation layer and the device drivers. For example, in the case of a heart rate monitor, device drivers must provide with a signal that inform the X73-kernel when a new sample-array (SA) is ready, and a method to access the data. In order to maximize interoperability it is preferable to create a framework that shall be used by all manufactures. To create this framework, the help of X73 world experts, experiences of other implementations, and the expertise of other SIG is key.

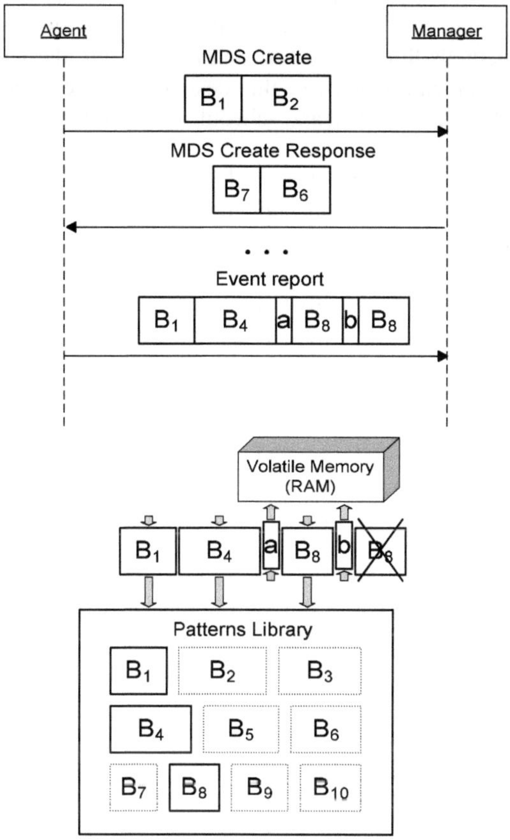

Fig.10. Synthesis of the X73 library

Open points

From this implementation results, several technical targets are opened, which are key objectives of CEN to advance on standard-based solutions for u-Health. These **open points** are:

Implementation of the protocols stack into micro-controller devices (X73-compliant MDs) and wireless devices (mobile X73-CE), considering their appropriate technologies of transport level and physical interface from handler layer (connections manager). For example, when several MDs with different physical interfaces (e.g. USB and Bluetooth) connect with the same CE, handler layer communicates in transparent mode with both MDs independently of each transport protocol. The designed architecture for handler layer, with the implemented methods and parameters, has to be completed with each new connection profile in order to manage, in real execution time, each service access interface. This implies the design of private program methods through *sockets* and *threads* into the handler layer to obtain a better management. Moreover, this design could be integrated with the implementation of allocation models and scheduling methods for particular MDs (under study from CEN).

Support of multiple connections between several MDs and CEs, optimizing the different MDIBs creation and interchange, and implementing a FSM states manager that can read the specific MD configuration parameters and add them to a database in order to guarantee P&P functionalities. This is directly related with the previous open point from X73-PHD perspective. This problem, also worked in CEN, requires a MDs adapter/concentrator to multiplex the communication of different devices. Thus, if a single MD is updated, changing the entire platform is not necessary due to the MDs adapter can connect via Internet to manufacturer site, download the required software, and send the correct parameters for creating the new MDIB of the updated MD. Anyway, if the MD is aX73-compliant device, this process is transparent into the micro-controller and the multiplex function is implemented directly in CE to integrate MDs that are not X73-compliant but needed in clinical routine.

Migration of the designed GUI to a completely interactive and customized user environment for being able to incorporate in the daily living of the patient. The environment has to be configurable regarding the device model (miniPC, mobile phone, smart phones, PDA, etc.), and in a transparent and modular mode. The designed platform as X73 demonstrator is a very useful tool for engineers and developers, but its commercial implantation requires an evolution towards a multimedia u-Health system. The design rules for the proposed architecture are ready for this evolution through Microsoft Foundation Classes (MFC), even through integrated graphic structures based Java, .Net, or Web 2.0, adapted for specific requirements of each application scenario, use case and OS (*Windows Mobile*, *Android*, *Symbian*, etc.) depending on the device model.

Conclusion

The need of standardization on middleware solutions has derived to an end-to-end X73-compliant platform that allows achieving a ubiquitous and plug-and-play solution, ready for its integration with wearable sensor networks. Besides, it can be seen as an X73-PHD tester to prove the challenges currently under discussion in the CEN: flow and errors control, errors and alarms management, multiple MD connection with one or multiple CEs, or implantation on micro-controllers.

Acknowledgment

The authors wish to thank X73-PHD Working Group, CEN, and Mr. Melvin Reynolds, *convenor* of the CEN TC251 WGIV, for the contributions to this research. We appreciate the contribution of Miguel Galarraga to the excellent results carried out during the last years, and also Adolfo Muñoz (*Instituto de Salud Carlos III*), Paula de Toledo (*Univ. Carlos III*), and Silvia Jiménez (*Univ. Politécnica de Madrid*).

References

[1] Stead, W.W., Miller, R.A., Musen, M.A., Hersh, W.R.: Integration and beyond: Linking information from disparate sources and into workflow. J. Am. Med. Inform. Assoc. 7(2), 135–145 (2000)
[2] Pedersen, S., Hasselbring, W.: Interoperability for information systems among the health service providers based on medical standards. Inform. Forsch Entwickl 18(3-4), 174–188 (2004)
[3] Kennelly, R.J.: Improving acute care through use of medical device data. Int. J. Med. Inform. 48(1-3), 145–149 (1998)
[4] Sengupta, S.: Heterogeneity in health care computing environments. In: Proc. Annu. Symp. Comput. Appl. Med. Care, pp. 355–359 (1989)
[5] Comiteé European Normalisation/TechnComm251 (CEN/TC251), http://www.cen.eu – http://www.cen.eu (Asoc. Española Normalización (AENOR/CTN139) (in Spain), http://www.aenor.es/desarrollo/inicio/home/home.asp) (Accessed, August 2008)
[6] DICOM. Digital Imaging and Communications in Medicine, http://medical.nema.org/ (accessed, September 2008)
[7] HL7. Health Level Seven, Devices Special Interest Group, http://www.hl7.org/Special/committees/healthcaredevices/index.cfm (accessed, September 2008)
[8] ENV13606CEN/TC251. Electronic Healthcare Record Communication. Parts 1, 2, 3 and 4, Pre-standard, http://www.medicaltech.org (accessed, September 2008)
[9] Galarraga, M., et al.: Standards for medical device communication. X73 PoC-MDC. Stud. Health Technol. Inform. 121, 242–256 (2006); Integrating the Healthcare Enterprise, IHE, http://www.ihe.net/ (accessed, September 2008)
[10] Continua Health Alliance web site, http://www.continuaalliance.org/home/ (Last access: 09/2008)
[11] Yao, J., Warren, S.: Applying ISO/IEEE 11073 standards to wearable home health monitoring systems. J. Clin. Monit. Comput. 19(6), 427–436 (2005)
[12] Warren, S., Lebak, J., Yao, J.: Lessons learned from applying interoperability and information exchange standards to a wearable point-of-care system. In: Conf. Proc. Transdisciplinary Conf. Distr. Diagn Home Healthcare (2006), doi:10.1109/DDHH.2006.1624807

[13] Clarke, M., Bogia, D., Hassing, K., Steubesand, L., Chan, T., Ayyagari, D.: Developing a standard for personal health devices based on 11073. In: Conf. Proc. IEEE Eng. Med. Biol. Soc., 6175–6177 (2007)
[14] Martinez, I., et al.: Implementation of an end-to-end standard-based patient monitoring solution. IET Commun. 2(2), 181–191 (2008)
[15] ISO/IEEE11073 Point-of-Care Medical Device Communication standard (X73-PoC). Health informatics. [Part 1. Medical Device Data Language (MDDL)] [Part 2. Medical Device Application Profiles (MDAP)] [Part 3. Transport and Physical Layers], `http://www.ieee1073.org`, See also the previous standards: IEEE 13734-VITAL and ENV13735-INTERMED of CEN/TC251, `http://www.medicaltech.orgh` (accessed September 2008)
[16] ISO/IEEE11073 - Personal Health Devices standard (X73-PHD). Health informatics (P11073-00103. Technical report - Overview] (P11073-104xx.Device specializations) (P11073-20601.Application profile-Optimized exchange protocol), IEEE Standards Association webpage: `http://standards.ieee.org/` (accessed, September 2008)
[17] Martinez-Espronceda, M., et al.: Implementing ISO/IEEE 11073: Proposal of two different strategic approaches. In: Conf. Proc. IEEE Eng. Med. Biol. Soc., pp. 1805–1808 (2008)

An Automatic Smart Information Sensory Scheme for Discriminating Types of Motion or Metrics of Patients

X. Ma and P.N. Brett

School of Engineering & Applied Science, Aston University,
Birmingham B4 7ET, UK.

Abstract Tactile sensing is a developing technology and can be used for detecting parameters describing contact between surfaces. It is of growing application as the technology progresses with increased possibilities for automatic perception. In this chapter the potential of the distributive sensing approach is discussed for monitoring metrics, motion and behaviour in people through the outcome of a series of experimental applications. These illustrate the ability to extract descriptions as information, rather than data on metrics or motion. The method uses an approach of discrimination to determine parameters describing contact conditions or for recognising the nature of contact. Using this approach, the distributive deformation response of a surface detected at a few sensing points leads to a device of mechanical simplicity. The approach has similarities with living tactile systems and offers the advantages of robust construction, greater resolution than the separation of sensing elements, and redundancy. The benefit of outputting information at source is the efficiency in storage and transmission and is a positive advantage for a sensing solution in the home. In homecare, the possibilities for monitoring people are numerous. The approach is discussed with reference to examples. Different techniques to derive describing parameters have to be applied to suit the different types of static or dynamic responses of surfaces in different applications. This approach to tactile sensing has an extensive future however the understanding of optimal design is at the developing stage.

Table of contents

K. Yogesan et al. (Eds.): Handbook of Digital Homecare, BIOMED, pp. 203–219.
springerlink.com

1. Introduction

Sensing systems that output information as opposed to data could offer a means to inform patients or medical practitioners of the changing state of the person or indeed how they are responding to treatment. The fact that the burden of processing data to find the meaning of the measurement is reduced will raise the efficiency of screening processes and widen access to such care. Further, if such systems are produced at low cost then there is a reasonable prospect of their being applied in the home to measure the patient in their normal living environment. In this chapter a new approach to discriminating the motion and behaviour of people through a mechanically simple tactile surface is described as an example that is currently being investigated. This approach has the potential to output a description of patient response or motion, even gait, that can be used to identify pathology or response to therapy directly. Working in terms of information as an output, rather than reams of data, offers benefit in terms of reducing demands on data storage or transmission requirements.

Tactile sensing is a developing technology for detecting parameters that describe the contact between surfaces. It is of growing application as the technology progresses with increased possibilities for automatic perception. In its most simple form tactile sensing could be described as the process of detecting and interpreting a single force to detect the intensity of contact between surfaces. It is often a useful control parameter used in the control of tool feed force. On more than one axis, contact force is measured to control surface following processes. More complex systems have been demonstrated in research studies. These aim to identify a range of parameters to determine more information on the conditions of contact. Often the objective is to provide additional information over that of vision for machine perception; to identify contacting objects through their surface characteristics and properties and to enable discrimination between types. There are further aims to determine a suitable construction that is robust and not complex to manufacture. With such qualities, solutions would be appropriate to the variable processes found in healthcare applications.

There are some interesting examples and methods in the application of tactile sensing in variable environments. (Khodabandehloo 1990) controlled a manipulator to cut meat from a carcass using a powered knife. This used forces detected at the handle of the knife to deduce trajectories relative to the invisible skeletal structure. Other types of tactile sensing in industrial processes use the force data to guide tool points over a surface. Where the size or shape of imprint of the object is to be retrieved, a matrix of point sensors has been used. (Raibert and Tanner 1989) describes an early integrated circuit type. Arrays are usually complex constructions, with the notable exception of the more recent innovation of (Holweg 1996) that reduced complexity. However, there is still the need to retrieve large volumes of data with many connections, and the data interpretation process can be computationally intensive. In contrast to the above examples, the scheme described in this paper is able to discriminate between different loading conditions and offers the potential to minimise data processing. By detecting a change in the estimated state of the load, the scheme can be used to determine, motion, deformation and slip (Tam et al. 2004) It can also be applied to recognise static objects and discriminate different groups of objects (Brett et al. 2003). Most recently the method has been applied to investigate the dynamic motion of human subjects.

The method is referred to as 'distributive' (as opposed to point-to-point) as it utilises the response of a continuous surface element that is monitored at multiple points within the surface from which to estimate the nature of the contact anywhere on the surface. An important characteristic is that sensor outputs are coupled through the deformation of the surface. This is illustrated in figures 1a and 1b which illustrate advantages, from a mechanical viewpoint, in contrast with array sensors. The distributive approach utilises few sensory points and consequently there are few connections and reduced computational load with respect to reading sensory values. As the surface is a continuous element, it responds with deformations over the entire area when loads are applied at any point. The deformation can be detected at strategically positioned sensing points. There may be as few as four active sensing positions required in some applications, and many more descriptors of contact can be derived than the number of sensing points deployed.

Through this simple mechanical construction, descriptions of contact can be derived through a computationally efficient process of discrimination between different conditions. The advantage of the technique is the ability to classify as range of features describing contact. First impressions of the approach may appear limited, however from the many interpretations of the combined static and transient signals it is possible to identify many states that can be used as descriptors correlating with objects and behaviour. The descriptors can be used to retrieve prominent values of the object, behaviour and motion, as well as to describe shape, size and orientation. The computational process to derive information from the few sensor points is efficient.

Such a technique has been used to sense contact force distribution in gripping devices (Ellis et al. 1994) and (Stone and Brett 1996) use this approach and employ a closed form interpretation algorithm to derive contact force information from the sensory data. (Evans and Brett 1996) and (Brett and Stone 1997) extended the application to detecting normal force distributions acting on soft materials in manufacturing and minimally invasive surgical devices, exploiting further opportunities found in the approach. More recently, the approach has been used to infer descriptions of contacting conditions at the tip of a flexible digit, as could be envisaged at the tip of a steerable endoscope (Tam et al. 2004). The shape of the digit and its relative motion, with respect to the tissues, as sliding contact can also be interpreted using the same three sensing elements. Building on potential advantages of the approach, this paper reviews the progress of this research study and describes some of the results achieved.

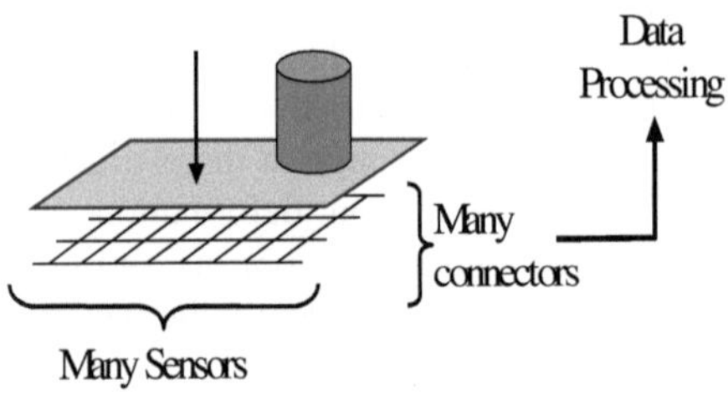

Fig. 1a. Tactile array sensors

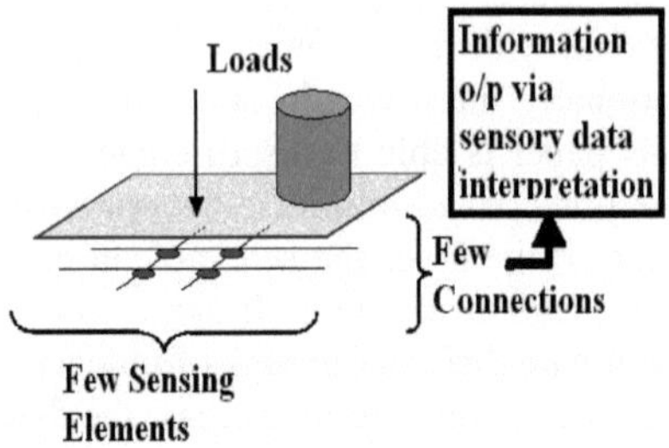

Fig. 1b. Distributive tactile sensing system

2. One dimensional performance study for a static load distribution

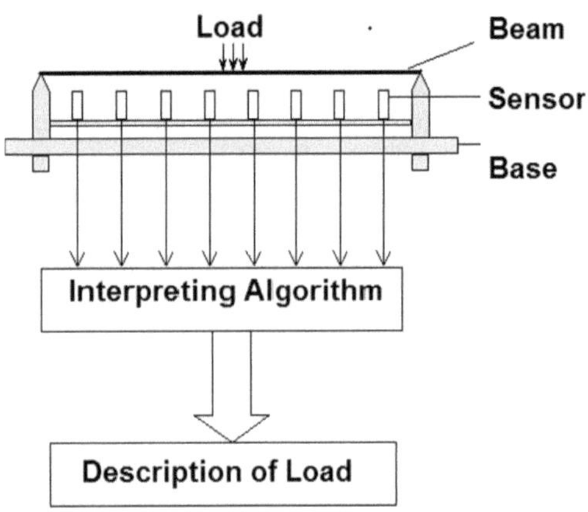

Fig. 2. A one dimensional surface example

In an initial study to understand factors influencing performance a simple 1-D version of a distributive sensor was constructed. The simply- supported beam sensing system shown in figure 2 was used to examine the effects of prominent design parameters on the performance of the approach. A variety of types of algorithm can be used to interpret the sensory data. Both fuzzy inference and neural networks have been applied successfully. Often it is found that a cascaded series of neural networks can be trained most readily in contrast to a single multi-input multi-output neural network (Table 1).

To test the system, known descriptions of forces were applied such that errors could be derived directly. For the sensing system there is advantage if a force can be represented by simple means, and therefore the function $f(z)$ given in equation (1) was selected to describe the load as a function of non-dimensional axial beam position z. The choice of function was arbitrary and convenient to apply in this application. The function incorporates the load position p, total load T and load width index c as follows:

$$f(z) = f_{\max}\ e^{-c^n (z-p)^n} \tag{1}$$

f_{max} is the peak load amplitude and z is defined non-dimensionally in terms of the position x along the beam of length L:

$$z = \frac{x}{L} \tag{2}$$

The total load T is given by the integral over the beam given in equation (3).

$$T = L\int_0^1 f(z)dz \tag{3}$$

Table 1. Systems error for two configurations of neural networks

Neural Network Configuration	**Output Load Parameters**	**Normalized System Error %**
Single Neural Network	Position, Width, Amplitude	4.2
Cascaded Neural Networks		
N.Network A	Position	0.1
N.Network B	Width	0.63
N.Network C	Amplitude	0.1

The other parameters are best described with reference to the typical distributed load function shown in figure 3. This function uses the parameters $fmax=290$ N/m, $p=0.2$m, $c=12$ and $n=8$. The sharpness of the curve is given by n, and the value of $n=8$ produces a sufficiently distinct step to define the boundary of the load. By choosing a greater value for n the sharpness can be increased further. The position of the load is centered at the value of $p=0.2$ along the beam.

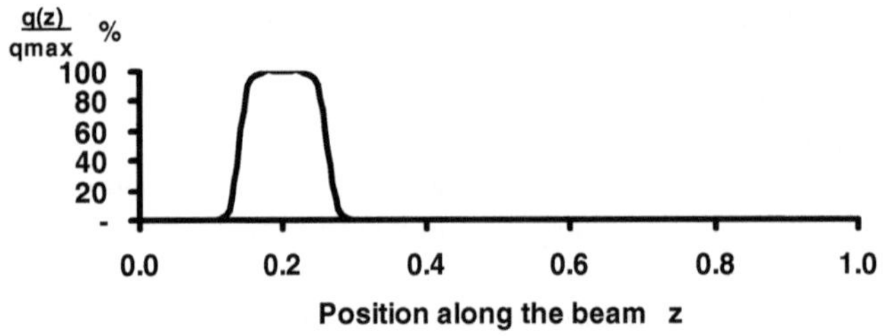

Fig. 3. Force distribution $q_{max}=290$ N/m, $p=0.2$m, $c=12$, $n=8$

By applying the cascaded Back Propagation Neural Networks (Figure 4) to interpret the load position from the sensory inputs provided by the 8 proximity sensors, detecting the static response of the beam, it was shown (Ma and Brett 2002) that the system could be used to determine the position of a point load to within an error of 3% over more than 80% of the length of the beam. Also the width and intensity of the load could be determined to within 4% of correct values. The results describing performance in evaluating these descriptors are shown in figures 5a, 5b and 5c for load position, width and value respectively. The errors shown are plotted as functions of non-dimensional position on the beam. Furthermore the tests showed that this performance could be achieved by using only 4 strategic sensing positions. The study has also been extended to a cantilever beam, where different distributions of load were also interpreted with great resolution (Ma et al. 2004) using three sensing elements. These investigations revealed the sensitivity that could be achieved with the approach in interpreting and evaluating a variety of descriptors from which information describing contact can be derived directly. These successful results have led to 2-D surfaces and most recently surfaces for discriminating dynamic motion of human subjects.

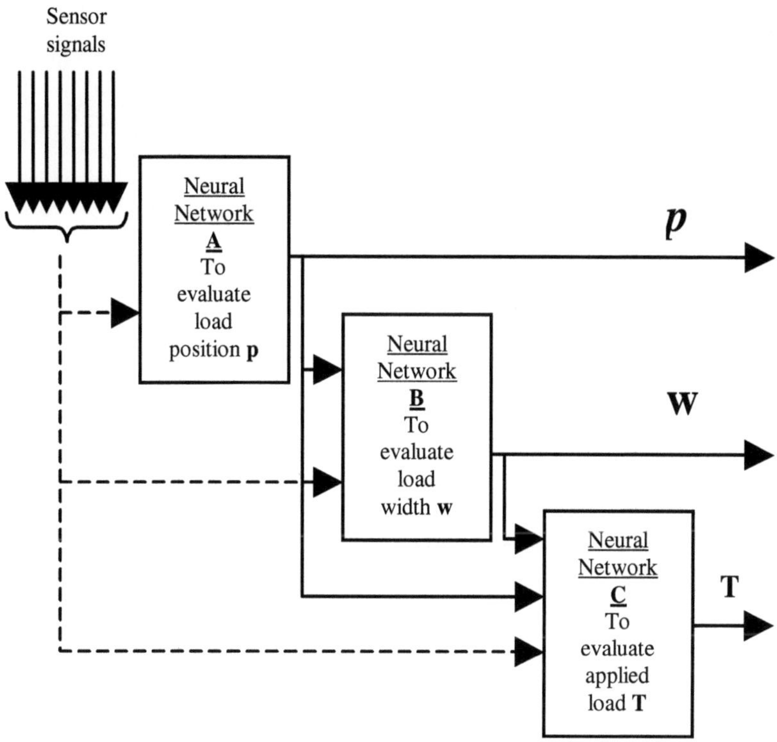

Fig. 4. A cascaded chain of neural networks to determine load parameters

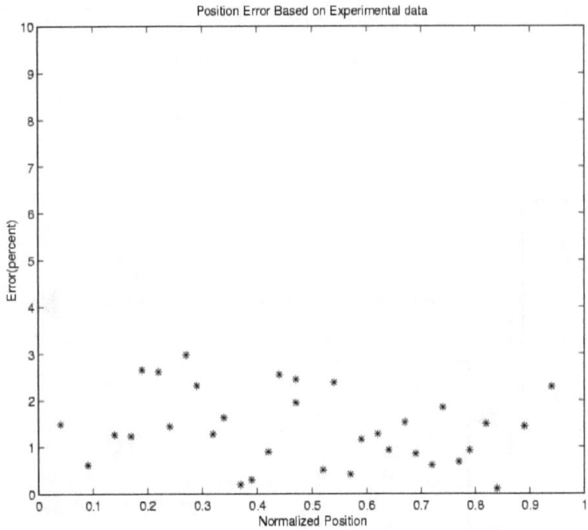

Fig. 5a. Error η_p in the determination of load center position

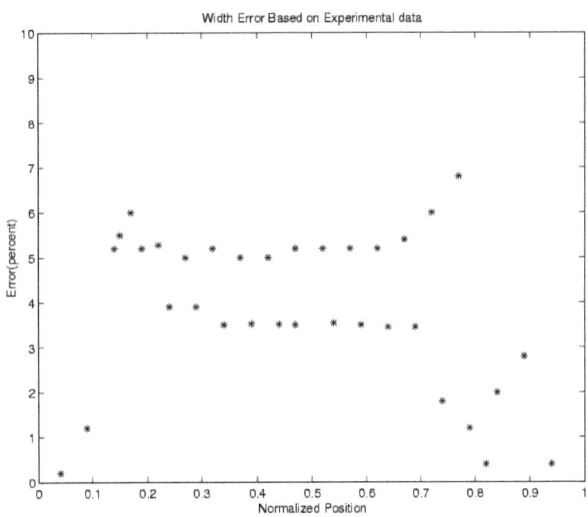

Fig. 5b. Error η_w in the determination of the width of the load

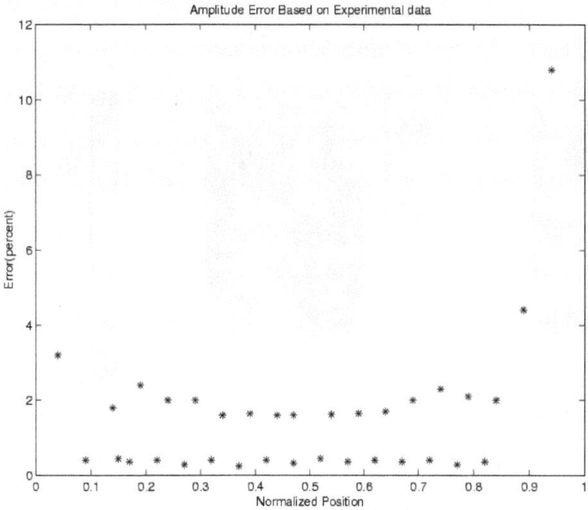

Fig. 5c. Error η_T in the determination of the total value of the load

3. Two dimensional performance study for a static load distribution

In two dimensions there are more aspects to be examined. In a number of studies, surfaces were simply supported at the edges over a sparse array of proximity sensors in a similar configuration to the 1 dimensional surface of figure 2. Figure 6 shows 2 contoured plan diagrams of the surface to illustrate the variation in positional error of a point load. The diagrams show error in the x and y ordinates respectively. As expected, errors were most prominent at the edges of the surface, although typically, positional accuracy was within 4% of the surface range.

Subsequent research on optimisation has shown that the array of sensing elements can be reduced to four placed in optimised positions (Tongpadungrod et al.2004). Provided the sensing elements have similar output characteristics, the error achieved is in the range of 5%. Studies have also shown that the system can also be used to discriminate different types and sizes of objects placed on the surface while determining an applied position and orientation figure 7. Least sensitivity is in evaluating the magnitude of applied loads.

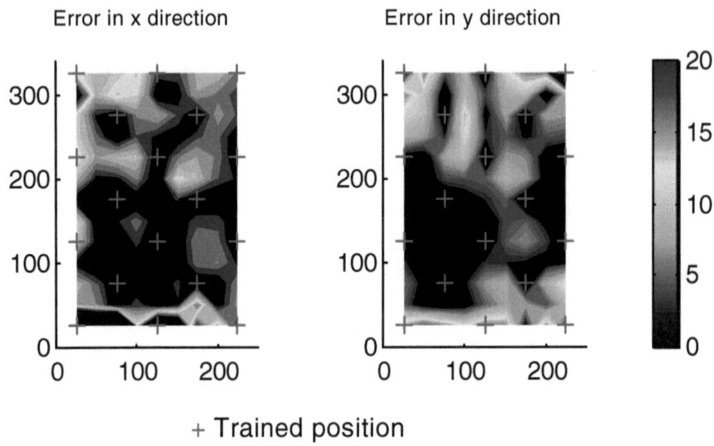

Fig. 6. Positional accuracy on a 2 dimensional surface (Dimensions in mm)

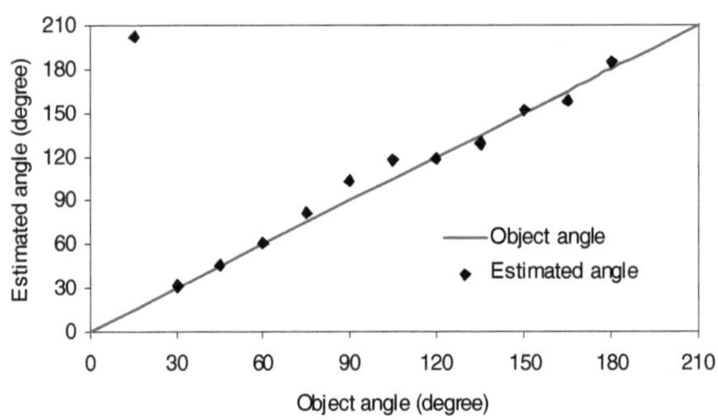

Fig. 7. Accuracy in discriminating object orientation.

These studies on discriminating types of objects, sizes locations and orientation (Tongpadungrod and Brett 2002) have shown that acceptable performance can be achieved within a range suited to the evaluation of human behaviour or motion. Both static and transient attributes are relevant. In this application, the challenge is to define a tactile sensing system able to distinguish different parameters describing the objective of the evaluation when presented with subjects that are similar in properties or behaviour and different in parameter values. Therefore care must be taken in defining the objectives. The sizing of feet is one simple possibility. A study revealed that a suitable performance can be achieved with 95% accuracy (Trace 1996). This performance compares with that achieved in the discrimination of fruit by type where accuracy greater than 90% was achieved (Tongpadungrod and Brett 2000).

These static examples have shown that contacting objects can be identified, even categorised by the shape of contact. Furthermore the studies have demonstrated that it is possible to infer such information over 80% of a surface such that evaluation is independent of position and orientation. To achieve this, it is most important to place sensors in optimal positions. This is likely to be dependent both on the interpreting algorithm used and the nature of the parameters to be resolved (Tongpadungrod et al. 2004).

4. Dynamic Loading studies

The dynamic response of surfaces is more complex to handle than the static case. There are different situations to consider and these depend on the disturbance type triggering the response of the surface. There can be periodic disturbances at the same point and at differing positions; there are also single event disturbances. The transient response of the surface can be captured at discrete positions and used to derive a description of the disturbance. Where the surface response is considered quasi-steady, then strategies implemented in the static case will apply. In addition there is the time dimension, where one can observe differences in the nature of captured transients and their relative timing to discriminate different conditions.

The ability to dynamically track the position of an object supported on a plate has potential applications in the area of measuring balance and posture in people. This is an important area of medical research, particularly in the elderly. For example, a key characteristic of Parkinson's disease is postural instability (Miller 2002) and this can increase the frequency of falls. (Adkin et al. 2005) produced results showing that trunk sway can be used to detect pathological balance control in patients with Parkinson's Disease, with the possibility of determining those at high risk of regular falls. (Lord 2003) has compiled evidence from several studies showing that the common occurrence of impaired vision in the elderly can be a predictor of increased sway and hence an increased likelihood of falling. The equipment currently used to measure the magnitude of sway and postural instability can be complex and expensive. Force plates are commonly used to measure sway (Freitas et al. 2005, Jonsson et al. 2004) which have a limited area in which the subject must stand and usually require a pair of plates to be used in most applications. Another method uses accelerometer (Hennksen et al. 2004) or velocity transducers (Adkin 2005), both attached to the subject using a large belt around the waist to measure the sway. The presence of this belt and the transducer box positioned on the lower back of the subject could potentially upset the subject's natural position and balance. The use of the distributive approach addresses many of these clinically based deficiencies in approaches to measurement.

4.1 Experimental study

In this section the results of an experimental study to investigate the application of the distributive sensing method for the measurement of sway using a surface based device are described. In this experiment a scheme for repeatable disturbance commensurate with a swaying person was applied to a surface. A surface of dimensions 0.9m x 0.53m was deployed with only three optical proximity sensing elements to detect surface deformation in locations selected to optimise performance of the method. The sensing elements were used to detect the response of the surface resulting from disturbances caused by the moving object in contact with the surface. The object used is a four legged frame supporting a pendulum swinging in the vertical plane and placed in random position and orientation, shown in figure 8. A 12 camera motion analysis system was used to track the position of the moving mass. This was used in the process of training the neural network implemented on a Field Programmable Gate Array (FPGA) and to verify the final output transients.

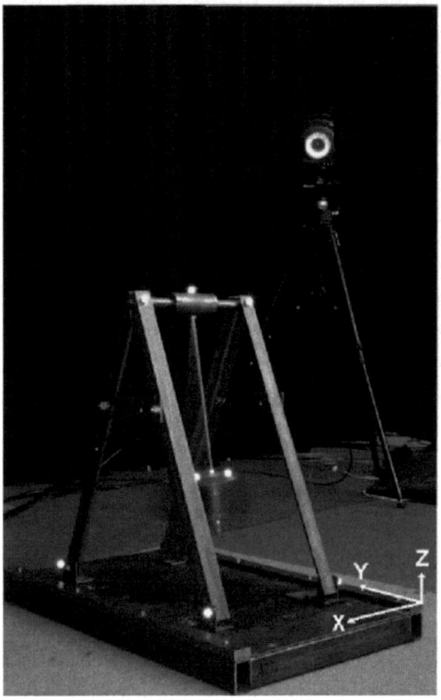

Fig. 8. Photograph of the experimental setup

Figure 9 shows the example of the results achieved by a cascade neural network configuration. The results compare the estimated position by the distributive sensing approach with the measurements by the VICON system for the cascaded configuration. The plot of tracking displacement as a function of time shows close agreement. The error is also plotted on the figure for each ordinate. The maximum error between estimates and measurements are listed in Table 2. A maximum tracking error of 5% of the motion on any axis is typical using this approach. Similar performance was found for each network configuration, although it has to be stated that having independent networks for each dimension produced marginally improved results.

Table 2. The maximum error of the estimated position of the pendulum by the distributive tactile sensing approach

Dimension	Percentage Error
X	3.8%
Y	2.1%
Z	4.7%

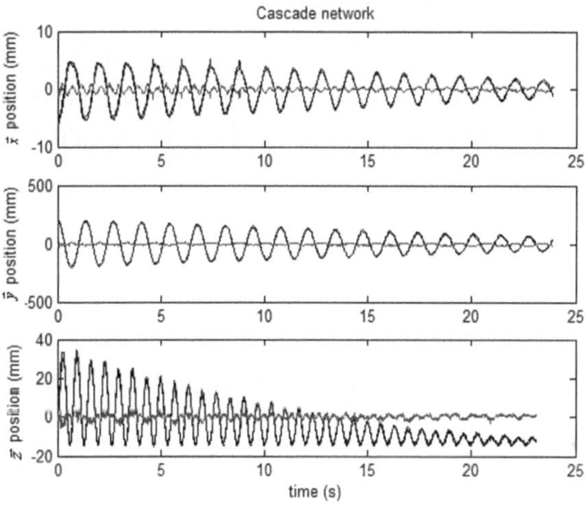

Fig. 9. Approximated (blue line) and vicon displacement (dark-green line) and relative error (red line) of using the Cascade networks

By using the distributive sensing method through an implementation with just three low cost sensors within the confines of the deforming plate it is possible to track the position of a swinging pendulum in real time with an error of less than 5%. Additionally, by using an FPGA based neural network we have shown that the distributive sensing method can be implemented successfully as a stand alone embedded system, operating without the processing input from a PC system. The accuracy of these results and the fact that output is independent to position an orientation shows that this is a viable approach for discriminating sway where output would discriminate the nature of sway and contrast with previous evaluations. Such a system could be implemented at low cost with low complexity, data storage and data transmission rates. For use in the home or central clinics.

4.2 Other applications

The above quasi-steady application of the distributive sensing approach has been used to discriminate differences in human motion both in simulated health and some sport applications. Here, rather than attempting to derive parameters associated only with spatial information, features captured in the time dimension have been used to delineate variations in motion or for sizing moving parts of the body rather than to determine the static parameters of say the size of feet.

Successful examples have been applied to sport, when determining variations in motion from the ideal or norm respectively. Examples selected were those where the human subject did not move their point of contact during motion, as illustrated in figures 10a and 10b respectively. These figures illustrate a sport application, and sway corresponding with the balance of the subject. Both applications use the same surface.

In a further study, the more complex application to intermittent contact, such as in the discrimination of parameters in gait (Figure 11), or indeed the grouping of gait by type, is showing promise. To achieve acceptable response, there is a need to match the dynamics of the sensing structure to the application. To illustrate the performance that has been achieved in terms of a tangible value, the positional error associated with foot impact position is less than 7% of the full surface range (Elliott et al. 2007).

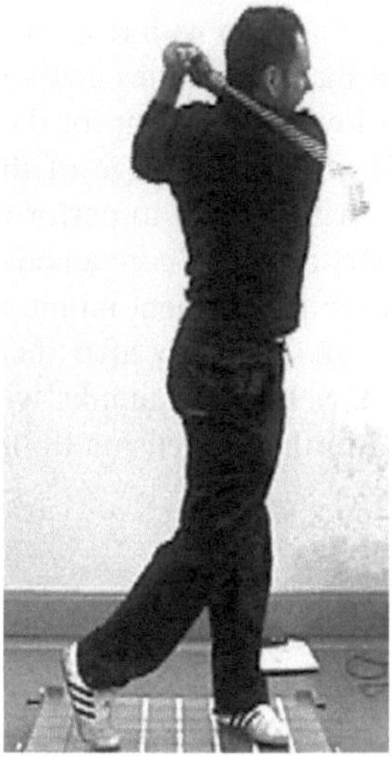

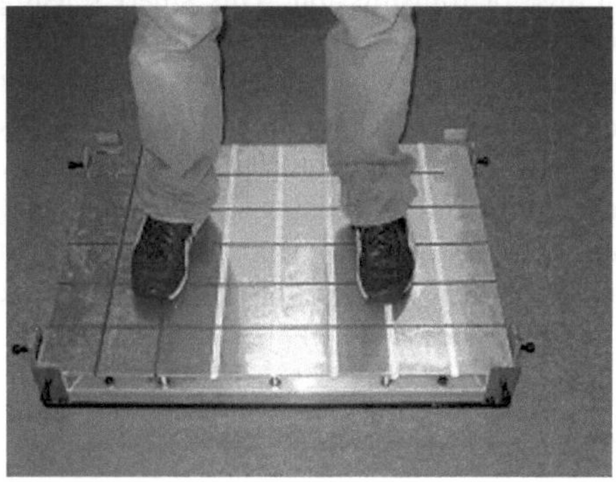

Fig. 10a. Sport Application **Fig. 10b.** Monitoring Sway

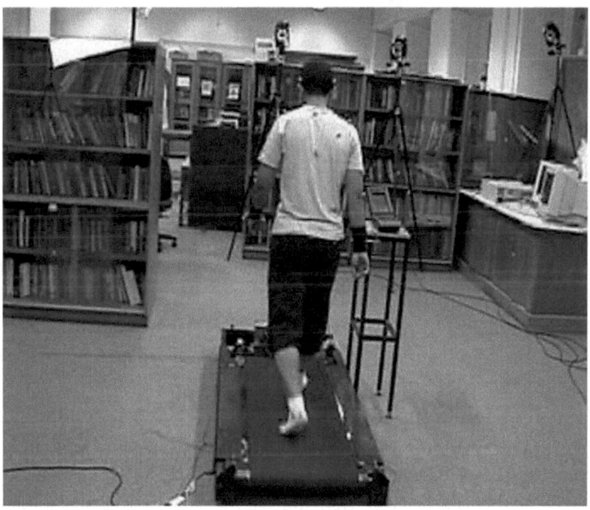

Fig. 11. A surface as part of a treadmill used to discriminate gait

5. Conclusions

This chapter has illustrated the merits and types of application of a distributive tactile sensing surface. A sensing system with appropriate attributes to retrieve information on patients in health monitoring and measurement has been demonstrated and the performance described. It is an ideal technology from the viewpoint of mechanical simplicity and robustness. This is especially so with respect to the practical nature of deriving information directly from data time series coupled through the deformation of a surface such that there is a low requirement for data storage or transmission. This smart sensing approach is at an early stage of the technology where the understanding of design strategies with respect to performance and nature of applications are beginning to be understood. For compunetics and care, there is significant potential for the approach in remote patient monitoring and for discriminating patient pathology, or response and recovery after therapy. In the future, sensing systems outputting information, as in this example, will add benefit to the efficiency of healthcare and will add a further dimension to the management of patient information with regard to health.

Acknowledgments

The authors would like to acknowledge the research on this topic by P. Tongpadungrod, M T. Elliott, I. Petra and D. J. Holding. The research has been partially supported by the Engineering and Physical Sciences Research Council in the UK.

References

Adkin, A.L., Bloem, B.R., Allum, J.H.J.: Trunk sway measurements during stance and gait tasks in parkinson's disease. Gait & Posture 22, 240–249 (2005)

Brett, P.N., Stone, R.S.: A technique form measuring the contact force distribution in minimally invasive procedures. In: Proc. IMechE Part H4, vol. 211, pp. 309–316 (1997)

Brett, P.N., Tam, B., Holding, D.J., Griffiths, M.V.: A Flexible Digit with tactile feedback for invasive clinical applications. In: 10th IEEE Conference on Mechatronics & Machine Vision in Practice, Perth (December 2003)

Ellis, R.E., Ganeshan, S.R., Lederman, S.J.: A tactile sensor based on thin-plate deformation. Robotica 12, 343–351 (1994)

Elliott, M., Ma, X., Brett, P.N.: Determining The location of an Unknown Force Moving along a Plate Using the Distributive Sensing Method, Sensors and Actuators, part A. Physics (2007)

Evans, B.S., Brett, P.N.: Computer simulation of the deformation of dough-like materials in a parallel plate gripper. In: Proc. IMechE, Part B, vol. 210, pp. 119–130 (1996)

Freitas, S., Wieczorek, S.A., Marchetti, P.H., Duarte, M.: Age-related changes in human postural control of prolonged standing. Gait & Posture 22, 322–330 (2005)

Henriksen, M., Lunda, H., Moe-Nilssen, R., Bliddal, H., Danneskiod-Samse, B.: Test-retest reliability of trunk accelerometric gait analysis. Gait and Posture 19, 288–297 (2004)

Holweg, E.: Autonomous control in dextrous gripping, PhD thesis, Delft University of Technology, Delft, Netherlands (1996)

Jonsson, E., Seiger, A., Hirschfeld, H.: One-leg stance in healthy young and elderly adults: a measure of postural steadiness? Clinical Biomechanics 19, 688–694 (2004)

Khodabandehloo, K.: Robotic Meat Cutting. In: IMechE Symposium on Mechatronics, Cambridge, UK (1990)

Lord, S.R.: Vision, balance and falls in the elderly. Geriatric Times 4(6) (2003)

Ma, X., Brett, P.N.: A novel distributive tactile sensing technique for determining the position, width and intensity of a distributed load. Transactions of the IEEE on instrumentation and measurement systems 51(2) (April 2002)

Ma, X., Brett, P.N., Wright, M.T., Griffiths, M.V.: A flexible digit with tactile feedback for invasive clinical applications. In: Proc. IMechE, part H, No: H3, vol. 218, pp. 151–157 (2004)

Miller, J.L.: Parkinson's disease primer. Geriatric Nursing 23(2), 69–75 (2002)

Raibert, M.H., Tanner, J.E.: Design and implementtation of a VLSI tactile sensing computer. In: Pugh, E. (ed.) Robot sensors: Tactile and Non-vision, Kempston, UK, vol. 2, pp. 145–155. IFS publications, North-Holland (1989)

Stone, R.S., Brett, P.N.: A novel approach to distributive tactile sensing. In: Proc. IMechE part B4, vol. 210 (1996)

Tam, B., Brett, P.N., Holding, D.J., Griffiths, M.: The experimental per-formance of a flexible digit retrieving tactile information relating to clinical applications. In: Proc. 11th IEEE Int. Conf. Mechatronics and Machine Vision in Practice, Macao, 30 November -1 December (2004)

Trace, M.: The sizing of feet by the distributive approach to tactile sensing. Thesis, Mechanical Engineering, University of Bristol, UK (1996)

Tongpadungrod, P., Rhys, D., Brett, P.N.: An approach to optimise the critical sensor locations in a 1 dimensional novel distributive tactile surface to maximise performance. International Journal of Sensors and Actuators, Permagon (2004)

Tongpadungrod, P., Brett, P.N.: Orientation detection and shape discrimination of an object on a flat surface using the distributive tactile sensing technique. In: Proc. 9th IEEE Conference on Mechatronics and Machine Vision in Practice, Thailand (2002)

Tongpadungrod, P., Brett, P.N.: The performancecharacteristics of a novel distributive method for tactile sensing. In: Proc. 7th IEEE Conference on Mechatronics and Machine Vision in Practice, Hervey Bay, Australia (September 2000)

User-Centered Design of Tele-Homecare Products

T.N. van Schie[1], M. Schot[1], M. Schoone-Harmsen[1], P.M.A. Desmet[2], A.J.M. Rövekamp[1], M.B. Van Dijk[2]

[1]TNO Quality of Life, PO Box 2215, 2300 CE Leiden, The Netherlands

[2]Delft University of Technology, Industrial Design Engineering, Landbergstraat 15, 2628 CE Delft, The Netherlands

Abstract Tele-homecare solutions tend to be mainly technology driven innovations. This means that the needs of patients easily come in second as it comes to these developments. This chapter proposes that, instead, people's needs should be the driving force of a development, and a basic approach for need-driven product innovation is introduced. The approach is based on the notion that all people share the same universal concerns. When people become ill, their every day life may change dramatically. They are no longer able to meet with specific concerns; a need is born. In an application study, gaps in the current assortment of tele-homecare products were identified by mapping the unmet concerns of ill people coming from this change in their life. The method proved to be a valuable addition to traditional methods inventorying people's needs like interviews or focus groups.

In the subsequent phases of the design process, generating ideas and forming them into products, the user can be involved in many different ways. Involving the user in the design process will lead to products that are a better fit for the needs of the user.

Keywords: tele-homecare, user-centered design, care-pull, concern, need, usability testing, design process, focus group.

Table of contents

K. Yogesan et al. (Eds.): Handbook of Digital Homecare, BIOMED, pp. 221–242.
springerlink.com

1. Technology pushed versus care-pull

There are different starting points for developing products. The starting point of a technology pushed strategy is to develop a product first and then find a market for it by identifying or creating a fitting need. A care-pull approach first identifies an existing need and then develops a product to fulfill the need.

The area of tele-homecare is primarily technology pushed. A care-pull approach means developing from the perspective of human needs. The goal of the care-pull approach of tele-homecare products is to develop 'care' that fits the user, and in this way improves the user's quality of life.

The development of products in healthcare is driven by many motives. Different parties have an interest in the product qualities from different perspectives, like budget optimization, cost-effectiveness, work-quality, care-quality, productivity, efficiency etcetera. This may lead to conflicting requirements. Patient organizations strive for more influence and empowerment of the patient in the development of healthcare products.

Good designers will always, from an early stage on, incorporate views and preferences of the targeted users into their design. Products that are designed and developed with the end user in mind will better comply with the final use situation. Those products will have a far greater chance to succeed and to fit the actual needs that patients have. Continuous interaction with the future user is crucial to stay focused and not end the design process with a product the user was not waiting for. Too often, at the moment the user is involved in the process, all major design decisions have already been made and the user's influence on the final product is negligible.

Conclusion

A user-centered approach of product design starts from the needs of users (care-pull) and strives for continuous interaction with users throughout the design process.

2. User-centered design: how to involve users

Product-development processes involve several stages. In each stage, user-centered design means something different and various techniques may be used to involve patients/end users. For our reflection five phases are distinguished: the exploration, analysis, idea generation, optimization, and realization phases

In the exploration phase, the problem is defined and articulated. A problem can be introduced by patients themselves, but also be derived from evaluation of health practice in literature or from discussions with care professionals, informal caregivers, healthcare researchers, etc. Finding the actual needs lying behind the formulated problems is a real challenge. Often people cannot articulate these deeper needs. Therefore a conceptual analysis of human needs, which can be mapped on the specific situation of the target group, is a powerful instrument. This approach is described in the first part of the chapter.

In the analysis phase, the developer/designer focuses on the selected need. Contact with the target group is essential to gain insight into this. Do users recognize this need? Interviewing techniques will help users to formulate their needs in more detail. Finally the need is operationalized and incorporated in design restrictions specifying the product idea. These restrictions set the boundaries of the solution space.

In the idea generation phase, a single need can be met with a variation of solutions. In the idea generation phase all sorts of creativity techniques can be used to generate solutions. In this phase open minded users may help to get new points of view and critically appraise ideas. Simple presentation techniques may be used to show the essence of an idea and confront users and other interested parties. Consensus on a final concept will be the starting point of the next phase.

In the optimization phase, the selected concept is detailed. This means that details are filled in tested with target group users. For this purpose simple and easy-made prototypes are useful. Ideally this phase is very interactive because the design is still open for iterations. Users participating in the focus groups must be able to grasp the ideas behind the prototype. An important aspect (especially for healthcare products) is the feasibility of the organizational context of a product.

In the realization phase, final design choices are made. The product definition may benefit greatly from interaction with users. Especially the look and feel of the product, user interface and handling can be optimized through interaction with the users in usability testing.

In figure 1, the described process is visualized in a schematic model. Note that in the actual design process, the steps are not necessarily strictly separated and elements of one phase may be used in the next. Also ongoing knowledge may lead to reconsidering earlier choices, so the process is in reality not linear but cyclic.

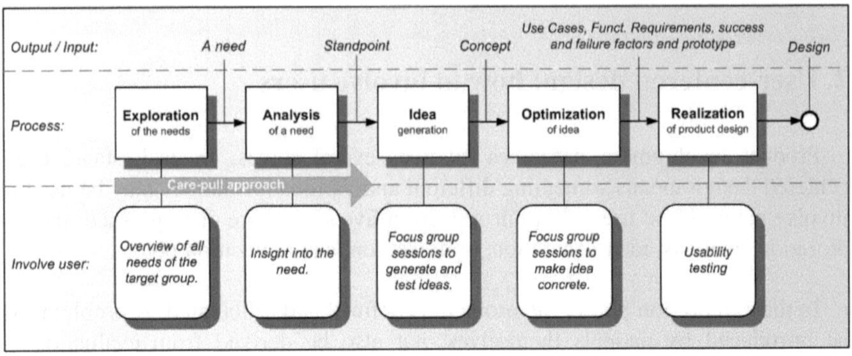

Fig. 1. User involvement during the design process

Conclusion:

Throughout the design process, involvement of the user is possible in many ways. Intensive interaction between the design team and intended users in each development phase will lead to products that better fit with these users' needs.

3. Phase 1 - Exploring the needs

A care pull approach requires a thorough study of the needs that people have. We start by providing some definitions:

A concern is a universal human principle. When the circumstances don't meet a concern, a need is formed. A concern is like a child, it's quiet as long as the circumstances match the ideal situation at certain level. As long as the child is satisfied, you won't hear it, everything is fine. But when the child starts crying, this indicates it needs sleep, food, or a new diaper. The crying stops when the need is fulfilled. In case of needs, it is the same. When the needs are fulfilled, the person won't be aware of them. When the circumstances deviate considerably from the condition of satisfaction, the concern suddenly becomes tangible. This results in a need. The existence of a need depends on the circumstances, and is therefore temporary. Basic needs, like food and shelter, will be present for lifetime. Others will only exist for a few minutes.

Concerns can either be met or not. When a concern is not met, the concern 'awakes' and the person will try to meet this concern; the person will develop a need.

To find out what concerns are unfulfilled in a certain target group, different approaches can be used. The most common way is to interview target group users. This approach is limited, however, because most people are not aware of all their concerns. According to Frijda (1988), the following events indicate an unfulfilled concern:

- Action: a person takes action to accomplish a certain situation
- Desire: a person expresses the wish to achieve a certain situation
- Emotion: a person shows an emotional reaction after a certain situation is achieved/ isn't achieved.

In case of a certain action or desire it might be clear which concern must be fulfilled. In case of an emotion, it will be much more difficult to understand, what concern is the cause of that emotion. So by interviewing people, probably, only the most obvious needs will be mentioned.

The ability to capture a more detailed overview of unmet concerns of a certain group can be facilitated by an overview of all human concerns in general. In the current project, various psychological theories were reviewed in order to assemble a complete overview of basic human concerns.

Studying different concern theories was the basis for creating a general profile of human concerns. The difficulty in understanding underlying concerns is that the number and the variety of human concerns is endless. Various typologies of concerns have been developed in the fields of organizational behavior (e.g. Maslow 1943), personality psychology (e.g. Murray 1938), social psychology (e.g. Rokeach 1973), and consumer behavior (e.g. Hanna 1980).

3.1 Human concerns

There is a large number of theories and models on human concerns. The most relevant theories about concerns used for the overview are: Maslow's Hierarchy of needs, the CIN model, Action Tendency of Frijda and Taxonomy of Human Goals of Ford & Nichols.

Hierarchy of needs

Maslow's Hierarchy of needs (Maslow 1979) is one of the best known descriptions of needs. It not only identifies five basic needs, it also shows how higher needs are not considered until lower-level needs are met.

Control Identity Novelty model

This is an interconnected model of the individual needs created by the authors of changing minds.org. What makes it really useful is the simple focus it gives to three key needs, and it shows how other needs are causally interconnected. CIN stands for Control, Identity and Novelty, which is the general priority order in which we experience them. Our Sense of Control tells us when we are safe and can bend our environment to our purposes. Our Sense of Identity tells us who we are, especially in relation to other people. Our Sense of Novelty tells us that we are learning, improving and evolving. It also helps us compete.

Action Tendency

Frijda developed a multiple theory centered on 'action tendency'. He defines emotions as a person's tendency to express a certain behavior, driven by certain concerns. Frijda (1988) divided concerns in three groups: 1) food, drinking and sex; 2) self-respect, and 3) appreciation of others.

Taxonomy of Human Goals

The Taxonomy of Human Goals (Ford and Nichols 1987) includes six different types of goals. Task goals represent desired outcomes of interactions with primarily non-social aspects of the environment. Social relationship goals represent desired outcomes associated with the ways we relate to other people. Some of those outcomes are primarily self-enhancing (self-assertive goals) and some are primarily other-enhancing (integrative goals).

The other three types of goals included in the Taxonomy focus on internal psychological states. Affective goals represent emotional and feeling states we might like to experience. Cognitive goals represent desired outcomes associated with perceiving and thinking. Finally, subjective organization goals represent psychological states that people may seek to experience involving a complex pattern of thoughts and feelings

These theories all identify a survival level, a self-respect level, and a growth level. Based on these theories, Schot (2008) has assembled a general profile of human concerns that was aimed to be both comprehensive (i.e. give a complete overview) and structured (i.e. give a clear overview). The profile includes three main concern layers:

- Concern for well-being. These basic preconditions are: physiological needs, intimacy, pleasure and autonomy. When these preconditions are out of balance in someone's life, the person will become physically or mentally ill.
- Concern for being. The 'growth' layer has been named the 'being' layer. This layer concerns the forming of a personality; self-development. Self-development consists of multiple facets: developing a personal identity, social relations, giving meaning to life, and task goals.
- Concern for control versus novelty. Compared to Maslow this model added a covering layer: the 'control versus novelty' layer. The need for control and novelty are the motives in daily life.

Schot (2008) developed a metaphor, shown in figure 2, to illustrate in what way the different concern layers play a role in one's life. The green and red characters on the person's shoulders respectively represent 'novelty' and 'control'. In every situation these factors involve a person's choices. The person walks his life path and meets different situations and events. 'Well-being' can be seen as the fuel to walk on. In case the fuel is disturbed the person's walk on the life path stagnates. The person focuses on the development of his or her 'being'. This influences the direction of the life path he walks.

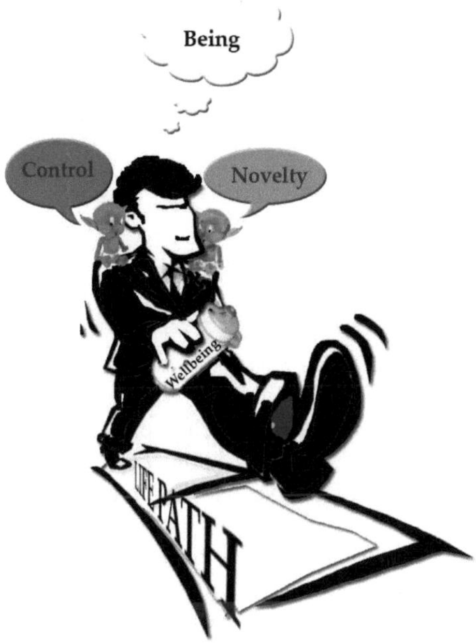

Fig. 2. Metaphor of role of concerns in one's life.

3.2 The profile of all human concerns

The profile of Schot, figure 3, shows an overview of all basic human concerns. The profile consists of three categories: the concerns that drive people (i.e. the need for control and the need for novelty);the concerns which relate to the outer world (i.e. the concern for meaning of life, task goals and identity in relationships); the concerns of wellbeing, which relate to the inner world (i.e. the concern to have pleasure, autonomy, physiological and intimacy).

People strive to have all the concerns fulfilled. It is not important how these concerns are fulfilled, as long as they are fulfilled in a way that is satisfying, which depends on the person and his/her specific situation.

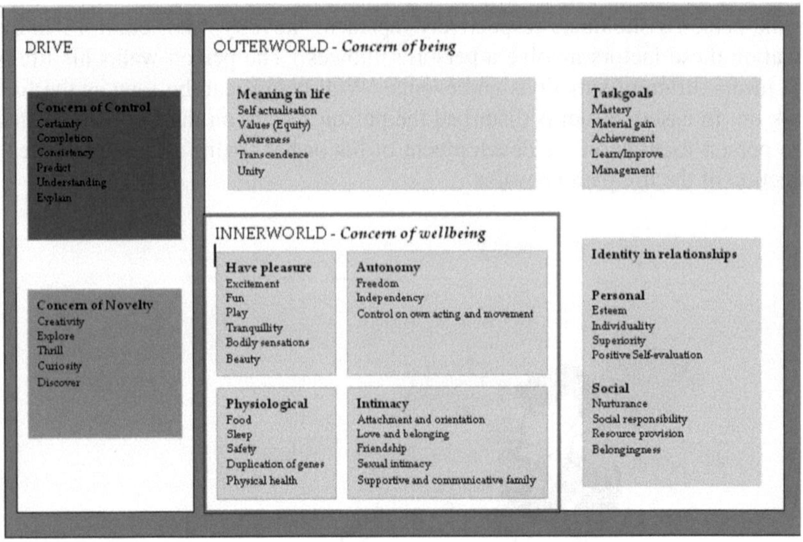

Fig. 3. Schot's profile of all human concerns (Schot 2008).

When people become ill, the circumstances of their every day life changes dramatically. As a result, not all concerns can be met in the way people were used to. A profile of all unmet concerns of ill people can be created by studying the changed situation.

First, the needs behind the different theories that measure 'quality of life' were analyzed. According to Veenhoven (1996) the quality of life reflects the degree to which needs are fulfilled. Furthermore people's experiences during their illness were researched to check whether the previously created image was complete. Based on these results, a profile of unmet concerns can be assembled.

3.3 How can quality of life be measured?

According to Hoeymans, Picavet and Tijhuis (www.rivm.nl), the quality of life is both objective and subjective. Quality of life consists of relatively objective aspects as well as subjective aspects. Objective aspects concern eventual limitations caused by the illness. Subjective aspects refer to how a person judges his own health. For example, the fact that someone is not able to climb stairs any more is not the only aspect. His own judgment of this restriction also plays a role.

Quality of life furthermore consists of different dimensions or domains. The most important are the physical, psychological and social domain. These can be subdivided in smaller dimensions, e.g. physical functioning and pain; both part of the physical domain of the quality of life. The psychological domain includes psychological problems, such as fear and depressed feelings. The social domain can be described as the degree in which an illness limits the ability to fulfill social roles, for example, the social role in a family, at work, among friends or during leisure time. (Essink-Bot and De Haes 1996). Aspects that are not directly related to illness or healthcare have been left out of consideration. Therefore the term 'healthcare related quality of life' is used rather than just 'quality of life'.

Three instruments to indicate quality of life.

- SF-36: The SF instrument indicates eight dimensions: physical functioning, restrictions in roles caused by physical limitations, physical pain, experienced health, vitality, social functioning, restrictions in roles caused by emotional problems, and mental health. De SF-36 is also known as RAND-36. (www.sf-36.org)
- EuroQol: The EQ-6D describes the quality of life for the following six dimensions: mobility, self care, daily activities, pain or other complaints, fear/depression and cognition. (www.euroqol.org)
- COOP WONCA to measure health as a functional status: The COOP/WONCA charts reflect the patients' assessment of his/her functional capacity at the given time. The charts measure six core aspects of functional status: physical fitness, feelings, daily activities, social activities, change in health and overall health. In addition, pain can be included as an optional aspect. (Weel 1995)

3.4 Adaptive Tasks

The Dutch Institute for Healthcare and Welfare has formulated an instrument to measure how people experience their illness. (Pool et al. 2003). The instrument measures the activities that someone has to undertake to give his illness a place in his life; this is called the adaptive tasks (Pool and Egtberts 2001). The principle of this instrument is finding balance. Four different Adaptive tasks are used:

- illness-related (e.g. finding a new balance between activities and rest),
- personal-related (e.g. adjust personal meaning of life),
- social related (e.g. keep social contact and learn to be alone),
- material related (e.g. taking care of aids and adjustments).

Conclusion

Different parties all approach illness by comparing it to the healthy situation and by looking to what activities people have to undertake to approach a healthy life. Looking to this on a higher level makes clear that this is about the concerns that are not met. The EuroQol, SF/Rand 36 and COOP/Wonca also ask people about their feelings and emotions. Feelings and emotions are an indicator for unmet concerns (Frijda1988).

3.5 Personal experiences of patients

A variety of information sources was used to formulate a vision on the experiences of ill people: autobiographic books, informative books (De pen als lotgenoot 2002; Bergsma 2000; Fest 2001), patient-websites, magazines, (Chronisch ziek 2007), television programs and literature. The following main topics were extracted from these sources: loss of control, feeling uncertain, having physical constraints, less social contacts, more dependent, emotional problems, lower esteem and illness forces to find meaning in life.

Conclusion

The data from the Euroqol, WONCA, Rand 36 and the adaptive tasks were translated into concerns. The experiences of the ill people showed that the overview of the unmet concerns extracted from the questionnaires was complete. Figure 4 shows the concerns that are awake in case of an illness.

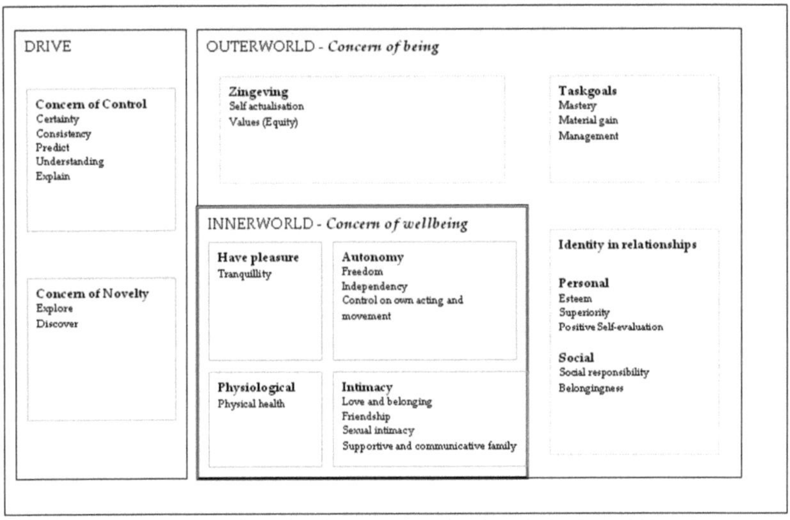

Figure 4. Overview of all unmet concerns of chronically ill people.

3.6 Tele-homecare products

We distinguish two types of tele-homecare products: tele-care and monitoring. Tele-homecare is about taking care of the patient (by for instance by a nurse) as well as prevention. Monitoring is mainly about diagnostics and curing. Figure 5 shows the position of tele-homecare products in healthcare.

Domotica is not a part of tele-products, but is related to tele-products, because it also supports the self management aspect. Domotica is the integration of high technological applications and services in someone's home, with the purpose to improve the quality of life and to support the target groups to be self-reliant.

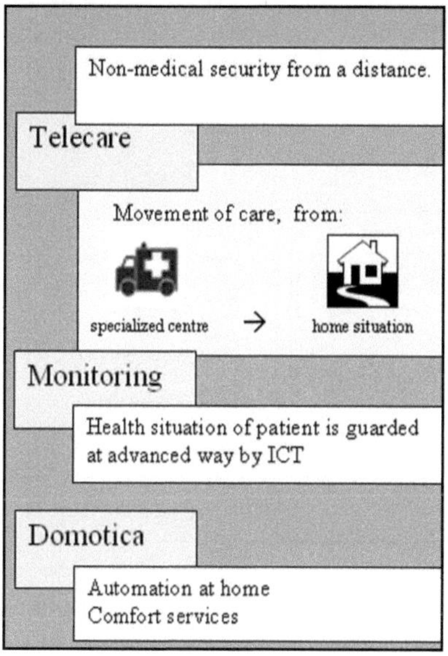

Fig. 5. Tele-homecare

Overview of concerns that are met by current assortment

Until now, there was no overview of the needs that are already fulfilled by the existing products and which are not. With such an overview, the development of the variety of products would be much more consistent with people's needs. This overview can be created by looking at the needs people have when they are confronted with illness or other physical or psychological limitations. This knowledge can give direction for a consistent, overall approach for further developments and shows the gaps in the existing assortment of tele-homecare products.

Therefore the assortment of tele-homecare products used in The Netherlands was studied. The purpose was to give an as broad and complete overview as possible. The products were categorized by their functionality and an interpretation was made to what concerns they meet. Almost all products can be categorized as tele-information, tele-consultation, tele-diagnosis, tele-treatment, tele-referring, tele-monitoring, tele-homecare and/or tele-aftercare.

Conclusion

Almost all products are developed to discover symptoms, to control and to treat them. Tele-products are used to guard the physical health. Camcare, Telekit and De Vertrouwenslijn are exceptions: they also partly meet the concern for Identity.

Figure 6 shows which awake concerns are met with currently available tele-homecare products (in blue), and which not (in white). The need for intimacy is partly met; patient-alarm makes it possible to contact the nurse very fast and some tele-products improve contact with fellow sufferers.

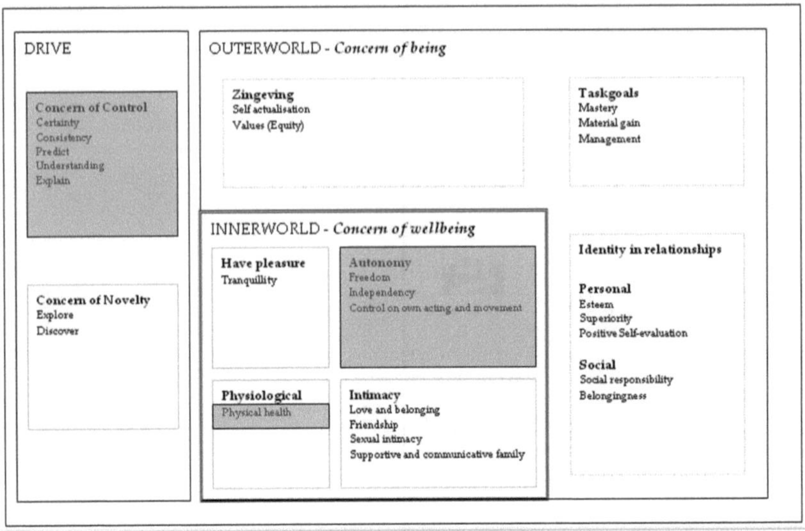

Fig. 6. Blue parts show which of all unmet concerns were met by current variety of tele-homecare products.

The areas where concerns are not yet met are interesting opportunities for product development. These unfulfilled needs can be the input for the next phase, the analysis of a single need.

4. Phase 2: Analysis of a single need

In a care-pull approach, a need is the input of the analysis-phase. That specific need can be brought forward by people working in the field, the target group, scientific research, etcetera. For the current study, it was decided to make an overview of the needs that were still unfilled despite the current available variety of products; see figure 6.

When a specific need is chosen to be the input for this phase, the analysis of a single need, it is important to get familiar with this need; to find out what the need means for the target group and in what way the need can be fulfilled in a way that is satisfying. Therefore, contact with the target group is very important, their stories and experiences will make clear in what direction the solution should be searched for. Questionnaires, autobiographic books, workbooks, diaries and interviews can be used to better understand their situation. Also assumptions can be proposed and discussed with the target group. The purpose of this phase is to understand the situation and to see relations between different factors in order to be able to form a vision. The vision can be summarized in a standpoint, which sets the abstract goal of the rest of the process. Besides focusing on the feedback of the target group it is also important to explore the context of the healthcare system from different perspectives to be able to end up with a feasible design.

During the analysis of this phase a set of design restrictions can be formulated. These restrictions set the boundaries of the solutions space.

Conclusion:

It is important to get in touch with the target group in order to understand the situation and to see relations between different factors in order to be able to form a vision.

Example:

The overview, figure 6, of all unmet concerns of chronically ill people was used as a basis for the development of new tele-homecare products. The analysis of the assortment existing tele-products showed which concerns were still unmet by the current assortment. An explanation of these gaps can be that it seems to difficult to come up with products that can fulfill these needs. By way of a graduation project of an interaction designer, TNO wanted to show that, actually every concern, could be used as input for a care-pull approach. Therefore, one of the unmet concerns, which was not covered by the current variety of tele-homecare products, was selected as input for a care-pull approach. The 'need for identity' was selected to be the input for the development.

During the analysis of the need, people were interviewed and the domain of chronically ill people was explored. This resulted in the vision that everybody has something to add to the world. The output of this phase was the standpoint: *to enable all individuals to use their potential to feel worthy members of society.*

The idea was to offer projects coming from society to a group of ill people. A group, with a lot of knowledge and potential. People can in their own way contribute to society.

The final concept was a radio show, functioning as a mediator between ill people and society. The radio show is their entrance to the world. It fills the living room with new impulses and offers opportunities to join society. During the daily broadcast, different clients offer new projects to the listeners (the ill people). The listeners can sign in on a project and become member of the project group. Every week, the project group shares their progress during the broadcast and the listeners can respond. This concept increases people's happiness in two ways. Joining the radio show and the project group helps people to meet their concerns of identity. Their new activities result in a flow experience.

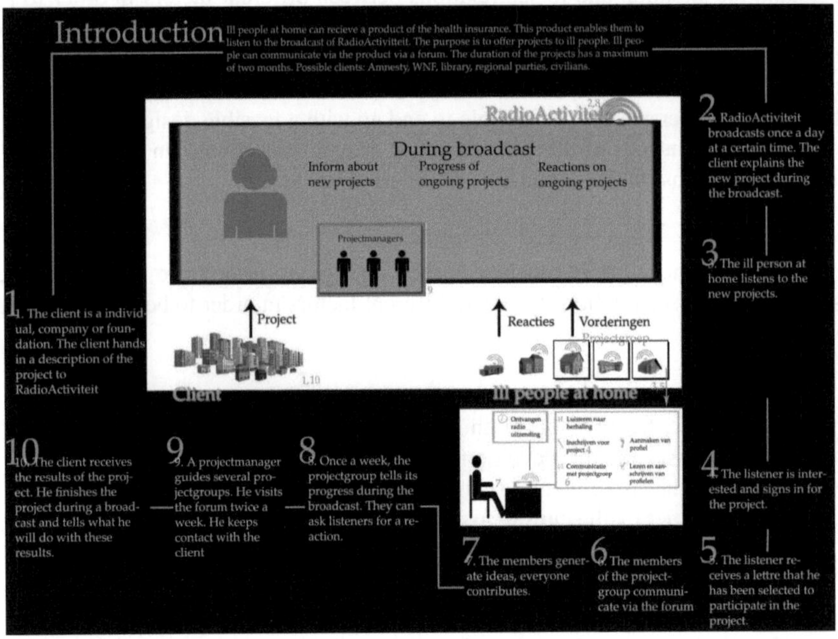

5. Phase 3: Idea generation

After the need is thoroughly analyzed and the design restrictions of the product are described, the creative phase of idea forming can start. Within the design restrictions, the single need can be met with a variety of solutions. In the idea forming phase all sorts of creativity techniques can be used to generate solutions. These creativity techniques may or may not include user involvement.

An inspiring form of idea generation is brainstorming. This may be done with any group of users or care professionals. This means relatively untrained people, as far as the creative process is concerned, but on the other hand people who have an inside knowledge and experience of the use situation and the use opportunities and restrictions. The development or design team can complete the ideas making use of more sophisticated creativity techniques like attribute listing, morphological analysis, story boarding, value engineering and such. For more suggestions see www.creatingminds.org/tools/tools_ideation.htm.

As soon as the first set of ideas is generated and visualized in writing, drawings or other forms of presentation, interaction with other parties outside the design team can be fruitful. Simple presentation techniques may be used to show the essence of an idea and confront users and other interested parties. Obtaining feedback on relatively vague ideas depends greatly on the ability of the designer to present ideas in an appealing way and of the ability of the persons involved to grasp still often abstract solutions and ideas behind ideas. Interaction with open minded users may help to get new points of view and critically appraisal of ideas.

It may require some investment to create a group of people to represent the target group, and to inspire these people into this creative thinking process. Once one or more of these groups are established, they may be of benefit in later stages with the usability tests and also they could be of use in subsequent development projects for the same target group.

The most promising ideas can be combined into one or more product concepts and discussion in focus groups may lead to consensus on a final concept. This will be the starting point for the next phase.

Conclusion

To involve users in the creative process is a challenge, but techniques like brainstorming can be used successfully. The success of user involvement in this phase depends on both the designer being able to present his or her ideas in an adequate way and the participating users to develop some flexibility towards creative thinking.

6. Phase 4: Optimization of idea

In the previous phase, the idea generation, focus group sessions were used to get feedback about proposed ideas. One concept came out as most promising. This concept is the input for the optimization phase, where the concept will be made more concrete. The results of this optimization phase are final functional requirements, a simple and easy-made prototype, use cases and success and failure factors. Like the idea generation phase, the optimization phase also uses focus group sessions.

For many people it is hard to think in an abstract way. Therefore possible functionalities for the concept need to be shown visually instead of describing them by telling. This will prevent miscommunication. The way of visualization can have different forms, depending on what suits the target group and the concept best. A demonstration can "trigger" people to make comments on the functionality that is shown, whereby the discussion starts. During this discussion, the demonstration of the prototype or the playact can be repeated if necessary (see 2. Prototype below).

The participants in the focus group sessions need to be chosen with great care, for they have to be representative for the target group. Adding extra focus group sessions with healthcare professionals, other employees of the healthcare organization and voluntary helpers will be a good enhancement to the overview of the target group and the relevant context.

Method

In the focus group sessions of the optimization phase, three questions will be answered:

- What should be the functionalities of the concept, to fulfill the existing need in an effective way? Deliverables: functional requirements and a prototype;
- What will the interaction with those functionalities look like? Deliverable: use cases;
- What factors would make the implementation and future use a success and what factors would make it fail? Deliverable: success and failure factors

The results of the optimization phase are the answers to these three questions.

Based on experience we found the answers can be categorized into the following four deliverables:

1. Functional requirements
This will be a list of specific requirements of the functionality. After each focus group session this list can be improved.

Example:
TNO wanted to optimize the ZorgGemak concept, which started out as:
"A system that is available in the home of elderly people that increases the empowerment of the healthcare consumer and enables efficient care to be given when needed. This way people can live longer in their own home and in their own social environment." (Rövekamp 2008)

The result of our focus group sessions were some interesting findings about relevant functionalities for ZorgGemak. For example the elderly people told us they would only use a health encyclopedia as additional information, and they could not imagine a health problem for which the encyclopedia would prevent them from going to the general practitioner. The elderly were very enthusiastic about functionalities that would enhance communication with family, friends and neighbors and they also mentioned security functionalities, such as using ZorgGemak video communication to see who stands at their front door, to make direct contact with the police and the possibility for the healthcare organization to open outside doors to let the healthcare professional in. The healthcare professionals we interviewed, urged us to use ZorgGemak for answering practical questions people have about their care, for questions like "When does the doctor or nurse visit me?" are frequently asked.

2. Prototype (demonstration)
The possible functionality needs to be shown in a demonstration, during the focus group session. This can "trigger" the interviewed people to make comments, whereby the discussion starts. A good way of demonstration is to show simple and easy-made prototypes. After each focus group session, the prototype can be re-

vised, based on the findings on which functionalities are relevant and which are not. It must be kept in mind that functionalities should not be set aside too easy, based on the comments of just one person in the session. The design team has to reconsider the functional requirements and the prototype carefully after each session. After the last focus group session in this phase, an easy-made prototype can be shown, that illustrates the definite functional requirements.

It could also be helpful to use paper prototyping. This is basically an example of the possible functionality by a simple prototype on paper. An advantage of this method is that it makes it easy to change the prototype during the focus group session. Also other visual aids are possible, such as illustrating on a white board during the discussion.

Another way of visual demonstration is to let (professional) actors perform a short role-play to show how the proposed product will be used. In this case, the product is fictional, but its functionalities become clear by the role-play (Sato 1999). The use cases are basically the script for the playact. When a playact is used to demonstrate functionality to a focus groups no real prototype is delivered at the end of the phase. The interaction with an imaginary product could sometimes be sufficient to gain a good idea about its functionality.

3. Use cases

A use case is a description of the interaction between an actor and a (computer) system. This actor can be a person, but also another system. A use case describes a series of events, from the actor's point of view (Jacobson 1992). In the optimization phase, simple use cases need to be written as a script for the demonstration with the prototype or the role-play. During this phase, the use cases will become more detailed, because more knowledge is gained about which functionalities are relevant and which are not. This means that some use cases will be discarded and others will be adjusted.

4. Success and failure factors

During the discussions, success and failure factors will be mentioned. These are factors that can improve or frustrate a successful implementation of the product and need to be taken in consideration during the further design, development and implementation of the product.

At the end, the output of this phase is a set of functional requirements, an easy-made prototype to represent the selected functionality, use cases to describe the use of the product and a set of success and failure factors.

Example:
In the earlier described ZorgGemak project, elderly told us they want a good instruction for the use of ZorgGemak. Also the video-helpdesk should be available 24 hours a day. Other failure factors would be too many wires in their homes and high costs for the use of ZorgGemak. The healthcare professionals stated that ZorgGemak would only work if it was integrated with

the electronic health records of the organization. They also mentioned that the video communication with the care consumer should be of good quality in order to do real consultation about health problems. A complaint the healthcare consumers had in a recently ended project, was that there was a lot of background noise and people walking around at the helpdesk during the video communication. This makes it difficult for the elderly to communicate. The interviewed also stated the importance of appropriate clothing of the healthcare professional during the video consult.

7. Phase 5: Realization of product design

The outcome of the previous phase, Optimization of idea, were final functional requirements, an easy-made prototype of the product, use cases and success and failure factors. These deliverables are the input for the realization phase, in which the product design will be developed further. Of course also technical requirements need to be made, but this will not be discussed here, because our focus is on actual user involvement.

To design a good (graphical) user interface, user involvement is necessary by usability testing. During the performance of several usability tests TNO found that elderly persons did not only have problems with the tested applications but also with some aspects of the used evaluation method as well. Therefore, a comparative study (Schie 2008) was performed on four well known methods for usability evaluation and their suitability for elderly persons. The methods are Pluralistic Walkthrough, User Walkthrough, Thinking Aloud method and the Questionnaire method.

Below, these four methods are briefly discussed and our considerations are given for their use when elderly people are involved in the context of telehomecare products. At the end we describe variations on these existing methods, to use with elderly people.

7.1 Pluralistic Walkthrough

With this method representative users, product designers and usability experts evaluate each screen of a user interface as a group. Before discussing a certain screen, each participant writes down his own findings about the usability (Bias 1991).

Considerations

When elderly people participate in such a session, they might have problems with switching between different kind of tasks (inspecting, writing down findings, talking and listening to other people). They also might feel a little insecure about the tasks they have to perform and their knowledge about the subject compared to the rest of the group. In that case, a pleasant atmosphere and some comforting words can help. To represent the group of elderly, a high level of imagination in the situation of the other is asked. Many people of this age find this difficult. Remembering what others said in the group discussion will give more problems than in younger groups. The required level of stress resistance, being able to hear/see and to be able to communicate (reading and writing) might give trouble as well. Other problems can be the formal setting, not being mobile enough to come and the required ability to express oneself.

7.2 User Walkthrough

In the method User Walkthrough the test person gets a test script with exercises and cases. Without any help (except for questions about the script itself or when the person gets stuck) he performs the test script while a test supervisor observes the human-computer interaction.

Considerations

Around the age of 65, test persons would probably not have many problems with the used method. Little problems that might occur have to do with concentration issues and the fact that it could be hard to switch between tasks.

Around the age of 80, the required level of imagination, to understand the situation of a case, might give big problems. Also continuous switching between reading, asking questions and interacting with the interface could give big problems. Some small problems that might arise have to do with the short-term memory of elderly, concentration issues, self confidence and the asked level of stress resistance. Also the required level for hearing/seeing, for communication by reading and for expressing oneself, might be too high.

7.3 Thinking Aloud

In literature, different variations of the Thinking Aloud method were found. We use the following definition of the method: the test supervisor asks a test person questions about the interface and to do exercises, while performing these exercises the test person is asked to think out loud (Nielsen 1993).

Considerations

Test persons around the age of 65 probably will not have many problems with this testing method. Perhaps small problems due to their level of self confidence and their level of being able to express themselves might occur.

For people around the age of 80, these two characteristics will probably cause bigger problems. Beside that, the switching between talking, listening, thinking out loud and interacting with the interface might give big problems, especially because of having to think out loud while performing certain tasks. Also small problems might occur because of the required level of being able to imagine a certain case and the required level of short-term memory, stress resistance and ability to hear.

7.4 Questionnaire method

In addition to a usability test the test person can be asked to give his opinion about the interface by answering a questionnaire. This questionnaire is multiple choice and contains some open areas for suggestions.

Considerations

Test persons in the age of 65 will probably not have many problems with this testing method. Concentration issues and the ability to express oneself might play a role.

Persons in the age of 80 might have more problems. One could find it difficult to switch between the tasks of reading, writing and inspecting the interface. Also their ability to see, the level of concentration and the ability to express themselves could play a role. A big problem could occur with reading the questions and writing down the answers.

This seems to be a very attractive method to use with groups of elderly, but the downside is that it won't test how they actually use the interface. One will only learn about their opinion.

7.5 Alternative

An interesting variation of the Thinking Aloud method is Constructive Interaction (Nielsen 1993). Instead of thinking out loud while interacting with an interface individually, this variation has two persons interact with the interface. The communication between those two people urges them to think aloud. For elderly people who might find it difficult to think out loud while performing a task, this variation could be an interesting alternative. The test supervisor can still hear their thoughts, but now in a more natural way (they talk to each other) which makes them feel more comfortable.

Conclusion

Usability testing of tele-homecare applications for elderly people is complicated by social, physical and psychological factors. The setup of the test should be such that a test group is selected that is representative for the target group. After that, the method that best suits the characteristics of the test group should be selected. These two should never be switched, otherwise the selected group might not be representative. In general, there is no perfect evaluation method available to apply to all elderly persons. Each method has its weaknesses, as previous paragraphs show. Based on a certain group of elderly people with certain characteristics, the most suitable method can be chosen and the weaknesses can be minimized by making some adjustments. An interesting example of such an adjustment is Constructive Interaction (Nielsen 1993).

8. Discussion

In this chapter we focus on user-centered design as one of the essential elements to influence the success in the use-phase of a tele-homecare product. The starting point is a care-pull approach focused on fulfilling actual needs of patients. We claim that intensive interaction with end-users in each development phase will lead to products that are more fitting the needs of these future users. Of course this is not the only factor influencing the success of a tele-homecare product. Especially in healthcare the end-user, i.e. patient, is surrounded by professional and informal care. Products for the patient must also be acceptable for their surroundings, and fit into the working pattern of caregivers.

Focusing on usability is essential as far as the part of the product is concerned that is directly used by the end-user, but a tele-homecare product consists of more than the user interface. Other parts of the product are for instance the interface at the side of the care organization and the whole organizational context. Feasibility study, taking success and failure factors of this organizational context into account, must be part of the early stages of the product development process.

This chapter shows that throughout the design process users can be involved in many different ways. Successful involvement can be achieved when design teams take initiatives to involve users in each phase of the design process. Finding users who are willing and able to take the challenge of thinking along in the design process is crucial. Depending on the phase, different methods and techniques are applicable. Essential is always that the product, from first idea to final form, is presented in a way that is appealing to the users involved.

User-centered design is a way to make a change in the success/failure ratio of tele-homecare products.

References

Bias, R.: Walkthroughs: Efficient collaborative testing. IEEE Software 5, 94–95 (1991)

Brede Inventarisatie Thuismonitoring Projecten en Mogelijkheden (2001)

Chronisch ziek, Magazine Week van de chronisch zieken (2007)

CIN: http://changingminds.org/explanations/needs/cin.htm
De pen als lotgenoot: ervaringen over het leven met een ziekte 5. Verzamenbundel. SWP: cop, Amsterdam (2002)
Desmet, P.M.A., Hekkert, P., Hillen, M.G.: Values and emotions; an empirical investigation in the relationship between emotional responses to products and human values. In: Proceedings of the fifth European academy of design conference, Barcelona, Spain (2003) (in press)
Domotica en telemedecine in het verzekerde pakket: naar nieuwe besluitvormingsprocessen? Een aanzet voor debat, TNO onderzoeksrapport, KvL/P&Z, 092 (2006)
Ford, Nicols: Taxonomy of human goals (1987)
Frijda, N.F.: De emoties: een overzicht van onderzoek en theorie. Bakker, Amsterdam (1988)
Jacobson, I.: Object-Oriented Software Engineering. Addison Wesley Professional, Reading (1992)
Maslow, A.H.: Psychologie van het menselijk zijn. Lemniscaat, Rotterdam, 4e dr (1979)
Monitoring thuiszorg. Deelrapportage Doelgroeponderzoek, TNO-Onderzoeksrapport PG/TG/99.136 (1999)
Nielsen, J.: Usability Engineering. Morgan Kaufmann, San Francisco (1993)
Questionnaires:
TERTZ- Scanformulier. Stap 3f. Kwaliteit van Leven
EQ-5D. Gezondheidsvragenlijst
SIP 68. Sickness Impact Profile
IMPACT: gevolgen van ziekte of handicap voor het dagelijkse leven. Tweede, ingekorte versie;mei (2006)
Rövekamp, A.J.M., et al.: Finding out What Elderly Think of the E-Health Homecare Project ZorgGemak. In: Med-e-tel proceedings 2008, vol. 1, pp. 152–155 (2008)
Sato, S., Salvador, T.: Playacting and Focus Troupes: Theater techniques for creating quick, intense, immersive, and engaging focus group sessions 6(5), 35–41 (1999) Interactions of the ACM, New York ISSN 1072-5520
van Schie, T., Rövekamp, A.J.M., Dumay, A.C.M.: Methoden voor usability evaluatie met senioren (in press, 2009)
Schot, M.: Graduation report: Design for happiness. To meet the concerns of ill people at home (2008)
van Weel, C., König – Zahn, C., Touw Otten, F.W.M.N, van Duijn, N.P., de Meyboom Jong, B.: Measuring functional health status with the COOP/WONCA Charts. A manual (1995)
www.rivm.nl/vtv/object_document/o2297n18749.html

A Multi-disciplinary Approach towards the Design and Development of Value$^+$ eHomeCare Services

Ann Ackaert(1), An Jacobs(2), Annelies Veys(2), Jan Derboven(3), Mieke Van Gils(3), Heidi Buysse(4), Stijn Agten(5), Piet Verhoeve(6)

(1) IBBT – UGent/IBCN, Belgium, 32 9 331 49 35, ann.ackaert@intec.ugent.be

(2) IBBT – VUB/SMIT, Belgium, an.jacobs@vub.ac.be, annelies.veys@vub.ac.be

(3) IBBT – K.U.Leuven/CUO, Belgium, jan.derboven@soc.kuleuven.be, mieke.vangils@soc.kuleuven.be

(4) IBBT – UGent/MIG, Belgium, Heidi.Buysse@ugent.be

(5) IBBT – Hasselt University – tUL/EDM, Belgium, stijn.agten@uhasselt.be

(6) Televic N.V., Belgium, P.Verhoeve@televic.com

Abstract *Do you need spells, magic potions or wizard's knowledge to approach the eHomeCare market in a successful way?* The design and development of eHomeCare services consumes a lot of effort, time and money. Needs and value chain aspects of the eHealth(care) market are complex and sometimes unexpected factors arise during the introduction and first use of technology in the homecare setting. Take up ratios of new products and services are furthermore critical in the return on investment curve. Within this chapter we want to elaborate and share the methodology developed within the IBBT eHomeCare projects Coplintho and TranseCare, used to design and develop ICT related products and services in the homecare field. This implies putting user research up front and working with an interdisciplinary team. This chapter does not claim to offer exhaustive and theoretical knowledge on the subject, but it gives an overview of the practical insights we gained during the passed years. Often references are given for further literature study. Feedback on the subject is greatly encouraged and appreciated.

K. Yogesan et al. (Eds.): Handbook of Digital Homecare, BIOMED, pp. 243–267.
springerlink.com

Table of contents

1 Get the picture right

1.1 Making a snapshot

An overall snapshot of the methodology deployed in the IBBT Coplintho and TranseCare projects on eHomeCare services can be viewed in Figure 1. Since the start of IBBT in 2005, user research has been put up front in collaborative R&D projects for application domains such as eHealth. This chapter will elaborate on the different aspects depicted in the drawing and we will try to share our methodology and experience with the reader. The scope, the team aspects and the need to look at the overall contextual mapping of eHomeCare services will be depicted in par 1. The user needs will be covered in par 2. The value net and value proposition can be found in par 3. The methodology used in the personas, scenarios and the script book are elaborated in par 4, while par 5 describes the need for a continuous evaluation design approach based on user centered design principles. How we elaborated on real life tests is written in par 6. The arrows show the interaction and feedback mechanisms at play in the different building blocks of the process. To conclude we describe a SWOT analyses for our methodology in par 7. Of course this is a snapshot in time as interdisciplinary R&D methodologies in itself are subject to research and continuous evolution.

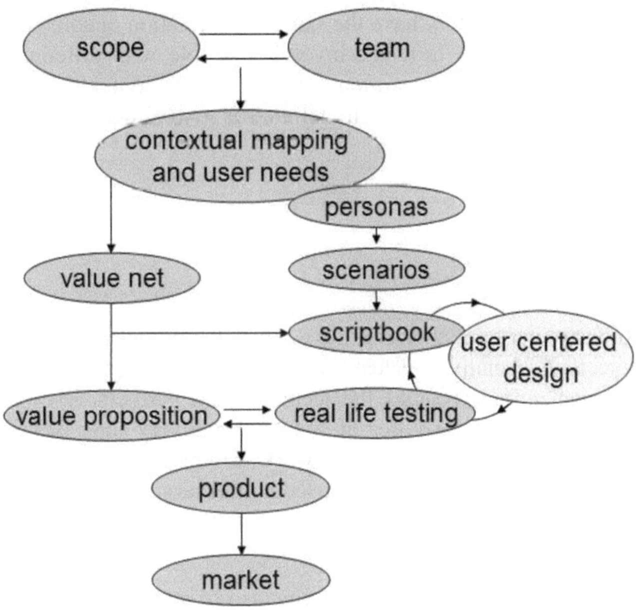

'Figure 1: Methodology deployed in the IBBT Coplintho and TranseCare projects

1.2 Setting the scope

The problems related to chronic disease management in combination with an ageing society are dominant in many countries (EU, US, Asia). eHealth is often stated as one of the factors that could milder the problems healthcare will encounter in the future. On the other hand however eHealth also comprises a lot of fuzzy ideas and definitions. What is eHealth exactly, what does it cover, what is left out of its context? Finding a concise definition of the concept is often a challenge in its own!

The definition of eHomeCare services used within the context of this chapter is highlighted in the box. This does not mean that this is the only valid definition of the terminology eHomeCare Service, but illustrates that it is important to start from a definition taken in consensus by the multidisciplinary project team!

> For the scope of this chapter the definition *eHomeCare Services* is used for "the delivery of (distant) (health)care services at home using ICT and involving (health)care professionals, the patient and the non-professional caregiver".

Just like getting the correct definition it is essential that you get a clear and a concise vision of what you want to realize. Take enough time to discuss the context and definition of your objectives and clarify the wordings. Cross checking that all team members really have the same interpretation of some key-wordings is very important, certainly in teams involving people with different backgrounds. Nearly identical terminology is often used in different contexts. It can save a lot of time at a later stage of the project to get a clear mutual understanding of the level and scope of the project ambition.

1.3 Find a good team

Multidisciplinary collaboration between industry and academia is inherent to IBBT-projects. Especially in eHealth-projects the inclusion of social science partners and organizations, besides the technological partners, is of utmost importance. In addition to the own area of competence, every actor has a specific common knowledge and jargon (e.g. a 'network' can be interpreted as a social versus computer network). Sharing this knowledge and jargon is thus a prerequisite for further communication and interaction throughout the project. The use and setting-up of a glossary in this context is important.

The mental process of both groups can also be stipulated as different. Technological partners seem to think in a very logic / rational way. Then they write down every problem schematically, almost in an 'if – then – else' way. They come up with technical use case scenario's, often based on their own experiences (or people they know) as potential users. On the other hand, social partners tend to discuss and evaluate all options before coming to a conclusion. For both partners it is difficult to handle these contrasting approaches. Social partners describe technological partners as "they put it too simple, they rationalize too much". On the other hand, technological partners describe the social research methodology as "beating around the bush". The project team should be aware of this hurdle, especially in meetings.

Another conspicuous point to take into account is that some social partners are not always aware of the technological possibilities. Currently they live in a communication world in which paper, telephone and face-to-face contacts are of great value. However, once they see the possibilities technology (or in this case ICT) can offer, they want a million things at once and have difficulties to articulate their ideas in a way the project team can implement them. Working with realistic real-life use-cases is hereby a solution. Convincing them is one hurdle, but even more important is keeping things simple and functional. A network going down, not having access to necessary (health-related) results / values is not acceptable in the healthcare setting end can be a reason to reject new supporting ICT-tools and going back to old habits. Thus, full technologically testing at different locations under different circumstances before testing the use-cases is of inestimable value (see also par 6).

Working with these types of interdisciplinary teams, involving people from different companies, organizations and research groups has proven to be both a challenge and richness to the IBBT eHomeCare projects.

1.4 Look at the contextual mapping

Independent living means more than staying at home. Quality of life for elderly people or chronically ill, often implies a good balance between proximity and autonomy in their daily life activities. Care networks and care needs are often complex and multi-dimensional.

Co-morbidity in many cases calls for a multi-disciplinary team surrounding and supporting the individual at need. Active life style coaching (regarding diet, physical activity, self-management etc.) has proven to be able to empower the chronically ill and prolong the stay at home. Safety and the feeling of being surrounded ("somebody will be able to come and help me at a time of need") seem to be pre-dominant factors for comforting elderly people. eHomeCare services are all about supporting the user within his/her own daily life context in a likeable and fashionable way. The adaptation and take-up ratio of these ICT services will largely depend on the seamless integration in existing life patterns and on the compliance with a real-needs-based approach.

eHomeCare applications could lead to a changing paradigm in healthcare practice, inducing a more "*need-based*" approach, in which applications are not solely focusing on medical purposes but also on care and social inclusion.
eHomeCare services should be designed in such a way that they put the ptient in the centre, offering adequate support at the place and time of need!

As homecare is multi-disciplinary and often involves several organizations, a paradigm shift towards a patient-centered needs-based approach will induce a change process for all actors involved. Specifically in healthcare the organizational mechanisms and value chain at place today are often complex and non-transparent. This implies that putting new eHomeCare services on the market could be blocked by these types of bottlenecks. It is important to identify potential obstacles for real market penetration from the beginning of the development process. Involving as many "actors" as possible from the beginning, or a least deploy a good communication and dissemination activity towards these actors can be very beneficial.

2 Investigate the needs

2.1 The who's and what's

Knowing that *user needs for new products and technology are very dynamic*, because of both internal and external mechanisms of change and stability [1] the investigation of those needs as a basis for a more user centered design approach is a complex endeavor in general. In healthcare the picture is even more complicated. Today the current paradigm in healthcare lies within the clinical validation of applications. Efficiency and productivity are both not enough to develop successful new homecare solutions. Other needs have to be integrated as well in this kind of applications to leverage the take up and smooth less integration in the current work field.

The choice who's and which kind of needs one wants to support with the technology under development has to be made explicit. To go beyond the medical centricity and look into the potential impact on the quality of life of people, patients and their caregivers, both formal and informal, more holistic approach is necessary. This is no easy exercise, since the healthcare sector is a complex institutional field, gathering different stakeholders with current habits, interests, power, roles, needs and expectations.

All those persons have to be considered as users of the system, though the person in need of care is the pivotal. Those users are not limiting the technological innovation, but are part of the solution offering insight in the evolution of future developments that fit into the daily worlds of the users to be [2]. To gain those insights, a *multi-stakeholder approach* is used, which is not limited to the fuzzy front-end of the process, but which is pursued throughout the project. Roughly three different angles can be named: a phase of limiting the projects aspirations (par 2.2), a phase of setting the stage by using the available knowledge on the user needs (par 2.3) and a phase of gathering through the project new insights on the unmet users needs and dreams (par 2.4).

2.2 Limiting the user group

A first phase aims to identify and to select potential patient groups for which the technology will be developed. The creation of a project is often based on an abstract concept of a target group active in people's head, or a kind of average user or somebody with needs they know personally. To gain a multi-perspective way of looking at your target group it helped us a lot to pursue the following method (a) gathering of epidemiological data, socio-demographic data; (b) identifying relevant inclusion criteria based on the project proposal to select patient groups;(c) qualitative weighing on the inclusion criteria to include potential patient groups in discussion with health care experts and (d) plenary discussion with all partners in the project [3], [4]. This exercise is so essential that it can not be recycled. Your can not just recycle your user groups of the previous project without questioning them, if you don't want to miss new opportunities for innovation. The first abstract description of the target group within the Coplintho project was chronically ill patients. Epidemiological data and expert interviews taught us how to make a rational choice between different pathologics. Based on the qualitative weighing, we limited ourselves to two groups of people: diabetics type II and people with Multiple Sclerosis (MS). At the other hand the project also learned, that one of the big challenges of eCare applications is to offer support for people having very dynamic needs, based on multiple pathologies. Therefore we started the TranseCare project by questioning the concept of dependencies in itself and we choose to define the user group starting from the operational definition of dependencies as used in the homecare sector in Belgium (so called Katz- or Weckscale).

2.3 Looking for the known needs fitting in their everyday practices

In practice, this first phase is concurrent with the second phase by doing what we call a *domain analysis*. This analysis is based on a search in literature, documents, having exploratory interviews with relevant stakeholders. Then the social scientists in the project team make an inventory of the different dimensions in everyday life of the (selected) target groups reflected in a reference document. For instance what is the effect on daily life activities for MS-patients, what are the peculiarities of this illness? This information is recombined with the visions and expectations of the project, and crystallizes in *social use cases* or so called work scenarios. In a group session the user researchers define some basic characters, describe a regular day or days in the users life, including details on their social life and degree of dependency (cfr. persona and scenario's described in par 4).

These stories are then used as an object of discussion from social, economical, ethical, legal and technical perspectives for all project partners, thus serving as a tool to prioritize the applications to be made. Within the Coplintho project it became clear that since MS is characterized by diminishing motor abilities, writing and typing are no viable options for every patient. Having an easy-to-use and time efficient voice-driven diary application was seen as an opportunity within technical reach of the research plans. After this prioritizing exercise a translation of the selected applications and services in technical use cases is made.

Because of the need for the project to have these scenarios as soon as possible, it is very difficult for the social scientist to dispose of more than an educated guess based on the available literature and expert information on some technical choices to be made. Therefore having iterations, through subsequent projects with more or less the same consortium, has proven to be a real advantage within the TranseCare project. Another approach, as developed in other IBBT projects, is to have an in-between user needs gathering phase by using more experimental methods, which will be described in the next section.

2.4 Looking for future needs in interaction with the current everyday practices

Since needs and wants are so dynamic (supra) and situated in the experiences one has already had with new technology, we also try to elicit new information on the future needs by experimenting with available prototypes and off-the shelf / on the market technologies, that approach the visions of the social use cases in the best possible way. We have called this approach proxy technology assessment, but it is also referred to as technological probing.

An example of this approach within the TranseCare project focused on the potential of camera use in the support of care of people with mild dementia. One of the options was a camera supported service allowing an informal caregiver to observe how their relative was doing at home and having the option to ask for a volunteer to watch their relative while leaving home for some time.

First to gain insight in the visions of the experts a focus group discussion with dementia nurses was held. Potentials, benefits and restrictions of video surveillance for (demented) elderly were discussed, as well as ways to inform the demented patient about video surveillance and ways to let them participate in an eHomeCare project. Because of the sensitivity of the topic, only one patient including his/her care network of family, care givers, volunteers and the care organization, volunteered to participate in the experiment. In-depth interviews were conducted with the informal caregivers, the dependent elder, the volunteer, and dementia nurse at three moments: pre introduction, during the experiment and after the agreed term of evaluation. In this way we started from the current everyday practices, attitudes and beliefs on both independent living and ICT solutions, trying to create a dialogue on the experience with this technology in interaction with the physical and socio-cultural surroundings. This experiment was, against general expectations, well received by all actors in this network. The informal care givers where released of some burden, because they had also a feeling of security and of more respect of their privacy, by having less frequent and less controlling visits. Also the volunteer and the relatives were very positive about the system. The need for formal agreements of the boundary of the work was formulated, as well as a longer relationship with the patient to diminish the feeling of violation of the patient's privacy. This was only one network which was willing to experiment, not averse to technology and with tight and harmonic family bonds. Further research is needed to gather insight in the ability to generalize the observations made in this case.

3 Match towards market opportunities and business strategies

3.1 The eHealth market place

From a business perspective eHealth is an emerging market with all uncertainties related to new applications and new customers. The only certain indication for the emerging market is the fact that society is ageing. All other business indications are based on assumptions to be proven in the future. The very nature of healthcare and care for people in general, result this market to be subjected to many existing regulations and institutionalizations, what renders it even more complex. As ICT systems can only be effective when they are the underlying tool for functional operational flows (for e.g. the (health)care for elderly people at home, this being a very multi-dimensional issue in itself), the problem often is that the organization of (health)care delivery first has to be fully aligned before the so-called eHealth service can prove its added value. Although all European countries have an established healthcare system, the different systems at hand are very diverse due to the historical and local nature in which they have evolved to their present state. Even on smaller scale (regions, provinces) rules and regulations, subsidies etc can be different. As a result, it is impossible to define a single eHealth solution that will fit the entire European market place, resulting in several small niche marketplaces.

To further illustrate the complexity, Figure 2 shows the money flows for a typical Belgian eHealth product. At the left hand side the different government levels are shown, each one generating specific money flows for different aspects of the solutions (a.o. based on the pathology, degree of dependency for the user, etc.). The middle of the figure shows the solution providers. At the right hand side the users which have to be interpreted broader than the mere patient but should also include the professional care givers and the family care givers (who can provide informal care themselves, and/or money for the eHealth solution).

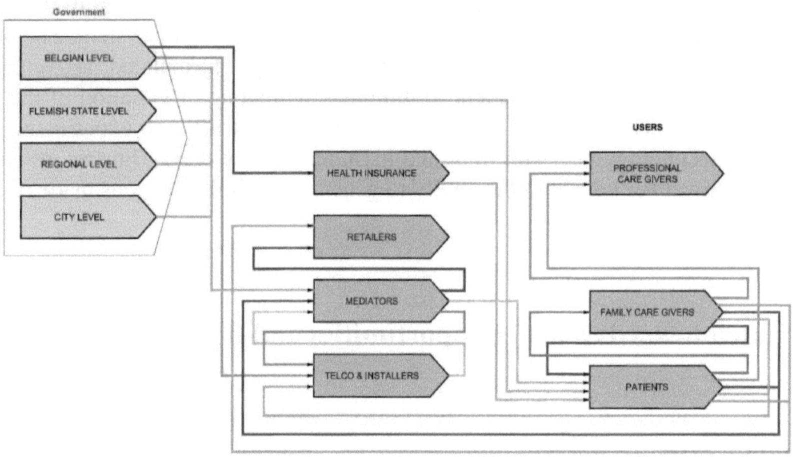

Figure 2: Money flow mechanisms in Belgian eHealth products

In addition to this business complexity of the eHealth market place, the user is not ICT-minded in general. For one, the care professionals are focusing on the caring act and the patient; thus considering ICT as a mere utensil like a car or a phone. This attitude is almost in contradiction with the typical tech savvy attitude of early adopters (consumers and companies) in the ICT marketplace. This implies that the well-accepted "diffusion of innovations model" from Rogers [7] is not readily applicable to the eHealth business model. Unpredictable or uncontrollable criteria can influence completely the uptake of your new service!

In addition, it is safe to state that the past decades ICT-solutions have promised a lot of efficiency but did not entirely fulfill these promises: the management collected more accurate information but the health practitioner itself ended up with additional administration and the burden of using the tools (meaning more work or less social interaction time with the patient).

3.2 How to find a solution?

From the above it is very clear that a technology-push approach is doomed to fail in healthcare, as it will hit the boundaries of the user domain requirements. The business models needed in health care are very particular, and more knowledge is needed about the particular social and economic dynamics in this field. Specifically in the health care sector a good understanding of the different types of users with their specific interests and expectations is needed (see also par 2). The technology developments have to be adapted to the very specific requirements and social characteristics of the field. On the other hand, in order to innovate and to make the health care sector more efficient, the sector needs innovative demonstrators, showing that ICT has an added value in delivering effective, qualitative and efficient health care, adapted to the prevailing norms and values of the different stakeholders.

In order to articulate the specific needs and transform them in convincing demo's and early products, the solution provider has to interact and collaborate closely with the future customer. Due to the large distance between the ICT and the healthcare domain, it is important that this problem identification exercise is done by means of a multidisciplinary team that can make the bridge. This approach not only makes it smoother to open a dialogue between two worlds with two different mindsets, it also strengthens the ICT-team since it will learn through *internal* discussion with other members of the multidisciplinary team how quickly misunderstandings can surface. Furthermore the ICT team will constantly face these aspects contrary to the traditional approach where it only surfaces during conversations with the end customer. The net result is that the whole team evolves toward a general attitude of better understanding. It becomes a better communicator and is better perceived by the healthcare actors so that an open dialogue culture can be developed, resulting in a constructive interaction to identifying the real problems and proposing innovative yet feasible solutions.

3.3 Taking a value proposition to the market

In order to take an innovative solution successfully into an emerging market like the eHealth market, it is important to define the market value in comprehensible terms for all actors involved. Although some actors (like a nurse in a big nursing organization) have no decision power, they can easily break the value of a solution by unwillingness to adapt or by practical concerns like the interaction time with a device, set up time for a connection or network bandwidth and coverage. No patient wants to have the *perception* that a nurse spends more time on an electronic device than spending time on the caring act itself. Therefore it is very important that the complete value network of the solution is identified and that the position of each actor in this network is looked at and cared for. An overall "win-win" situation should be the target!

It is important to note that the whole value network is actually bigger than the partners needed from a pure operational viewpoint. As explained in [5] and [6], the value network also includes complementors (i.e. parties that are not an operational part of the solution but can have benefit from or add value to the solution envisaged). Last but not least, the government is also part of the value network, due to the highly regulated nature of the healthcare market place.

4 Assemble the puzzle

4.1 Personas and scenarios

As an outcome of the user research (see par 2) we define personas. These are imaginative people that act as future users of our new service. To optimize the inclusion of all aspects (context, social, acceptability, likeability) from the start of the design, we describe these personas as realistic as possible. Learn to talk about these personas as they were real people, gives them real faces, real families and real lives. Learn to understand the situation they live in, and what their needs are! Are they reluctant towards the use of new technologies and tools, do they have friends to help them out, to motivate them? The picking out of personas at first instance seems to limit the potential "design-for-all" principle, but it has proven induce just the opposite effect. Projection of abstract requirements into technical design principles tends to create a distance between the designer and the future user. This concept has proven to be useful and lead to successful and likeable services [8], [9], [10].

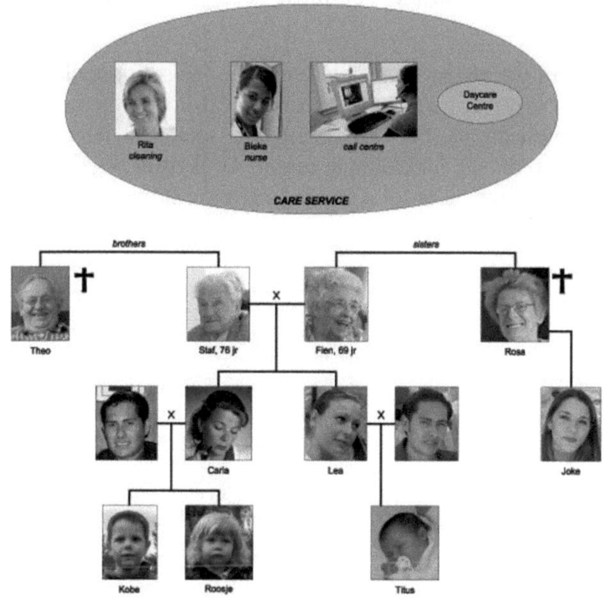

Figure 3: Example of persona description

Figure 3 illustrates such a persona description. In this project Staf and Fien are the main users of the eHomeCare services under development. We describe explicitly what they like, what they don't like, what they can do independently, what they need assistance for. We also describe the social and care context in which they live. Persona descriptions can be a few pages, so that designers really can understand how Staf and Fien will use the services.

4.2 Script book – dream or reality?

After the personas have been defined, a day out of the life of these people is written down in detail. It describes how the eHomeCare services will be naturally incorporated in the activities of daily life. It is a future projection of the domestication of the services under development. This story is then split up in little comprehensible parts (for e.g. called tasks T.1 until T.x), defining step by step how the new eHomeCare services under construction are included in the daily activities. Make sure that these tasks only cover one set of technical actions at the level of the end-to-end service delivery. For every task you can now explicit the technical requirements, the pre-requisites needed, the hard and software components to be developed. Within the script book you can also define the preconditions in view of regulation (what conditions do you need to certify to be in line with for example privacy issues), in view of compatibility with other in-house technologies or networks (does eHealth related Internet traffic need priority in case of limited bandwidth?), etc.

At the level of the tasks you should complete the script book into as much detail as possible. Describe the technical scenario (also what is running in the background of the application), list and specify the technical interfaces between all components involved. (see for example Figure 4). Writing a good script book consumes effort, but it is the basis for a good integration strategy!

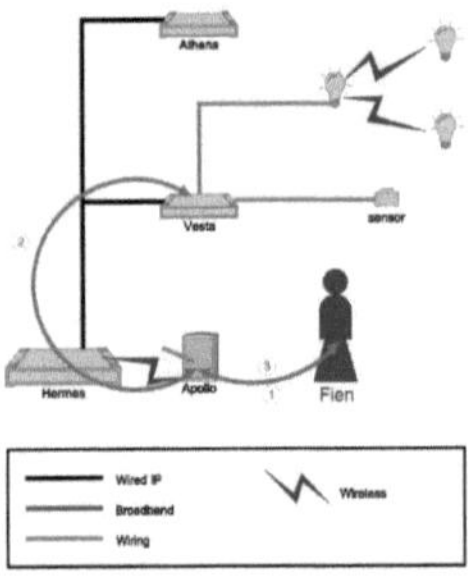

The task depicted at the left is the scenario when Fien wakes up at night. She needs to go to the bathroom. She uses the mobile device 'Apollo' to put on an indoor light street. This assists her in getting to the bathroom and back into bed, minimizing the danger of falling on the way. Such an explicit technical implementation is detailed for all tasks in the script book.

Figure 4: Excerpt out of a script book for the development of a eHomeCare Service.

4.3 The I-strategy

What seldom seems to work within the interdisciplinary context of eHealth service development is the "I will do it all alone" strategy; a more sensible way is putting priority on the establishment of a good integration strategy. Integration begins at the start of your project and implies focus on communication and interfacing, on version control, on build approaches [11], [12]. A good skeletal system for the overall architecture is THE enabler for a good integration strategy. Be aware that this skeletal overview should eventually line up with the business model and value chain that you have worked out before (see par 3.3). Subsystems of your service should be supported by identified stakeholders in your value network. If nobody will enable a specific subsystem, your service will not run. If interfaces of one subsystem are spread over several stakeholders you are in trouble too!

As soon as the top level system architecture is fixed, interfaces need to be defined and frozen. A software integration tool can be used to assign tasks to specific people, and create the environment for the management of the integration and testing procedure [13]. Do assign the task of integration and continuous testing to a specific team member! First handle the interaction of the architectural components at subsystem level, than start adding functionality. Set up test sequences and identify critical test paths (the most important, frequent and useful manipulations of the system).

Progressing in your project through the aid of a script book, underpinned by a good integration strategy allows you to improve the overall outcome of your project. Perhaps you will not realize all dream-scenarios listed in the script book, but you will have realized a set of operational building bricks that will be valid for further expansions!

5. Test and evaluate from the early start

5.1 Introducing the UCD principle

Within the Coplintho and TranseCare projects, we implemented the user centered design (UCD) methodology which has proven to give valuable results. The methodology consists of two distinct phases, an analysis phase and a design and evaluation phase. Both phases and their main components are depicted in Figure 5. The first phase gathers all the data needed to build a functional and intuitive user-based application. In the second phase, this information is processed into the end product in two complimentary, iterative phases. In the next paragraphs, the main UCD components are briefly introduced and clarified with some practical examples. The input from the social investigation of the user needs (par 2) is an in feed to the start of this UCD iterative process. This means that the target user group and specific user needs have been identified within the context of the project boundaries.

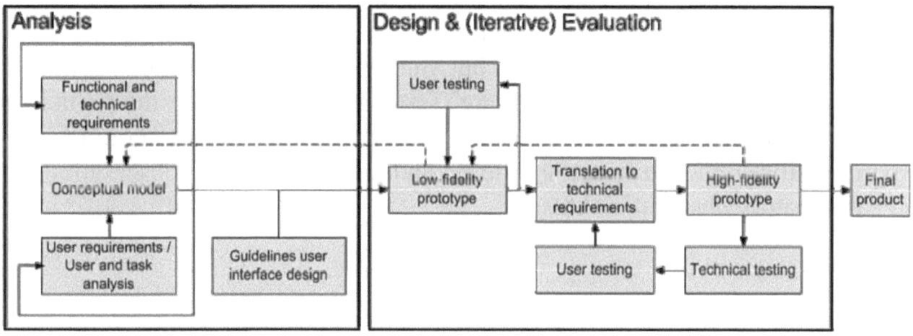

Figure 5: Schematic overview: from analysis to end product

5.2 User and task analysis: gathering information on the end user

Initial analysis of the end users and their current tasks is performed in a user and task analysis. A common approach in such an analysis is conducting contextual inquiries. This is a technique in which potential end users of the product are observed during the execution of their normal tasks in their normal working or living environment. In essence, the observed people are asked to tell the observer what they are doing. For instance, in developing an eCare platform like the Coplintho or TranseCare platform, it is useful to observe the use of communication devices in the daily environment of potential end users. A contextual inquiry, in any case, is not an interview, in which the observed people only tell something when they are asked a question [14].

Such an analysis can be very important to gain insights in the daily life of the elderly, ill or disabled users as they have different information needs and might have various limitations (e.g. visual, auditory and tactile). However, when observing disabled persons or elderly it is often difficult to have people talk about what they are doing while they are doing it. Especially when working with older users, asking questions can make it hard for them to reorient themselves to what they were doing [15] and can therefore compromise the observation.

As an alternative, the contextual inquiry can be replaced by pure observation, completed with expert interviews. For instance, in the TranseCare project, elderly people were observed while playing board games in group in a day care centre. The elderly were not disturbed while playing: no questions were asked, and no interventions were made. To complete the observations with some more information, additional interviews were held afterwards, both with the elderly themselves, and with the therapists in the care centre.

Participatory observation, a different technique in which the researcher participates instead of observes, can be a second alternative to the more standard contextual inquiry. In the project mentioned above, researchers merely observed people while they were playing in group, but, during another observation session, they also actively joined in a 'brain training' session aiming to keep the participants' memory fit. This way, both a 'detached' observational view was combined with expert opinions obtained from interviews, and more 'immersed' observations from the participatory observation session.

5.3 Conceptual model and the transition to a first design

Starting from both functional requirements and the information on the end users from the user and task analysis, a conceptual model can be constructed. This model offers a conceptual overview of the product functionality, its structure, and the way it should be made available to the end user. This conceptual model is the main input for the development of a first prototype.

Together with the conceptual model, basic guidelines for user interface design are considered another input source for the creation of a low-fidelity prototype. These 'design-for-all' rules guide the developer to build a final product that corresponds to both standard user interface expectations and non-standard user requirements, because, as Fisk states,"[...] age-related effects on, [for instance,] cognition lead to fundamental design guidelines." [15]. Several characteristics of the elderly have to be taken into account, as elderly cope with heterogeneous limitations. Taking into account specific visual and cognitive limitations will, for instance, lead to user interfaces with only basic, limited information shown onscreen, in rather large, high-contrast typefaces.

As an addition to these design-for-all guidelines, some interfaces need special adjustments for the medium they are designed for. For example in the Coplintho project the communication software was designed to be displayed on both computer and television screens. One of the adjustments that had to be made for the computer screen version was for example the menu navigation that also had to support arrow navigation instead of only point-and-click interaction.

It is important to note that the translation of the conceptual model and the basic user interface guidelines to a prototype (i.e., the translation from analysis to design) is not always a trivial step to take. Sometimes, conceptual model and basic interface rules may be slightly conflicting. We noticed this in the TranseCare project. Recommendations stating that all information should be easy to reach and clearly visible onscreen conflicted with basic user interface guidelines and common sense indicating that font and button size should not be too small and overview should be kept by providing enough distance between distinct user interface elements, and not showing too much content in one screen. This is only a simple example on how several goals and recommendations can conflict. It is clear that in these cases inventiveness and common sense should lead to a compromise.

5.4 Testing the prototype

Very basic prototypes without any functionality (i.e., low-fidelity prototypes consisting only of mockups), but giving a realistic impression of the new product, can and should be tested in a controlled environment in early stages with potential end users. As a result, the prototypes can be evaluated and adjusted relatively fast/up-front in the development process compared to changes made to an (almost-)final product. If major changes are necessary to the prototype, it is even possible to return to the conceptual stage of the design, without losing a lot of time and money.

When testing prototypes with older users, it is crucial to take into account the user characteristics from the user and task analysis. For instance, Lazar describes user and task analyses taking more time than analyses conducted with 'regular' people. "Instead of scheduling five user observations, you may have to schedule 10 sessions for seniors, each half as long as sessions for younger users who do not tire as quickly as seniors" [16]. Obviously, the same remark holds true for user tests, in which people have to focus on a – for them – entirely new product. Additionally, user characteristics other than age or disability can also be very relevant as well. For example computer illiteracy can influence the feedback collected from user tests.

5.5 Translation to technical requirements

The translation to technical requirements can start when the low-fidelity prototype is considered finished. Deciding whether a prototype is finished can be discussable but the number, nature and priority of changes that are suggested by the user tests of the first prototype is a good indication on the status of the mockup. At this stage of the development, the first step will be to decide which technology is the most suitable for successfully implementing the end product. This choice is greatly influenced by the functional requirements that have been determined in an early stage of the design. The technologies that will be used have to support the functionality of choice. Although the decision on which technology to use is often already thought over at the 'functional requirement' stage, it is possible that the implementation technology has to be reconsidered based on the feedback from the low-priority prototype testing. Once a technology is decided on, this choice should be respected after every iterative evaluation of the high-fidelity prototype. In the TanseCare project a web-based alarm central was designed. The choice for a web application was partly made before the creation of the low-fidelity prototype, because of some advantages like maintainability and ease of distribution. After iterative user tests of the low-fidelity prototype, the choice was confirmed and the underlying code structure could be developed to support all desired functionality.

Together with each translation to technical requirements, a list of features is composed based on the low-fidelity prototype or the user test results, depending on the current stage of the development chain. For each listed feature, a new inventory of alternative implementations is created, each with the advantages, disadvantages and impact on the existing technical design. When all feature implementations have been decided on, a (new) high-fidelity prototype can be created.

The high fidelity-prototype is a working design that converges with the final product in every iteration. Because of the low-fidelity prototype iterative approach, major design and user interface issues were already detected and resolved earlier in the development process. Apart from detecting more usability issues, the goal of iterating user tests with this more advanced prototype is also to track flaws in the functionality of the application. In some cases it might be necessary to go back to the low-fidelity prototype if important functionality appears to be missing during the user tests or questioning.

Experiences from the Coplintho project have learned that the test audience for high-fidelity usability testing can be varied according to the technical implementation status of the product. Early iterations of high-fidelity prototypes, in which the product is not entirely stable and technically reliable yet, can best be tested with test participants that do belong to the target group of the product, but are least frail (elderly that are not as easily fatigued, or disabled persons that can still function quite normally). A technical testing or debugging phase after the implementation of each high-fidelity prototype must ensure relevant results and conclusions after the user tests. This debugging will be based on feedback of the designer's testing of the prototype, as well as on technical issues that arose during previous user tests.

More frail test users, and more heavily disabled persons can be involved in the user tests in a later stage, when the product is technically more stable: this will put less strain on people that already have certain difficulties. This approach also allows for testing the actual user experience of the target audience, which is much more difficult or even impossible when the prototype still suffers from major flaws.

In the Coplintho project, the functional prototype was submitted to user tests twice (see Figure 6) with remarkable functional differences between the high-fidelity prototypes that were tested. The biggest lesson learned in these iterations was to provide a decent amount of dynamic textual and visual feedback concerning application specific events like for example incoming notifications. In a non-functional prototype, it is possible to display a feedback message in a mockup, but it is much harder to simulate the appearing and disappearing of different types of feedback messages. This is where the high-fidelity prototype complements the low-fidelity prototype.

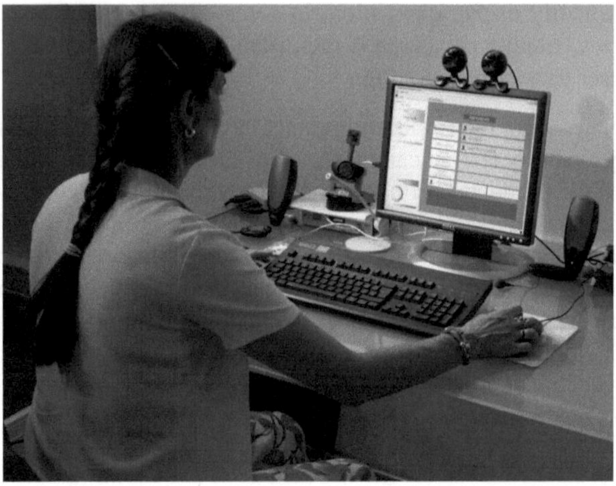

Figure 6: Usability testing for the COPLINTHO project

5.6 Final product?

The final product is considered the last iteration of the high-fidelity prototype, although in this design model one could always decide to do another iteration of user tests and translate the results to a better end product. In the end, one might even conclude that in an iterative UCD cycle, a product is never quite finished.

6 Do the proof of the pudding

6.1 Checklists

The proof of the pudding for eHomeCare services is of course in testing them in a real life environment with real life users. In that context eHealth also calls for specific measures and attention. Some relevant items to keep in mind are:

* Coping strength of elderly people and/or patients is often limited.
* Real life situations are often complex and comorbidity can be present.
* Existing care networks are work over-loaded and embedded in routines.
* Field trials consume a lot of time, effort and money.
* The healthcare world asks for "statistical evidence" that eHealth is worth the "pain of change".

It is thus of primary importance that you think through the objectives and the methodology of your field trial into detail before starting off. Collaboration and support from patients, patient organizations and/or care organizations is precious and should not be over-consumed. You seldom get a second change for a field trial for the same purpose! So a bullet-proof methodology should be explored from the start in order to optimize the usefulness of your test results.

A checklist and implementation scenario should be outlined and defined within the consortium. A range of questions you need to get answered before you initiate your field trial are:

√ What do we want to measure or to learn out of the field trial (acceptability of your service, technical stability, end-to-end service delivery, impact on care or on quality of life, etc.)?

√ What are the inclusion criteria for the testgroup?

√ Is the trial compliant with the local and national regulation (privacy protection, patient protection [17]?[1]

√ What about ethical committees and liability?

√ What about patient information and support (informed consent, single point of contact in case of problems or questions)?

√ What are the preconditions for the test situations?

√ What are the evaluation criteria and mechanisms?

√ How do you round-up the field trial (user-feedback, handling the expectations of the test persons)

√ Who write the user-manuals and supports the field installation process?

√ ...

Inclusion criteria for the test group (level of disease or disability, level of coping with new situations, supporting informal caregivers and follow up) should be defined a few months before the kickoff of the field trial. Recruitment of test sites and people takes time! Be aware that a drop out rate of 10% is always possible due to unexpected life events, sickness, de-motivation of test persons. Make sure you have an adequate support team able to respond within the necessary time limit when failure, questions or problems occur. Install a single point of contact for the test sites and people involved. Give spontaneous and open feedback to all actors involved in case of questions. Be aware that you will need to handle expectations (and eventual disillusions) of test persons. You do need an inter-disciplinary team to conduct a field trial in a good and profound way!

---

[1] In US the HIPA (Health information protection act) is valid in view of health information. A comprehensive and useful checklist according to the HIPA act can be found at: http://www.health.gov.sk.ca/hipa-checklist

A bottleneck within eHealth is that there is a cry for "statistical" evidence for the new applications. As field trials are cumbersome and not easily deployed for a high number of patients it is essential that you apply a good methodology for this test phase. An optimum route is to try to align your approach with the methodology used in other local and/or national eHomeCare projects, so that the combination of test results of several small field trials could end up as more convincing statistical proof. A good idea is therefore to get in touch with similar projects and consortia in your region or elsewhere. Exchange of ideas and combining strength can lever your project results to a wider extent.

6.2 Stage gate process

As coping strength of people involved in the field trials is often limited, and field trials are expensive the first thing you should make sure of is that the service you want to test is 100% stable and operational in the selected test environments. Every tester knows this is wishful thinking, but you can optimize the success rate and minimize the problems by evolving towards the field trial in a so-called stage-gate process.

L-stage (lab stage): Test early prototypes of your service in a controlled environment (technical lab, living lab) with selected testers (see also par 5). Do an internal and/or external evaluation of these test results. Dare to question your initial design and adapt if needed. Include critical path testing in your test cycle. Induce stress conditions onto your application (fool-proof testing, compatibility with other applications, resilience in case of power failure). A single successful demo is no guarantee that your application will run in a real home environment!

PHT-stage (pre-home trial stage): The results from the lab-test should lead to a more profound and adapted solution of your service. This prototype solution should then be installed and tested in preliminary home tests. The PHT is done to assess acceptance, usability, technical stability, compatibility with home environments and operational issues. The people in the PHT environment should be considered as "innovators" within the defined target group, and thus should have an interest in the services envisaged and have enough coping strength to deal with new and changing situations. Next to the initial testers attention should be given to the supporting network of people surrounding these testers. Active involvement of (in)formal caregivers and family and/or friends can offer extra means of feedback and test results to your project.

HT-stage (home trial stage): For the final home tests of the developed eHomeCare service, careful selection based on the inclusion criteria listed in the script book should be made. Motivational feedback and support is very important to avoid high drop-out rates. However life events can often result in test people stopping the co-operation during the field trial. Interviews should be conducted at several stages of the field trial and evaluation mechanisms should be as objective as possible to give a correct view.

I-strategy: The key-word from the beginning of the process is the integration methodology. (see also par 4.3). At this time the effort investigated in a dedicated integration methodology pays off. When adaptations are needed in the different test stages mentioned above, the I-strategy allows you to keep an overview of an often complex process of changes.

6.3 Happy endings?

Field trials come to an end! Explain this in advance to the people involved in the field trial (at the time of selection of the test persons!). Often the eHomeCare services appeal to real needs of the people involved, so you have to avoid disappointments when you have to stop the testing period. Discuss in advance with the consortium if the application could stay in place when test persons ask for it, and how this could be done (Continuous support? Cost involved?)

Be sure to document your field trial from the early start to the end phase for future reference. Your faults can be very valid to others in the future! Be willing to share your experience with others and or with future projects.

7 SWOT analyses

As a conclusion we want to share with the reader the overall view of the consortium on the weaknesses and strengths of the projects run using the described methodology. What did we achieve already? What are the hurdles taken? Were did we trip over? What is next to come? What are the booby traps ahead?

7.1 S for Soul mates!

- The willingness to create mutual understanding within projects aiming at the successful combination of social, economical, and technical aims/expectations.
- Self-evaluation led to better project-planning, goal definition, communication and interaction.
- The user needs were studied starting from a holistic perspective (not just solving a punctual problem!).

7.2 W for We are not perfect

- The applied methodology to create a user centered approach is time and resource consuming. Large number of partners co-operating within the project makes optimum technological integration a challenge. All user iterfaces should be uniform in look and feel!

7.3 O for Other things to do?

- Patient empowerment should be made real through more active participation in the design choices made and by having more iterations.
- Cumulative knowledge and experience should lever these user centered research approaches.

7.4 T for Try to stop us!

- Availability of resources in the care organization to participate in these type of projects is often limited and will probably diminish even more due to increasing workload and budgetary constraints.
  - √ Regulatory frameworks are not always in favor of possible technological solutions.
  - √ The care sector's skepticism about technological innovation can be intensified by technical problems that disturb the user's initial experience with innovative products.

Acknowledgments The authors would like to thank all the consortium members and the IBBT and the IWT for partial funding of the two related eHomeCare projects: IBBT - Coplintho (Innovative communication platforms for interactive eHomeCare), 2005 – 2007, https://projects.ibbt.be/coplintho/ and IBBT and IBBT - TranseCare (Transparant ICT platforms for eCare), 2007 – 2009 https://projects.ibbt.be/transecare/.

8 Reference list

[1] Molotch, H.: Where the stuff comes from. Routledge, NewYork (2003)

[2] Frissen, V.: De domesticatie van de digitale wereld' Rede uitgesproken bij de aanvaarding van het ambt van bijzonder hoogleraar ICT en Sociale verandering, Erasmus Universiteit Amsterdam, June 25 (2004)

[3] Veys, A., Jacobs, A.: Elderly, who (e)-cares? eHospital; IT@Networking Communication 1(4), 3 (2007)

[4] De Rouck, S., et al.: A methodology for shifting the focus of e-health support design onto user needs. A case in the homecare field' Int. J. Med. Inform. 77(9), 589–601 (2008)

[5] Brandenburger, A.: Business strategy: Getting beyond competition, Harvard Management Update Newsletter, U9612B (1996)

[6] Anderson, J., Narus, J.: Business marketing: Understand what customers value. Harvard Business Review, 98601 (November-December 1998)

[7] Rogers, Everett, M.: Diffusion of Innovations, 5th edn. Free Press, New York (2003)

[8] Cooper, A.: The Inmates are Running the Asylum, SAMS (1999)

[9] Carroll, John, M.: 2000 Making Use: Scenario-Based Design of Human-Computer Interactions. MIT Press, Cambridge (2000)

[10] Pruitt, J., Adlin, T.: The Persona Lifecycle: Keeping People in Mind Throughout Product Design. Morgan Kaufmann, San Francisco (2006)

[11] `http://www.martinfowler.com/articles/continuousIntegration.html`

[12] Duvall, P., et al.: Continuous Integration: Improving Software Quality and Reducing Risk. Addison-Wesley Signature Series (2007)

[13] `http://www.intland.com/`

[14] Beyer, H., Holtzblatt, K.: Contextual Design: Defining Customer-Centered Systems. Morgan Kaufmann Publishers, Francisco (1997)

[15] Fisk, A.D., et al.: Designing for Older Adults. CRC Press, Boca Raton (2004)

[16] O'Connell, T.A.: The Why and How of Senior-Focused Design. In: Lazar, J. (ed.) Universal Usability. Designing Computer Interfaces for Diverse Users. John Wiley & Sons Ltd., Chichester (2007)

[17] Verhenneman, G., Van Gossum, K.: Privacy and Digital Homecare, Allies not Enemies. In: ICMCC book on digital homecare (2009)

[illegible]

Changing Role of Nurses in the Digital Era: Nurses and Telehealth

Sisira Edirippulige

Centre for Online Health
University of Queensland

Abstract Being the largest contingent of the healthcare workforce engaging in diverse care activities, nurses play a very important role in the health care sector. However, the shortage of nursing population has posed serious challenges to the nursing services. Both developed and developing countries are facing a critical shortage of nurses. Mal-distribution of nurses has contributed to the disparity of care. The emergence of new diseases, rapid increase of chronic diseases and the growth of aged population have aggravated the problem. The challenges have demanded a review of the way care services are traditionally provided. Nurses have shown a remarkable flexibility and adaptability amidst these challenges. Nurses are among the first groups to embrace telehealth to provide care. This chapter provides an overview of the current practice of telenursing. The discussion will also include the advantages and the barriers to the expansion of telenursing.

Table of contents

K. Yogesan et al. (Eds.): Handbook of Digital Homecare, BIOMED, pp. 269–285.
springerlink.com

Introduction

Nurses are the largest group of carers in the healthcare sector. According to recent statistics, there are about 12 million nurses worldwide. (1) In the United States, the registered nurses constitute the largest health care occupation, with 2.5 million positions. (2) The number of nurses in Australia is about 260,000.

Nurses play a critical role in almost every sphere of healthcare such as primary, community and tertiary care. Nurses, regardless of specialty or work setting, treat patients, educate patients and the public about various medical conditions, and provide advice and emotional support to patients' family members. Nurses are responsible for recording patients' medical histories and symptoms, help perform diagnostic tests and analyse results, operate medical machinery, administer treatment and medications, and help with patient follow-up and rehabilitation. Teaching patients and their families how to manage their illness or injury, explaining post-treatment home care needs, diet, nutrition, and exercise programs and self-administration of medication and physical therapy are also some important duties of nurses. Among others, providing care to people at home is also one of the traditional roles of nurses. Research has shown that there is a clear relationship between the number of nurses and the quality of care. Studies have also found the co-relation between nursing care and the speed of healing process, length of hospitalisation and stress level of patients and families.

The role of nurses in health care settings is rapidly evolving. New terms such as district nurses, health visitors, school nurses, GP practice nurses, nurse consultants, clinical nurse specialists and home health care nurses are added to the list showing the diversity of practice that nurses are undertaking.

One well documented problem relating to nursing is the shortage of nurses. It is evident that the overall shortage of nurses is staggering. According to recent statistics, all Organisation of Economic Cooperation and Development (OECD) countries have a growing shortage of nurses. A US Federal Government study predicts that hospital nursing vacancies will reach 800,000, or 29 percent, by 2020.(3) Australia projects a shortage of 40,000 nurses by 2010. (6) Shortage of nurses in developing countries is daunting. Lack of resources to produce qualified nurses has aggravated by the rapid exodus of nursing staff from developing countries.(4) According to WHO statistics, Sub Saharan Africa is short of 60,000 nurses to meet Millennium Development Goals.(5)

In addition to shortage, mal-distribution of nurses is a serious problem. There is a significant disproportional distribution of nurses within and among countries. For example, while the United States have 773 nurses per 100,000 population, the number of nurses in Uganda for the same size population is 6. (6) Disparity of nurses in urban and rural communities is a significant problem in both developing and developed countries. The World Health Report aptly expressed the acuteness this problem, as 'the most critical issue facing healthcare systems is the shortage of people who make them work'. (7)

Growing shortage of health workforces (nurse included) has compounded by several other problems. Emergence of new diseases and the increase of chronic diseases have challenged the health systems around the world. HIV/AIDS is just one example. The increasing incidence of chronic diseases (such as cancer, coronary heart disease, diabetes and dementia) and growing number of aged population have added to the pressure on healthcare systems worldwide. The World Health Organisation (WHO) projects that chronic disease will be the leading cause of disability by 2020 and will be the most expensive problem facing healthcare systems.(8) For example, type II diabetes mellitus is becoming the most common chronic disease in the United States. It affects 7% of the adult population. Congestive heart failure affects about 5 million Americans each year accounting for around 20% of hospitalised patients over 65 years. Studies show that caring for people with chronic diseases consumes approximately 78% of all health care spending in the United States – more than $1 trillion annually.(9) The Centres for Medicare and Medicare Services estimated total national health expenditure for home care was $40 billion in 2003, an increase of almost ten percent over the previous year. An additional $111 billion is spent on nursing home care. With the ageing of the population, this rate of growth will only accelerate.

Undoubtedly, these tendencies have put additional pressure on the already overburdened nursing community around the world. Therefore addressing these urgent needs demands new ways of delivering services more efficiently and effectively.

Despite these challenges nurses have shown remarkable flexibility and adaptability. The nursing profession has been the first group to embrace telehealth which offers an alternative to providing care to patients at home and health care settings. This chapter will focus on the role of nurses in telehealth practices, the benefits of telehealth for both patients and providers, current practice and future opportunities. In our discussion we will also pay some attention to the existing barriers to the expanded use of telehealth.

ICT and nursing

Telehealth is an emerging discipline focusing on the use of information and communication technologies (ICT) to deliver health services. A number of different terms and terminologies have been associated with this discipline. For example the terms such as telehealth, telemedicine, health informatics and e-health, have been used interchangeably. The use of ICT in nursing practice has widely known as telenursing or nursing informatics. According to the official definition of American Nursing Association (ANA), nursing informatics is: the speciality identifying, collecting, processing, analysing and managing data. Although this definition solely concentrates on the information, it is believed that nursing informatics should also incorporate the aspects of the delivery of care. It is apparent that the definitions are continuing to evolve. In broader terms telehealth is a tool for healthcare delivery, diagnosis, consultation, treatment, and transfer of medical data/images and education by using ICT (i.e. interactive audio, visual, and data communications) at a distance.

Brief history

The exchange of health information and the delivery of healthcare at distance have a long history. In the mid 19th century telegraphy (signalling by wires) was used in the American Civil War to transmit casualty lists and order medical supplies. Later developments permitted the transmission of X-ray images. When the telephone was invented doctors were able to use it to transmit sounds from a stethoscope through the telephone network. Later on, telephone networks were used to transmit electrocardiograms (ECGs) and electroencephalograms (EEGs). Today ordinary telephone networks are used to send faxes for medical purposes, while the use of telephone lines to access the Internet has become widespread.

Another landmark development in the history of telehealth was the use of radio in the late 19th Century. Healthcare providers initially used radio to send information by Morse code and this was soon followed by voice transmission. Radio has been widely used in providing medical advice to seafarers. In 1920 the Seaman's Church Institute of New York became one of the first organisations to provide medical care using radio. Subsequently, many other nations established radio-medical services. The International Radio Medical Centre (CIRM) in Italy was set up in 1935 and still continues to provide services to thousands of patients. In addition, in-flight medical assistance is provided to passenger aircraft mainly by radio.

The next important technological development, which affected telehealth, was television. In the late 1950s developments in closed circuit television and video communication were used in medical and clinical applications. In 1964, a two-way closed circuit television link was set up between the Nebraska Psychiatric Institute in Omaha and the state mental hospital in Norfolk, 180 km away. This permitted interactive consultations between specialists and general practitioners, and facilitated education and training at the distant site.

Telehealth has also been used in space. Satellite based communication has been used to provide medical services to remote communities and to coordinate relief efforts following natural disasters and war.

Telehealth covers a very wide range of healthcare interactions for many different purposes. These interactions can be classified:

by participant e.g. nurse-to-doctor, nurse-to-patient
by type e.g. realtime, non-realtime
by information transmitted e.g. audio, video.

Telehealth can involve a wide range of participants. The nature of the communication in health can be:

patient with practitioner
practitioner with practitioner
patient with patient (that is mutual support)
practitioner or patient accessing educational material (that is sources of health information).

Types of telehealth interaction

The interaction in telehealth can be classified as either real-time or store and forward.

Real-time

The closest alternative to a conventional, face-to-face consultation is a real-time telehealth consultation, otherwise known as synchronous or interactive. Parties involved in real-time consultation communicate simultaneously via a telecommunication network. During a videoconference, both sound and vision are transmitted. During a telephone consultation, only voice is transmitted. In an Internet chat room, only text messages are conveyed. The primary advantage of real-time telehealth is that there is no time delay between the information being transmitted and received, that is the parties concerned can interact as though they were present in the same room.

Real-time telehealth has been proven to be effective for providing specialist consultations to rural health workers and for educational purposes.(10) Videoconferencing has also been used for home nursing. (11) There is evidence that videoconferencing in fields such as dermatology, geriatrics, speech therapy and psychiatry can be effective. (12, 13)

It is commonly assumed that real-time telehealth consultation is expensive, and certainly high quality videoconferencing equipment can be costly. However, videoconferencing is also possible with low cost equipment. For example low cost videophones used over the public telephone network can enable community nurses to provide care and support to patients at home. (14)

Store and forward

Store and forward telehealth involves the non-interactive transmission of information from one site to another. (15) Store and forward telehealth, which is sometimes referred to as asynchronous or pre-recorded, involves information being captured and then transmitted to the other party for advice, opinion or specialist consultation. The main advantage of this method of working is that the parties involved can work independently from one another that is they do not have to be present at a pre-arranged time. Those who send the information can do it when it is convenient to them, while those who view and use the information can do so at their own convenience.

In addition, store and forward telehealth is usually inexpensive in comparison with real-time telehealth. If real-time telehealth requires sophisticated and expensive equipment, store and forward communication can be carried out with relatively cheaper technology. Examples include the transmission of ECGs using a simple fax machine(16) or obtaining a second opinion by email.(17)

Not all consultations can be done by store-and-forward telehealth. Store and forward interaction is ideal where specialists rely on image interpretation, such as in radiology, dermatology and pathology. Digital images of microscopy specimens, radiographs, wound and skin lesions can be stored on a computer and then transmitted via email to a specialist. A number of studies prove the feasibility of this approach. Acquisition of information stored in websites on the Internet can also be considered as asynchronous telehealth and there are increasing numbers of websites with health related information. (18)

The major disadvantage of store and forward telehealth is that the specialist is entirely dependent on the information that the referrer sends, so if a poor quality picture of a dermatology lesion is sent, for example, it may be impossible to make a diagnosis.

Whether the telehealth interaction is in real-time, or store-and-forward, the technology required for the telehealth system will comprise three main components:

equipment to capture the information at each site
communication equipment to transmit this information between the sites
equipment to display the information at the relevant sites.

Four types of information are common in telehealth:
audio
text

still images
moving images (video).

Audio and visual transmission does not allow a consultant to access aspects like touch, smell and physical feeling. However, a consultant can see the patient closely, wounds and skin lesions from different angles, close ups of different field on the microscopic specimen, ultrasound recording. This seems to be sufficient for many consultations.

Audio: The most common form of audio transmission is for speech. It is also possible to transmit heart or breathing sounds using an electronic stethoscope.

Text: messages can be transmitted by use of a fax machine. Better quality transmission can be achieved if the documents can be transmitted in digital form. If the information already exists as a computer file this is easy. Alternatively, printed documents can be digitised using a flatbed scanner or a digital camera and then transmitted as still images.

Still images: may be transmitted for various health purposes such as diagnosis, management and education. Low-cost digital cameras are capable of capturing good quality images that can be transmitted to specialists for consultation. A flatbed scanner can be used to produce digital images of charts such as ECG traces. X-ray films can also be digitised this way, although when high quality diagnostic images are required, the equipment involved can be costly.

Video: Commercial videoconferencing equipment can allow a high quality online meeting where a specialist can see and communicate with the patient almost naturally. Setting up a sophisticated videoconferencing studio can be expensive although equipment costs can be expected to reduce in the future. It is important to understand that videoconferencing is not the only mode of communication in telehealth or even necessarily the best. The suitability of a system depends on the needs, which will vary from one application to another.

The reliability of the technology is a critical factor in a successful telehealth implementation. Analogue telephone transmission is not appropriate for many telehealth purposes, since signals may be degraded because of noise on the lines and low bandwidth. Digital signal transmission is preferable, since digital signals can be transmitted over networks for long distances without degradation and bandwidths are usually much higher.

Telenursing

In general terms telenursing is the use of ICT for delivering health care services at distance by nurses. Telenursing can be used in both healthcare setting or a non-institutional setting – that is at home or in an assisted-living facility. (19) Telenursing application may include real time techniques, for example videoconferencing or telephony and store and forward techniques, for example email or web-based applications. Through interactive video systems, patients can contact on-call nurses and arrange for a video consultation. This kind of applications is particularly helpful for children and adults with chronic conditions and long term illness. Telenursing can also help patients and families to be active in care, such as self management of chronic conditions.

In addition to real time telehealth applications, various devices such as alarms, sensors and monitoring equipment are being used in telenursing applications. (20) The use of systems that allow nurses to monitor physiological parameters such as blood pressure, blood glucose, respiratory peak flow and weight management are becoming commonplace. Telenursing techniques help provide accurate and timely information and support while making more frequent contacts available compared to traditional home visits.

There are signs that interest in telenursing is awakening. Recent data shows that 20% of American based home health agencies employ some kind of telehealth in their day to day operations and another 20% plan to offer telehealth services in the next 12 months. (19) The last few years have seen an increase in the number of manufacturers of home telehealth equipment in the US (mainly) and elsewhere. It is believed that in the United States almost half of the on-site nursing visits could be replaced by telenursing. (21) The situation is similar in Europe and other developed countries. An increase has also occurred in the number of home telehealth episodes. During 2001-2003 the number of Medicare home health users increased to 2.6 million and the number of episodes rose to 36 million. At the same time, the average number of visits per episode fell slightly to 17.3. (19)

In the following section we briefly review some telenursing studies in reference to the improvement of quality of care and benefits for both consumer and provider.

To support the patient in the home

The main bulk of studies in telenursing have focused on delivering care at home or non-health care settings. These studies have examined the efficacy and effectiveness of telenursing to provide care at distance. A number of studies have tested the use of telephone to provide nursing care while some studies have examined the effectiveness of 'video-visits'. For example, a study comparing the use of telephone for diabetes mellitus care management showed that both communication tools had similar effect on glycemin control. (22)

Several significant studies have examined the effect of telehealth on wound care management. The access to specially trained wound care nurses is limited. For example the number of specialist wound care nurses in the US is about 4300 (0.2% of RNs). A pilot investigation used a combination of real-time consultation and the capture of digital wound images to provide specialist wound care. Outcomes included earlier assessment of patients by a specialist wound care nurse, a reduction in healing time, fewer in-person home visits and an increase in productivity. Additional benefits included improved education of patients and improved education and professional development in the use of wound care protocols for generalist home care nurses. The study concluded that home telehealth is an alternative means of delivering the knowledge and expertise of a wound care nurse to underserved patients.

A study examining the feasibility and acceptance of teledermatology for wound management of patients with chronic leg ulcers by home-care nurses found that teledematology was accepted both by patients, home care nurses and wound experts. They concluded that teledermatology offers great potential for chronic wound care. (23)

A randomised control trial to determine the effect of telehome care on hospitalisation, emergency department use and mortality showed patients in the telehome care groups had a lower probability of hospitalisations and emergency department use compared to the patients in the control group. Results also showed greater reduction in symptoms for patients using telehome care compared to control patients. The study concluded that technology enables frequent monitoring of clinical indices and permits the home health care nurse to detect changes in cardiac status and intervene when necessary. (24)

One year pilot study evaluated the feasibility of videoconferencing between hospital and family homes to provide support to children with special health care needs. This study showed the effectiveness of this system. (25)

Another development in patient in-home support is the smart-home concept. This idea focuses on autonomy and independence with the aim to give people (and those caring for them) added security, safety, quality of life and access to medical care without an in-patient admission. (26) In some cases it may delay or avoid institutionalisation.

In the mid 1990's, smart-homes were equipped with sensors that turned on lights at night when movement was detected, turned off stoves if overheating or left on, unlocked doors and turned on lights if smoke was detected, alerted staff if residents were out of bed for prolonged periods and, for wandering people, alerted staff if external doors were opened. (27)

Newer developments in smart-home sensors include detectors worn by the resident to alert staff if a fall occurs (28) or if a resident at risk of falling, sits-up in bed and to monitor the mobility and subsequent health status of residents. (29)

In telenursing - remote monitoring has been identified as a growing area. Studies have demonstrated that telehealth modalities can be used to monitor patients stationed at home. With the global aged population growing demanding increased care, telenursing can be an alternative way to provide services. A Japanese study showed that using monitoring devises can help keep contact with elderly people at home which leads to better care. (30)

A study focused on feasibility and efficacy of integrating home monitoring into a primary care setting installed telehome care units with 1 or more peripheral devices (e.g. blood-pressure monitor, weight scale, glucometer) in patients' homes. This pilot study demonstrated that telehealthcare monitoring in a collaborative care community family practice is feasible and well used. The study also concluded that home telemonitoring can improve access to high quality care.

A study conducted in Hong Kong showed the effectiveness of care services to residential nursing homes from hospital based geriatric outreach service using videoconferencing. (32) The study showed that travel time of nurses, patients and consultants were saved.

Another randomised control trial tested the impact of telehome monitoring on hospital readmission, quality of life, and functional status in patients with heart failure or angina. The study showed that telehome monitoring significantly reduced the number of hospital readmissions and days spent in the hospital for patients with angina and improved quality of life and functional status in patients with heart failure or angina. (33)

To support remote nurses

For example in the United Kingdom (UK) nurse practitioner units have been established to provide care to patients with minor injuries. Telehealth is used in these units as a support for nurses. (34) They can use videoconferencing to contact emergency medicine specialists for advice and support. This has effectively reduced the need to refer patients to the tertiary emergency medicine department and to the local general practitioner, saving time and reducing costs. Home telehealth can assist nurses to expand their role, to access direct clinical support for this expansion, and to reach more patients and provide more services. (35)

One nurse practitioner in the USA uses home telehealth to support other nurses in a remote medical facility by conducting patient consultations online. (36) This allows the nurse practitioner, working with the remote nurse, to complete patient histories, assess patients using peripherals such as a stethoscope, a camera for viewing eardrums, nasal mucosa, mouths and throats as well as a dermascope used to view and magnify skin lesions. The nurse practitioner can remotely print prescriptions for the patient, order additional investigations or refer the patient to specialist care.

To promote and support self-care

The role of home telehealth in helping patients to mange their own health is another growing area. Many elderly people live with at least one chronic disease or condition, such as diabetes or heart disease. On discharge from hospitals (particularly if the patient is newly diagnosed) patients need extensive support to manage their condition successfully. Traditionally this has been done with routine home nursing visits. However, home telehealth provides an opportunity to interact with and instruct patients at home. This may improve self-care, reduce subsequent readmissions and to allow people to stay in their own familiar environment.

Telehealth units are available with the ability to add peripheral monitoring devices for tracking a patient's physiological status and providing this information to them as part of an ongoing education and self-management program. Peripheral devices can include blood glucose meter, blood pressure cuff, pulse oximeter and other measuring/monitoring devices. Multimedia materials can also be integrated into home telehealth units. These materials may be used to remind patients to track their weight daily, to alter their fluid intake or increase their activity levels.

Home monitoring studies for people with multi morbidity have shown effective. A study carried out at home and nursing home setting showed significant savings of hospital bed days and nursing hours. Increased involvement of the patients in their own management provided them a better understanding of their conditions, resulting in increased reassurance and reducing the need for GP visits. (37)

To improve medication management and compliance

There is also a growing body of literature on the value of home telehealth in medication management. Medication-related complications are a contributing factor in accidents and illnesses that lead to hospitalization. (38) Research has shown that patients with greater than nine medications have at least a 22 percent incidence of medication errors which in turn contribute to adverse reactions and hospitalisation. (39) Home telehealth in medication management has proven effective. For example, a study by the Veteran's Administration in the USA demonstrated a 30 percent improvement in medication compliance after telehealth implementation. (40) Medication reminders, interactive voice response (IVR) systems and telemonitoring solutions can improve medication management and enable nurses to improve the quality of care provided.

Cost saving

There is certainly not a great deal of evidence on cost effectiveness of telenursing. This may have also resulted the reluctance of public and private sector investment in telenurisng. However, there are several studies showing that telenursing can offer cost savings to health providers, governments and consumers.

A study within Kaiser Permanente Tele-Home Health Research Project aiming to evaluate the use of remote video technology in the home health setting showed the effectiveness of this tool, patient satisfaction while maintaining quality of care and potential for cost savings. (41)

Another study aimed to determine whether home telehealth (when integrated with the health facility's electronic medical record system) reduces health care costs and improves quality of life outcomes relative to usual home healthcare services for elderly with complex co-morbidities. This study concluded that telehome care reduces resource use and improves cognitive status, treatment compliance and stability of chronic disease for homebound elderly with common complex morbidities. (42)

Another randomised control trial was to compare the outcomes and costs when home health care is delivered by telehealth as opposed to traditional means for patients receiving skilled nursing care at home. This study showed virtual visits between a skilled home healthcare nurse and chronically ill patients at home can improve patient outcome at lower cost than traditional skilled face-to-face home healthcare visits. (43)

In a recent study the Centre for Information Technology Leadership in the United States aimed to investigate the cost savings by telehealth encounters. The telehealth services were provided by store and forward, real time and hybrid systems. The simulation made by the study predicted savings of $4.3 billion per year if hybrid telehealth systems were to be implemented in emergency rooms, prisons, nursing homes facilities and physician offices across US. Savings were mainly due to the reduction of transfer of patients, prisoners and nursing home residents to and between emergency departments and from facilities to physician offices. In addition, there were savings by reduced health care utilisation, specifically from fewer face to face appointments at physician office and emergency departments. There was also a significant reduction of a duplicate and unnecessary testings. (44)

Telehealth offers a number of advantages, the main one being its potential to make specialist care accessible to underserved people and communities. In the context of nursing profession, telehealth offers patients an alternative ways to access nursing care. Reduced travel time, expenses, and inconvenience for patients and their families are also significant advantages offered by telehealth.

Telehealth can be advantageous for health professionals too. Telehealth has helped dispel professional isolation, particularly for those practitioners in geographically isolated areas. It helps them to communicate and obtain specialist advice, update their skills and knowledge. Telehealth can facilitate continuing medical education for isolated practitioners, allowing them to update their knowledge and skills and avoid interruptions in their practice, transportation costs and inconvenience. There is evidence that healthcare professionals accept telehealth as an essential part of the healthcare sector.

Barriers

One frequently cited barrier is the lack of information about the cost-effectiveness of telehealth. In order for telehealth to become integrated into mainstream healthcare, convincing evidence for its cost-effectiveness is required. Depending on the perspective, the financial benefits of telehealth applications may vary. Cost shifting is a common situation in telehealth. For example, the savings are made by the patients (who can avoid much travelling) while the costs accrue to the hospitals (which must pay for telehealth equipment and communication).

In line with other developments in health care, education and training is a key factor in uptake. Like advances in medical imaging, ongoing education and training are critical for patient safety and for staff to use telehealth systems efficiently and effectively.

Very little attention has been paid to education and training in telehealth. Research has shown that despite the fact that health practitioners are familiar with computers and other electronic devices the practice of telehealth requires systematic education and training. (45) The lack of knowledge of telehealth, its basic concepts and application is a result of the absence of systematic education. (46) Unless students are given education in basic concepts, principles and the variety of applications available, then it is unlikely that telehealth will become a part of their practice. The potential benefits of telehealth can only be realised if students are provided with formal education as part of their curriculum.

In addition, integrating telehealth into ongoing professional development is important. Health and medical professionals must be supported to acquire (at least until telehealth is integrated into mainstream curricula) and maintain their knowledge and practical skills in telehealth through continuing professional development (CPD) programmes. For this to occur, these courses will need to be recognised by relevant professional bodies through formal accreditation process. Financial and other relevant support must be provided to the health professionals by employers to attend telehealth CPD programmes.

References

1. Gostin, L.O.: The international migration and recruitment of nurses. JAMA 299(15), 1827–1829 (2008)
2. Occupational outlook handbook, USA (2008-2009), http://www.bls.gov/oco/ocos083.htm
3. Health Resources and Services Administration, Bureau of Health Professions, National Center for Health Workforce Analysis. Projected supply, demand, and shortages of registered nurses: 2000-2020, http://bhpr.hrsa.gov/healthworkforce/reports/rnproject/default.htm
4. Kingma, M.: Nurses on the move, Migration and the global health care economy. Cornell University Press, Ithaca (2004)
5. The World Health Report (2006), http://www.who.int/whr/2006/en/
6. Summary- Global shortage of registered nurses. The global nursing review initiative, International Council of Nurses, Geneva (2005), http://www.icn.ch/global/summary.pdf
7. The World Health Report, The Global Health Workforce Crisis (2003), http://www.who.int/whr/2003/chapter7/en/index4.html
8. Belfield, G., Colin-Thome, D.: Improving chronic disease management. Department of Health, UK National Health Service (2004), http://www.dh.gov.uk/en/Publicationsandstatistics/Publications/PublicationsPolicyAndGuidance/DH_4075214 (Retrieved October 20, 2007)
9. Information Technology Association of America e-Health Committee: Chronic care improvement: How Medicare transformation can save lives, save money and stimulate an emerging technology industry, ITAA (May 2004), http://www.itaa.org/isec/docs/choniccare.pdf (Retrieved October 20, 2007)
10. Callas, P.W., Ricci, M.A., Caputo, M.P.: Improved rural provider access to continuing medical education through interactive videoconferencing. Telemedicine and e-Health 6, 393–399 (2000)
11. Tran, B.O., Buckley, K.M., Prandoni, C.: Selection and use of telehealth technology in support of homebound caregivers of stroke patients. Caring 21(3), 16–21 (2002)
12. Hakan, G., Thoden, C.J., Carlson, C., Harno, K.: Realtime teleconsultations versus face to face consultations in dermatology: immediate and six month outcome. Journal of Telemedicine and Telecare 9(4), 204–209 (2003)

13. Chambers, M., Connor, S., Diver, M., McGonigle, M.: Usability of multimedia technology to help caregivers prepare for a crisis. Telemedicine Journal and e-Health 8(3), 343–347 (2002)
14. Loane, M., Wootton, R.: A review of telehealth. Medical Principles and Practice 10(3), 163–170 (2001)
15. Srikanthan, V.S., Pell, A.C., Prasad, N., Tait, G.W., Rae, A.P., Hogg, K.J., Dunn, F.: Use of fax facility improves decisionin making regarding thrombolysis in acute myocardial infarction. Heart 78(2), 198–200 (1997)
16. Vassaleo, D.J., Hoque, F., Patterson, V., Roberts, M.F., Swinfen, P., Swinfen, R.: An evaluation of the first year's experience with a low-cost telemedicine line in Bangladesh. Journal of Telemedicine and Telecare 7(3), 125–138 (2001)
17. Swinfen, P., Swinfen, R., Youngberry, K., Wootton, R.: A review of the first year's experience with an automatic message-routine system for low-cost telemedicine. Journal of Telemedicine and Telecare 9(suppl. 2), 63–65 (2003)
18. Ball, M.J.: Welcome to e-Health. In: Healthcare Informatics, pp. 45–49 (October 2001)
19. Wootton, R., Kvedar, J., Dimmick, S.L.: Home Telehealth: Connecting care within community. Royal Society of Medicine Press, London (2006)
20. Darkins, A., Dearde, C.H., Rocke, L.G., Martin, J.B., Sibson, L., Wootton, R.: An evaluation of telemedical support for a minor treatment centre. Journal of Telemedicine and Telecare 2(2), 92–99 (1996)
21. Agency for Health Care Research and Quality. The Characteristics of Long-Term Care Users. Rockville, M.D: AHRQ (2000)
22. Chang, K., Davis, R., Birt, J., Castelluccio, P., Woodbridge, P., Marrero, D.: Nurse practitioner-based diabetes care management: Impact of telehealth or telephone intervention on glycemic control. Disease Management and Heath Outcomes 15(6), 377–385 (2007)
23. Hoffman-Wellenhof, R., Salmhofer, W., Binder, B., Okcu, A., Kerl, H., Soyer, H.P.: Feasibility and acceptance of telemedicine for wound care in patients with chronic leg ulcers. Journal of Telemedicine and Telecare 12(suppl. 1), 15–17 (2006)
24. Dansky, K.H., Vasey, J., Bowles, K.: Impact of telehealth on clinical outcomes in patients with heart failure. Clinical Nursing Research 17(3), 182–188 (2008)
25. Cady, R., Kelly, A., Finkelstein, S.: Home telehealth for children with special health care needs. Journal of Telemedicine and Telecare 14, 173–177 (2008)
26. Rialle, V., Rumeau, P., Ollivet, C., Hervé, C.: Smart homes. In: Wootton, R., Kvedar, J., Dimmick, S. (eds.) Home Telehealth: Connecting care within community, pp. 65–75. Royal Society of Medicine Press, London (2006)
27. Bjorneby, S.: Smart houses: can they really benefit older people? Signpost 5, 36–38 (2000)
28. Gibson, F.: Seven Oakes: friendly design and sensitive technology. Journal of Dementia Care 11, 27–30 (2003)
29. Prado, M., Reina-Tosina, J., Roa, L.: Distributed intelligent architecture for falling detection and physical activity analysis in the elderly. In: Proceeding of the Second Joint EMBS/BMES Conference, vol. 3, pp. 1910–1911 (2002)
30. Kawaguchi, T., Azuma, M., Ohta, K.: Development of a telenursing system for patients with chronic conditions. Journal of Telemedicine and Telecare 10, 239–244 (2004)
31. Liddy, C., Dusseault, J.J., Dahrouge, S., Hogg, W., Lemelin, J., Humbert, J.: Telehomecare for patients with multiple chronic illnesses. Canadian Family Physician 54, 58–65 (2008)

32. Chan, W.M., Hjelm, N.: The role of telenurisng in the provision of geriatric outreach servicesto residential homes in Hong Kong. Journal of Telemedicine and Telecare 7, 38–46 (2001)
33. Woodend, K.A., Sherrard, H., Fraser, M., Stuewe, L., Cheung, T., Struthers, C.: Tele-home monitoring in patients with cardiac disease who are at high risk of readmission. Heart & Lung 37(1), 36–44 (2008)
34. Darkins, A., Dearde, C.H., Rocke, L.G., Martin, J.B., Sibson, L., Wootton, R.: An evaluation of telemedical support for a minor treatment centre. Journal of Telemedicine and Telecare 2(2), 92–99 (1996)
35. Kawaguchi, T., Azuma, M., Ohta, K.: Development of a telenursing system for patients with chronic conditions. Journal of Telemedicine and Telecare 10, 239–244 (2004)
36. Reed, K., White, P.: Telemedicine: Benefits to advanced practice nursing and the Communities they serve. Clinical Practice 17(5), 176–180 (2005)
37. Taylor, D.M., Capamagian, L.: Experience with planned and coordinated care using telemedicine. Journal of Telemedicine and Telecare 13(suppl. 3), 86–87 (2007)
38. Joanna Briggs Institute: Strategies to reduce medication errors with reference to older adults. Australian Nursing Journal 14(4), 26-29 (2006)
39. Ahrens, J., Feldman, P.H., Frey, D.: Preventing medication errors in home care. Centre for Home Care policy & Research Policy Brief 12, 1–6 (2002)
40. Kobb, R., Hilsen, P., Ryan, P.: Assessing technology needs for the elderly: finding the perfect match for home. Home Healthcare Nursing 1, 666–673 (2003)
41. Johnston, B., Wheeler, L., Deuser, J., Sousa, K.: Outcomes of the Kaiser Permanente Tele-home health research project. Archives of Family Medicine 9, 40–45 (2000)
42. Noel, H.C., Vogel, D.C., Erdos, J.J., Cornwall, D., Levin, F.: Home telehealth reduces healthcare costs. Telemedicine Journals and e-Health 10(2), 170–183 (2004)
43. Finkelstein, S.M., Speedie, S.M., Potthoff, S.: Home telehealth improves clinical outcomes at lower cost for home healthcare. Telemedicine and e-Health 12(2), 128–136 (2006)
44. Cusack, C.M.: The value proposition in the widespread use of telehelath. Journal of Telemedicine and Telecare 14, 167–168 (2008)
45. Edirippulige, S., Smith, A.C., Young, J., Wootton, R.: Knowledge, perceptions and expectations of nurses in e-health: results of a survey in a children's hospital. Journal of Telemedicine and Telecare 12(suppl. 3) S3, 35–38 (2006)
46. Edirippulige, S., Smith, A., Beattie, H., Davies, E., Wootton, R.: Preregistration nurses: an investigation of knowledge, experience and comprehension of e-health. Australian Journal of Advanced Nursing 25(2), 78–83 (2007)

Dr Sisira Edirippulige PhD (Moscow), PhD (Auckland), MSc (Moscow), GradCert Health Sciences (UQ)

Coordinator - Graduate Programmes in e-Health care

The University of Queensland Centre for Online Health

Dr Edirippulige's main responsibilities involve teaching and include the coordination of all undergraduate and graduate courses in e-health care and continuing professional development courses in telehealth. His research interests include the development, promotion and integration of telehealth education and telemedicine applications into the health care sector. Before joining the University of Queensland, Sisira taught at Kobe Gakuin University in Japan and at the University of Auckland in New Zealand. He has extensive experience in development studies working in number of countries including Russia, Sri Lanka, South Africa, Japan and New Zealand.

Sisira Edirippuligé
Coordinator e-Healthcare Programs
Centre for Online Health
University of Queensland
Level 3, Foundation Building
Royal Children's Hospital
Herston Road, Herston 4029
QLD Australia

Tel: +61 7 3346 4887
Fax: +61 7 3346 4705
Web: www.uq.edu.au/coh

A Multi-Modal Health and Activity Monitoring Framework for Elderly People at Home

Andy Marsh (a), Christos Biniaris (a), Ross Velentzas (a), Jérémie Leguay (b), Bertrand Ravera (b), Mario Lopez-Ramos (b), Eric Robert (b)

(a) VMW Solutions Ltd
9 Northlands Road – Whitenap
Romsey - Hamsphire SO51 5RU – UK
{firstname.name}@vmwsolutions.com
tel. +44-(0)1794-500 145
fax. +44-(0)1794-522558

(b)THALES Communications
System Engineering Architectures
160 Boulevard de Valmy - BP 82
92704 Colombes Cedex – France
{firstname.name}@fr.thalesgroup.com
tel. +33-(0)1-46132346
fax. +33-(0)1-46132686

Abstract Since the population of elderly people grows absolutely and in relation to the overall population in the world, the improvement of the quality of life of elderly people at home is of a great importance. This can be achieved through the development of generic technologies for managing their domestic ambient environment consisting of medical sensors, entertainment equipment, home automation systems and white goods, increasing their autonomy and safety. In this context, the provision intelligent interactive healthcare services will improve their daily life and allowing at the same time the continuous monitoring of their health and their effective treatment. This paper presents a multi-modal health and activity monitoring framework that enables abnormal event detection and long term evaluation of the health of the elderly people at home. We describe its integration with a Residential Gateway and provide details on the demonstration scenario developed, involving different kinds of sensing modules. This work is supported by the INHOME Project EU IST-045061-STP, http://www.ist-inhome.eu.

Keywords: Healthcare Services, Elderly, Patient Monitoring, Assisted Living at Home, Network Architecture and Design

K. Yogesan et al. (Eds.): Handbook of Digital Homecare, BIOMED, pp. 287–298.
springerlink.com

Table of contents

I. Introduction

Europe's ageing population is a challenge for both its social and health systems. By 2020, a quarter of Europe's population will be over 65. Spending on pensions, health and long-term care is expected to increase by 4-8% of GDP in coming decades, with total expenditures tripling by 2050. Similarly, by 2050, elderly people aged between 65-79 years old are expected to make up almost a third of the population which is a rise of 44 per cent compared to the start of the century. As for very elderly people (80+), their share of the total population could grow by 180 per cent over the same period. The majority of older people do not yet enjoy the benefits of the digital age such as low cost communications and online services that could support some of their real needs; only 10% use the internet. Severe vision, hearing or dexterity problems, frustrate many older peoples' efforts to engage in the information society. According to findings of the Center for Disease Control, nearly three quarters of elders over the age of 65 suffer of one or more chronic diseases. The majority of the growing elder population worldwide requires some degree of formal and/or informal care either due to loss of function or failing health as a result of ageing.

The cost and burden of caring for elders is steadily increasing. If given the choice, many elders would prefer to lead an independent way of life in a residential setting with minimum intervention from the caregiver. Ambient Assisted Living (AAL) programs are intended to address the needs of this increasing elderly population, to reduce innovation barriers of forthcoming promising markets for the various target group populations, but also to lower future social security costs on the long run. The major challenges of AAL research programs are to extend the time elderly people can spend in their home environment by ameliorating their level of autonomy and assisting them in carrying out simple or even more complicated everyday activities.

It is a challenging issue for someone to deal with the special needs of elderly people especially in the home healthcare monitoring and treatment. The goal of the INHOME project is to provide the means for improving the quality of life of elderly people at home by developing generic technologies for managing their domestic ambient environment, consisted of white goods, entertainment equipment and home automation systems with the aim to increase their autonomy and safety [1], [2]. Monitoring of different types of chronic diseases of elderly people at an in-home environment relies heavily on patients' self-monitoring of their disease conditions [3]. In recent years, telemonitoring systems, that allow the transmission of patient's data to a hospital's central database and offer immediate access to the data by the care providers, is of a great importance [4], [5].

From the healthcare delivery system point of view, an evolving picture of the patient at any given time will be produced, taking into account diagnoses and treatments, successes and setbacks [6]. The system would assess the current level of functionality and interactively coach the patient to higher levels of functionality. The consistency of continuous monitoring would eliminate much of the inaccuracy from the current random interactions between patients and physicians [7], [8]. Periodically and as determined by medical parameters and health plan factors, this data would be reviewed by trained professionals to such evaluation process.

The User Group is provided by the Health Centre of Vyronas (HCV), which is specialised in the provision of medical services to elderly people at home. The medical personnel are also involved in the requirements specification for aged people. The institute offers some of the houses under surveillance to be used as application testbeds and assist in the evaluation phase of the INHOME technology. This paper presents the overall network architecture, discusses the health and activity monitoring framework, describes the A/V streaming and personal data acquisition by medical devices within the home environment, and finally summarises project's current conclusions.

II. The overall network architecture

The project identified the need for several devices, sensors and terminals to be integrated for enabling the different kinds of identified services for the elderly people. The overall network architecture with all involved device categories and intermediate network entities is shown in Figure 1. The concept of a centralized gateway as communication and interworking entity is utilized. In this scenario, the gateway is the only device directly connected to the Internet and external service providers with the rest of the home devices connected to the gateway. All messages issued by the devices are routed through the gateway and there has not been envisioned direct communication flow between the devices for this project. The residential gateway undertakes the role of coordinating information requests, it establishes the connection to appropriate content servers and forwards the requests of the service applications. The architecture is also enhanced with the introduction and usage of a Multi Service Terminal which acts as a repeater, increasing the limited coverage of the Bluetooth devices and sensors. The gateway processes as well as forwards the information either to WAN and to LAN entities [9].

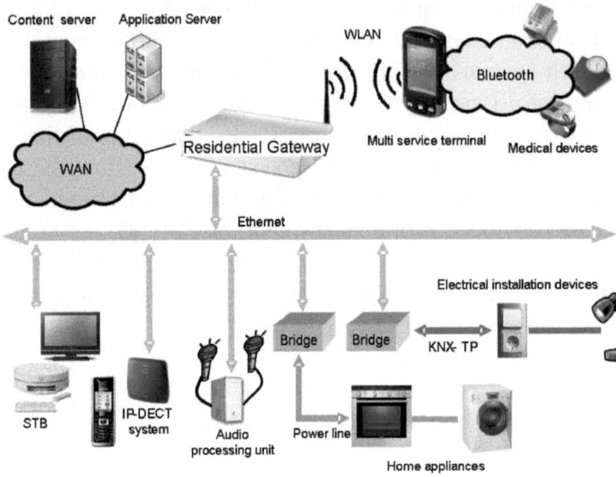

Figure 1. The INHOME Overall Network Architecture

Ethernet, Wireless LAN (WLAN) and Bluetooth are used as communication technologies. Since most devices are equipped with Ethernet sockets and pre-configured cabling is available, the installation procedure becomes rather easy. Also, nearly all the gateways available on the market are equipped with a build-in wireless network interface. The dominating technology for WLAN communication follows the IEEE standards 802.11 a, b, g or n.

The INHOME services are communicating both internally within the home network as well as with the external world. This means that communication must not be limited to in-home data flows only. Depending on the service, communication must be secured to guarantee a level of intimacy. Only user authentication and authorisation can grant access to personalized services. The INHOME residential gateway is the central entity in the home networking environment, deploying the services and facilitating the communication with the external world. The gateway simultaneously functions as both client and server to the other nodes on the network. The peer node functionality is supported by OSGi, which is capable to host both server parts (Web Servers, Custom Servers etc.) and client parts (UPnP, Web Services, custom clients, HTTP clients etc.). Additionally, the residential gateway is hosting data such as related to the user (user profiles, policies etc.), multimedia data (photos, videos etc.), etc.

Services composition involves the user and a service synthesis environment interacting for the production of a personalised service specification. This specification is consistent with the capabilities of the service execution platforms in use and the user profile stored in the identity management module of the residential gateway and will be produced by a Service Synthesis module located on the Residential gateway. The service composition functionality is being used by the application level of the INHOME gateway for providing AAL services to elderly people. Figure 2 depicts the architecture of the INHOME Residential Gateway and the services supported.

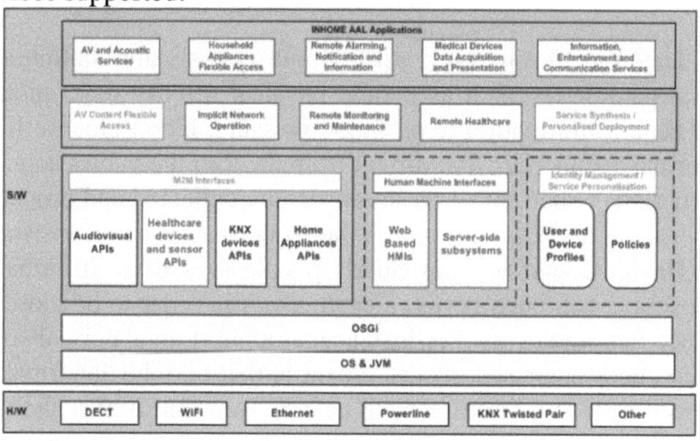

Figure 2. INHOME Residential Gateway and Services

III. Health and activity monitoring framework

The health and activity monitoring system that we present in this work enables people living in a monitored home to be assisted by a specialist (emergency hospital department or private health security center) in case of abnormal events. This system is adapted to aged, disabled or diseased people. More generally, the idea behind this appliance is to collect all the kinds of data that would help monitoring health of people or that would benefit to other appliances to make smart decision making. Two kinds of monitoring activities are performed by this appliance:

- Activity monitoring: By activity, we refer to people physical activity (frequency, duration and intensity of their movements) or to the consequences of their actions on their environment (e.g., temperature in a room, change on the daylight in a room because the curtains have been closed). This information by itself (e.g., a very high temperature in a room) or after combination with other information (e.g., a suddenly closed curtain) can plot abnormal behaviours that could be of interest to record as well as for further investigation on the elderly people's health.

- Health monitoring: This monitoring activity includes parameters such as the vital signs which consists in physiological statistics (i.e., body temperature, pulse rate, blood pressure, respiratory rate) often taken by health professionals in order to assess the most basic body functions. This activity could include any other parameter that would be useful to trigger alarms or to monitor on a long term basis.

Concerning specifically the health of people, the proposed monitoring appliance has two main purposes:

- Abnormal event detection: A variety of sensing sub-systems are continuously monitoring several parameters such as people physical activity (e.g., motion, ambient light) or health information (e.g., blood pressure, blood glucose level, heartbeats). Abnormal events (i.e., that differs from the average values acquired during a training period) issued by all these sensors are collected and processed by the system in order to take decisions upon the requesting or not of assistance from an external Health Center or from elderly people's relatives. Information received from sensors is validated between each others in order to be more accurate and to reduce false positives. For instance, at night if an abnormal sound activity is detected and a heart beat measurement is that may be abnormal, an alarm will be immediately send to a medical center. To refine further the relevance of the information provided by the system, different level of alarms can be defined (e.g., notice, warning, alarm, emergency) and mapped to different actions.
- Long term monitoring: The aforementioned sensing modules will also enable to assess the state of the person based on its behavior and medical parameters. Thus, the Health Center will be able to refer to history data to better choose future prescribed medications.

Whereas such integrated system has already been studied by several projects, INHOME project is to validate the concept of an evolving health and activity monitoring service based on a home gateway. The following section details the multi-modal monitoring system that we have developed in INHOME for that purpose.

IV. Framework architecture

This section details the framework that we propose to be used which offers coordinated operation of activity monitoring and medical monitoring for both abnormal event detection and long term evaluation of the health of the elderly people.

A. Overview

Figure 3 depicts the different entities composing the INHOME health and activity monitoring appliance that we have developed. The medical analysis sub-systems in charge of the gathering of the vital health parameters of elderly people is connected to the INHOME gateway. Besides this, a processing unit connects the two different activity sensing modules that we have integrated for our demonstration: the audio sensors and the networked motion sensors.

This processing unit performs high-level analysis of the parameters gathered from the sensing sub-systems and is able to detect abnormal events. It interacts with the INHOME gateway by initiating events and/or receiving queries for measurements from the audio and motion sensors. The INHOME gateway is based on a Residential Gateway (RG) concept, using the Open Service Gateway initiative (OSGi) platform [10].

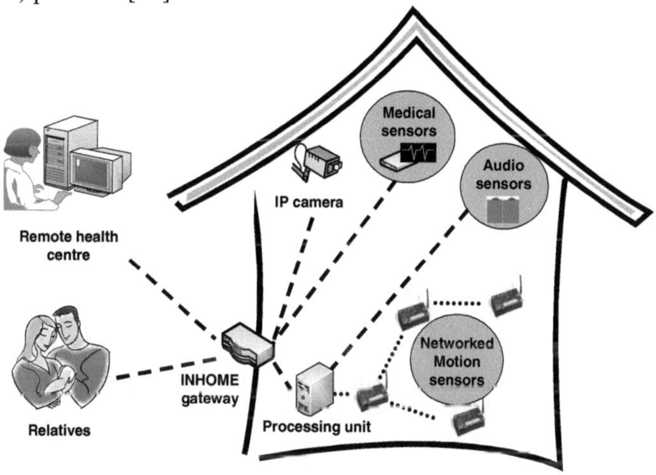

Figure 3. INHOME Health and Activity Monitoring

We propose to use two different sub-systems for activity monitoring function depending on the time of the day: A sensor-network based motion detector using a wrist lace or a necklace that elderly people wears at day time and an audio monitoring system mainly used at night in the bedroom. Both systems trigger alarms which are first processed and then exposed to the rest of the system through the activity monitoring processing unit. These two sub-systems are described with more details in the following sections.

B. Sensor-network based motion detector

We propose an activity monitoring service running on Crossbow MICAz [11] sensors equipped with a MTS310 sensor board attached to their serial port which offers a variety of sensing modalities such as light, pressure, acceleration, temperature and acoustic. MICAz nodes have very limited capacity in memory and processing power as they only embed an Atmel ATmega128L microcontroller with 4KB of RAM and have 128KB of programmable flash ROM.

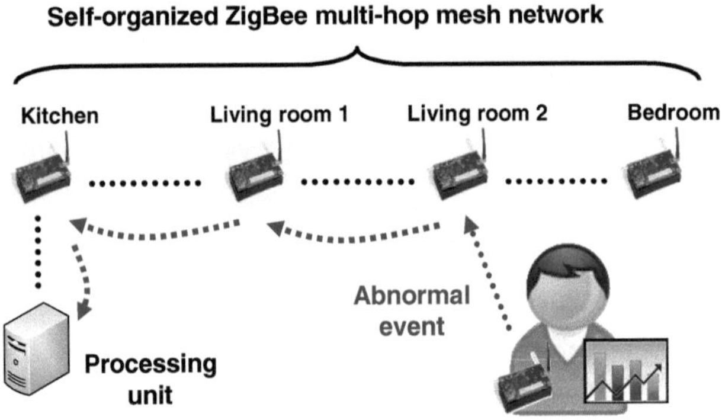

Figure 4. Sensor Network Based Monitoring Service

As shown by Figure 4, sensor nodes are divided in two categories: infrastructure nodes which form the ZibBee-based mesh communication network and sensing nodes which are worn at day time by people. Infrastructure nodes run a routing protocol to enable multi-hop communications. Such network organization allows auto-configuration and eases the extension of the network as users would just have to deploy a new relay to cover a new room or to adapt to new room layout. On sensing nodes, the sensing service is related to the accelerometer. It offers the possibility: (1) to get the latest values of the accelerations over the z and x axis, (2) to be notified periodically of these values and (3) to be notified of these values whenever an abnormal event occur.

The fact that infrastructure nodes are static after deployment provides a very simple positioning system which allows adding location information to alarms: the data packets issued by the sensors are tagged with the id of the first node of the infrastructure. A simple mapping between sensor's identifier and rooms helps to locate where the elderly person was when the alarm occurred. The monitoring service stack implemented in TinyOS [12] rests upon the IEEE 802.15.4 interface, also known as ZigBee, and a queuing management module which has been implemented to handle incoming and outgoing packets.

C. Audio monitoring system

The purpose of this application is to detect any audio event which does not belong to the audio background related to non activity ambiance. Figure 5 shows the sound processing chain required by our audio monitoring system. A microphone network, associated with a pre-amplifier and a sound-board, is used to measure the audio activity of each monitored room in real time. In its first version, the system does not intend to model abnormal audio event but just to analyse current audio energy level and the difference form the previously trained model. Yet, the audio analysis algorithms implemented on the processing unit could later be enhanced to enable more elaborate capabilities. If significantly different from the average values usually experienced (the threshold can be defined) an alarm is raised by the processing unit. A home sound cartography is also computed by the processing unit and possibly provided on demand to the Health Center through the residential gateway.

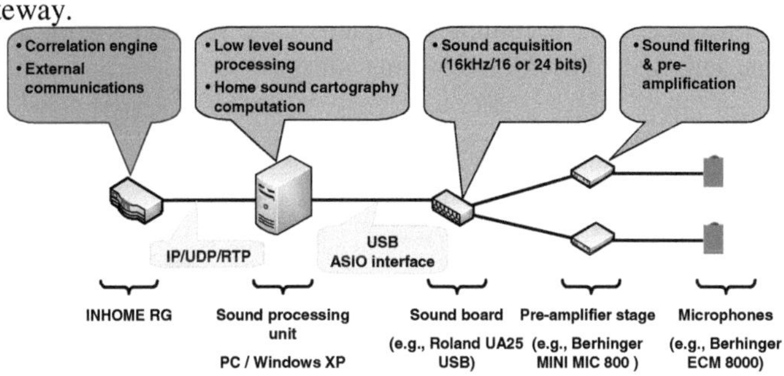

Figure 5. Sound Processing Chain

D. Health monitoring subsystem

The health monitoring subsystem develops a real time, interactive, home health care service based on the wireless or wireline acquisition of medical data from devices operating at the user's home environment. Interconnecting the health monitoring subsystem with the activity monitoring subsystem at the home gateway, the overall system becomes an integrated, adaptive, reactive, customisable, with extendable intelligence health care system

The health monitoring subsystem acquires the data from the medical devices, checks for possible alarm conditions, takes action is necessary, relates and/or presents the measurements values, stores the measurements for post-analysis and archiving purposes, The elements participating in this subsystem are illustrated in Figure 6 and highlighted as:

- The medical devices, which are used to perform measurements such as blood pressure, cardiac pulse, body weight etc.
- The INHOME terminal which is responsible to communicate with the devices for acquiring those measurements.
- The residential gateway which is responsible to run services based on the data produced by the medical devices.
- The TV device which is responsible to display the measurements in a user friendly manner.
- The DECT phone which enables the user to contact his/her physician.

There are two different communication interfaces utilised, the Bluetooth and 802.11. The Bluetooth communication is used to directly transfer the medical information to the gateway or at the INHOME terminal. The INHOME terminal is used as an intermediate collection point due to the fact that it could be carried by the user and it can be in the proximity of the medical devices. It can be extended with the ZigBee interface, thus becoming also part of the sensor network and a bridge between the activity and health monitoring subsystems.

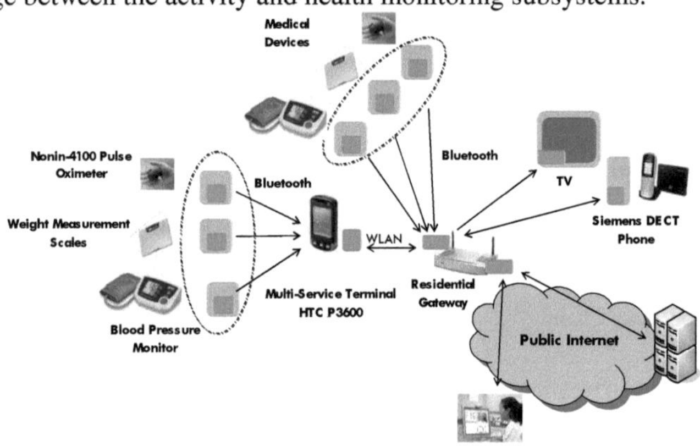

Figure 6. Health Monitoring Subsystem

The INHOME terminal and the 802.11 interface are used as the Bluetooth connectivity would not be always guaranteed, since the medical device could be out of the Bluetooth coverage of the gateway. After having acquired the data from the medical devices, the INHOME terminal sends this data through a WLAN communication to the residential gateway, which in turn processes this data.

Some key processing is related with the identification of alarm values based on the normal range for each type of measurement, the user profile and updates that can exist from the doctor. The service execution in the gateway is also responsible to send the data to the TV, enabling the user to view the values and assisting the elderly people as vision capabilities are reduced. Upon the detection of an alarm condition, the service in the gateway is also responsible to take appropriate action according the medical case and user. For example, it may require additional information from the activity monitoring subsystem, discover the phone number of the relevant physician, which maybe stored locally or at a remote location, send the phone number to the DECT phone allowing the user to avoid the manual dialing of the number or even call directly the doctor, etc.

The implementation at the INHOME terminal is based on J2ME (Java2 MicroEdition) which is capable of communicating with each medical device and acquiring the relevant data over Bluetooth. The alternative approach of direct communication with the residential gateway and alarm/action logic were performed with the development of communication

V. Conclusion and future work

The proposed framework offers coordinated operation of activity monitoring (motion detection & audio in our case) and medical monitoring for both abnormal event detection and long term evaluation of the health of the elderly people.

Continuous interaction, collecting of information, detailed patient status and appropriate user profiling would be the key issues to address the needs of both the elderly users at home as well as the experts at the Health Care centers. In this paper, an interactive healthcare services environment for assisted living at home was presented, identifying the underlying technology employed such as adaptive audio monitoring algorithms, self-organized ZigBee multi-hop mesh networks, OSGi, Java and Web Services.

These technologies have not yet fulfilled their full potential and according to the model presented at this paper, utilising them as integrated and interacting technologies, they may provide solutions and services that would be influencing the way that home networking and home health care architectures are provided in the future.

Acknowledgement

This work was performed under the INHOME research project (An Intelligent Interactive Services Environment for Assisted Living at Home), funded by the European Commission under the Sixth Framework Programme (Proposal/Contract no.: IST-2005-045061/STP).

References

[1] INHOME Deliverable D-2.2: INHOME Architecture Specification, http://www.ist-inhome.eu
[2] INHOME Deliverable D-2.1: Architecture Requirements & Showcases, http://www.ist-inhome.eu

[3] Rialle, V., Lamy, J.B., Noury, N., Bajolle, L.: Telemonitoring of patients at home: a software approach. Computer Methods and Programs in Biomedicine 72(3), 257–268 (2003)
[4] Lee, R., Chen, H., Lin, C., Chang, K., Chen, J.: Home Telecare System using Cable Television Plants – An Experimental Field Trial. IEEE Transactions on Information Technology in Biomedicine 4(1), 37–43 (2000)
[5] Maglaveras, N., et al.: Home care delivery through the mobile telecommunications platform: the Citizen Health System (CHS) perspective. International Journal of Medical Informatics 68(3), 99–111 (2002)
[6] Kyriacou, E., et al.: Multi-purpose HealthCare Telemedicine Systems with mobile communication link support. Healthcare Engineering OnLine 2(7) (2003)
[7] Pattichis, C.S., Kyriacou, E., Voskarides, S., Pattichis, M.S., Istepanian, R., Schizas, C.N.: Wireless Telemedicine Systems: An Overview. IEEE Antennas & Propagation Magazine 44(2), 143–153 (2002)
[8] Engin, M., Yamaner, Y., Engin, E.Z.: A biotelemetric system for human ECG measurements. Measurement 38(2), 148–153 (2005)
[9] Vouyioukas, D., Maglogiannis, I., Vergados, D., Kormentzas, G., Rouskas, A.: WPAN's Technologies for Pervasive e-Health Applications – State of the Art and Future Trends. Journal for Quality of Life Research 3(2), 198–204 (2005)
[10] OSGi Alliance. About the OSGi Service Platform - Technical Whitepaper Revision 4.0 (2005), http://www.osgi.org/documents/
[11] xBow MICAz: Wireless measurement system, http://www.xbow.com/Products/Product_pdf_files/Wireless_pdf/MICAz_Datasheet.pdf
[12] Hill, J., Szewczyk, R., Woo, A., Hollar, S., Culler, D.E., Pister, K.S.J.: System architecture directions for networked sensors. In: Architectural Support for Programming Languages and Operating Systems, pp. 93–104 (2000)

Digital Homecare Experiences: Remote Patient Monitoring

Dr Helen Aikman (a), Phillip Coppin (b)

(a) LaTrobe University, Bendigo
Mobile 0419 510 762, Email: Helen.aikman@lmha.com.au
(b) Loddon Mallee Health Alliance
Telephone 03 5454 8456, Email: Pcoppin@bendigohealth.org.au

Abstract Digital home care provides exciting opportunities to overcome the difficulties of distance and lack of access in the delivery of health care. This chapter describes experiences encountered by "*Connecting Clients* [2] *Care*", a project designed to implement Remote Patient Monitoring (RPM) and conducted by Loddon Mallee Health Alliance in Victoria, Australia. RPM is discussed in terms of the need for the project, objectives, equipment and systems used, implementation, maintenance of the project and evaluation. To enable the experiences of this project to be described from multiple viewpoints, two case studies are included from clients who used RPM. Benefits have included: increased client and carer confidence in managing and interpreting symptoms, increased quality of life, increased healthy behaviour, decreased nursing visits and travel time with resultant efficiencies and increased capacity for agencies to cater for clients that would not otherwise have been catered for.

K. Yogesan et al. (Eds.): Handbook of Digital Homecare, BIOMED, pp. 299–327.
springerlink.com

Introduction

Loddon Mallee Health Alliance (LMHA) is one of five Rural Health Alliances throughout the state of Victoria, Australia that are charged with representing the information technology interests of health agencies in their regions. LMHA, with funds from Multimedia Victoria, has partnered with five agencies in the Loddon Mallee region to install seventy Remote Patient Monitors (RPM) in the homes of chronically ill clients with chronic obstructive pulmonary disease, heart failure, and diabetes. This was a part of a larger project entitled "*Connecting Clients* [2] *Care*".

The objectives of the RPM project were to:

- Enhance client care with more frequent and comprehensive assessment,
- Increase agency capacity to maintain chronically ill clients at optimal levels of health in their own homes,
- Investigate the technical and clinical feasibility of using high technology telecommunications services to enhance client care, and
- Determine the economic efficiencies that RPM may offer.

The project purchased the RPM equipment from an Australian company, TeleMedCare. TeleMedCare is the only Australian supplier of this type of equipment designed for installation in the client's home. The equipment has peripheral devices that allow chronically ill clients and/or carers to measure blood pressure, temperature, blood sugar level, oxygen saturation, spirometry, lead I ECG, heart rate, weight and answer online health questionnaires. These measurements are then transferred over the internet to nurses at the participating agencies. These measurements assist:

- Nurses in provision of client care,
- Clients and carers in making choices about healthy behaviour and
- Doctors in managing medical regimes.

In addition, the client can see their own measurements on the monitor in graph format, can enter short details about health activities and visits, and can access relevant health websites allocated to them by the nurses.

The RPM project commenced in April 2007. A comprehensive and academically rigorous evaluation will be conducted using baseline, six and twelve month data collection points with the data compared to data from a control group not participating in RPM from the same agencies. Evaluation will be complete by December 2008.

Early data indicates that RPM has been very successful, with many positive client outcomes. Anecdotal evidence indicates the availability of the RPM devices has increased client and carer confidence in managing and interpreting symptoms, increased quality of life, increased healthy behaviour, decreased routine nursing visits and travel time with resultant efficiencies and increased the reach of agencies to cater for clients that would not otherwise have been catered for.

Background

Remote Patient Monitoring is yet another service that has been made possible by the advent of the internet. It uses a computer terminal located at a client's home that peripheral devices can be attached to. Data measured by the peripheral devices is stored on the computer for transmission over the internet to a server. A secure site on the server can be accessed by health care professionals who then use the client data for clinical decision making. The most immediate advantages are that the health care professional does not have to be with the client when the measurements are taken eliminating the time required and the cost of travel for client and/or professional and that the client can record the measurements when they need to and as often as desired.

With the knowledge that equipment for RPM existed, LMHA embarked upon an initiative to implement a project whereby RPM would be installed in the homes of clients throughout the Loddon Mallee region.

LMHA is a not-for-profit information technology organization that services the needs of health care agencies in the Loddon Mallee region. At the time of implementation of the RPM project the Alliance serviced 26 agencies, which included hospitals, community health centres and several small community based health services offering service to special groups like the intellectually disabled and career respite services. The core services provided to agencies by the Alliance include: IP telephony, internet, video conferencing and the provision of a fully managed wide area network. The Alliance also offers a hosted email service plus shared service aged care application. Additionally, the Alliance has initiated several special projects in the telehealth space with funding from the Victorian and Commonwealth governments. The objectives of LMHA are to:

- Strive for excellence in the provision of ICT services and support to the health sector across the Loddon Mallee region.
- Demonstrate achievements and identify ways to improve through program review and the analysis of data
- Build alliances throughout the health and community sectors to create better health ICT systems.
- Encourage the provision of services to health clients across the Loddon Mallee region wherever they live, whatever their background, with special needs and those disadvantaged in our society using ICT.

Funding for the RPM project was obtained from Broadband Innovation Fund administered by MultiMedia Victoria which is a section of the State Government Department of Information Communication and Technology. The purposes of the Broadband Innovation Fund are to:

- Accelerate the implementation of broadband by government agencies,
- Quantify the impact of broadband on improving cost and administrative efficiency and service delivery,

- Test innovative business and technology models for the rollout of broadband in Victoria,
- Identify the impact of accelerated provision of broadband on the broader community, and
- Identify any associated economic and community development benefits.

The genesis of this initiative lay in the desire of LMHA to improve the delivery of health care to residents of the Loddon Mallee region, using a telehealth initiative. LMHA had already assisted with IT initiatives aimed at the acute health sector such as building the managed network, developing hosted mail services and deploying patient management systems, but identified an opportunity to make a contribution to the care of the chronically ill at home and in the community. Personal knowledge of the difficulties faced by the chronically ill was a driving force and knowledge of geographic, demographic and workforce issues in the region heightened the need for a solution.

This region comprises approximately 25% of Victoria's land mass and is Victoria's most sparsely populated region. Weekly household income is less than the median for Victoria, $795 vs. $1,022 (ABS, 2007a, ABS 2007b) and the population is older with 15.6% of residents being 65 years or over as compared to 13.7% for Victoria (ABS, 2007, ABS 2007b).

Like most regional areas, the Loddon Mallee has a shortage of medical and allied health professionals. Although the region has 6% of Victoria's population, it only has 4.1% of the state's allied health professionals. The average general practitioner to population ratio across the three Federal electorates in the Loddon Mallee region is 1:1485.

Within this large, sparsely populated area, there is a higher burden of disease than in metropolitan areas for cardiovascular disease and chronic respiratory disease (among other conditions). In Victoria, cardiovascular disease, chronic respiratory disease, and diabetes are significant contributors to the burden of disease, accounting for 17%, 7% and 3.7% respectively, or a total of 28.7%, of all burden of disease (DHS, 2005)

Coexisting with this situation is an increased emphasis on ambulatory care and the delivery of health care in the home. There is also a state focus on prevention of unnecessary presentations at Emergency Departments and prevention of readmissions to hospital for this client cohort, through programs such as Hospital Admission Risk Program (HARP). These programs are often reliant on the nursing workforce, which is also under significant pressure. There is predicted to be a statewide shortfall of 8,300 Division One FTE nurses and 2,874 Division Two FTE nurses by 2011 (DHS, 2004).

To date, avenues for addressing the problem of caring for the chronically ill in sparsely populated and other areas, have hinged on administrative solutions and reorganization/redefinition of services that already existed. Telehealth initiatives have an important role to play in the Australian health care arena. Optimal use of information technology can improve the quality of health care, clinical decision making and reduce wastage of resources.

This initiative implemented an innovative solution based on new technology by introducing RPM into five agencies in the region. A premise for the project was that home monitoring would reduce nursing effort to manage a given group of clients, thereby allowing the take-up of more clients with the same sized workforce.

The objectives of the project were to:

- Trial the implementation of a telehealth solution to manage chronically ill clients in their own homes.
- Develop an understanding of the clinical efficacy of the RPM technology,
- Gain insight into the technical capabilities of the RPM technology in Australian rural health environments,
- Understand the factors concerning practitioners about introducing this technology and develop effective change management process to address concerns,
- Develop new work practices to deliver improved clinical outcomes, organisational efficiencies and productivity gains through the use of RPM
- Share the finding with clinicians, health care organizations and government leading to a greater understanding of the benefits of RPM technology in the clinical setting.

Remote Patient Monitoring Equipment and Systems

The monitors used in this project were manufactured and supplied by an Australian company, TeleMedCare Pty Ltd. The RPM units selected are depicted in Figures 1 and 2. The monitors were installed in client's homes. They are not designed to be portable and do not involve the wearing of any devices on a continuing basis. Specifications of the equipment are listed in Table 1. The monitors have a laptop sized processing unit that the measurement devices connect to. The operating system is Microsoft Windows xp. The touch screen, which controls functions, is positioned on top of this unit. The monitor system requires power and connection to a standard telephone line or to broadband. The system is approved for use by the Therapeutic Goods Administration, and uses the highest quality equipment available.

Table 1. Specifications of RPM equipment used by Connecting Clients [2] Care

ECG module	
Single channel	Leads: I (RA-LA)
	Input range: 10mVpp
	Resolution: $\pm$ 1.25μV
	Input device: Dry- Ag/AgCl electrode TMC ECG
	Plate or PEG Clamp Electrodes

Pulse Oximeter Module	
Display	Oxygen saturation
	Pulse rate
Display range	SpO2: 0%-100%
	Pulse rate: 20-250 bpm
SpO2 Accuracy	%SpO2 ± 1SD
SpO2 Accuracy Adults:	70%-100% ± 2 digits
	0%-69% unspecified
Pulse Rate Accuracy	50-250 bpm ± 3bpm
Personal Weight Scales	
Maximum capacity	150kg
Minimum display	50g
Battery life	Approx. 2,000 measurements
Memory	31 measurements
Auto power off	Yes
Blood Pressure Module	
Measurement method	Oscillometric and auscultatory linear pressure release 3- 4 mmHg/sec
Displays	Systolic, mean, diastolic, pulse rate
Data recorded	Pressure, auscaltatory signal, oscillometric signal
Patient range	Adult, Adult Large, Child
Pressure display range	10-300 mmHg
Measurement range	Systolic 60-250 mmHg
	Diastolic 40-200 mmHg

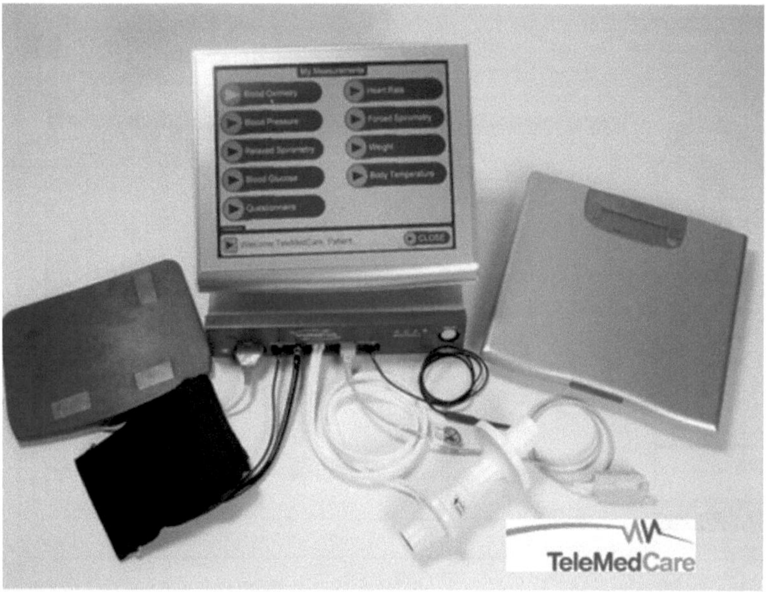

Figure 1: A Remote Patient Monitoring unit with measurement menu displayed and peripheral devices for clinical measurements attached.

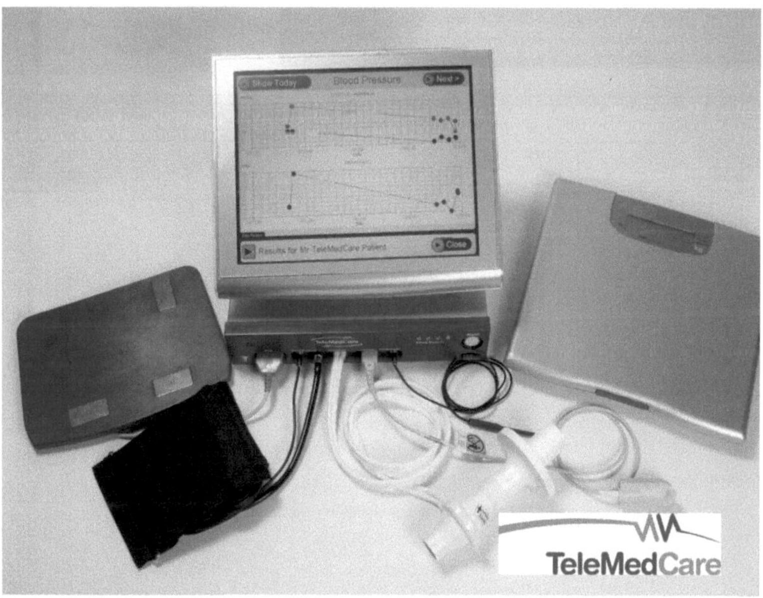

Figure 2: The monitoring unit with the client's view of one of their measurements, blood pressure.

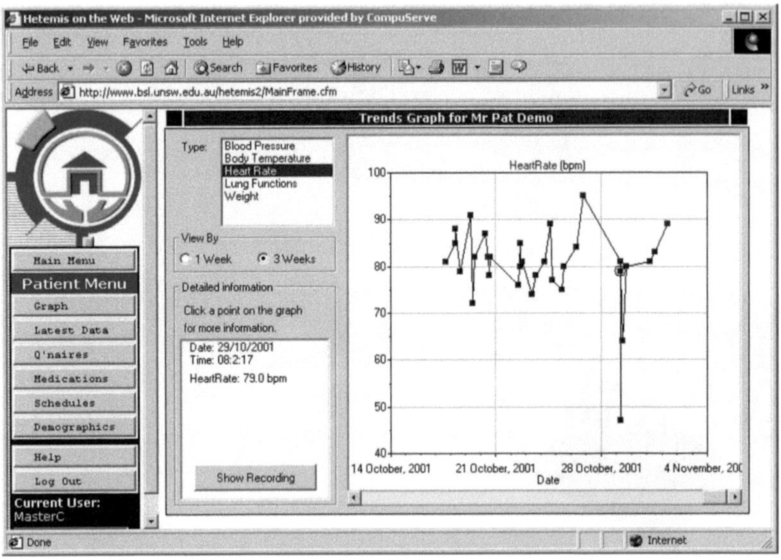

Figure 3: A clinician's view of a client's heart rate data as it appears in graph format on the website. Client data is also available in table format.

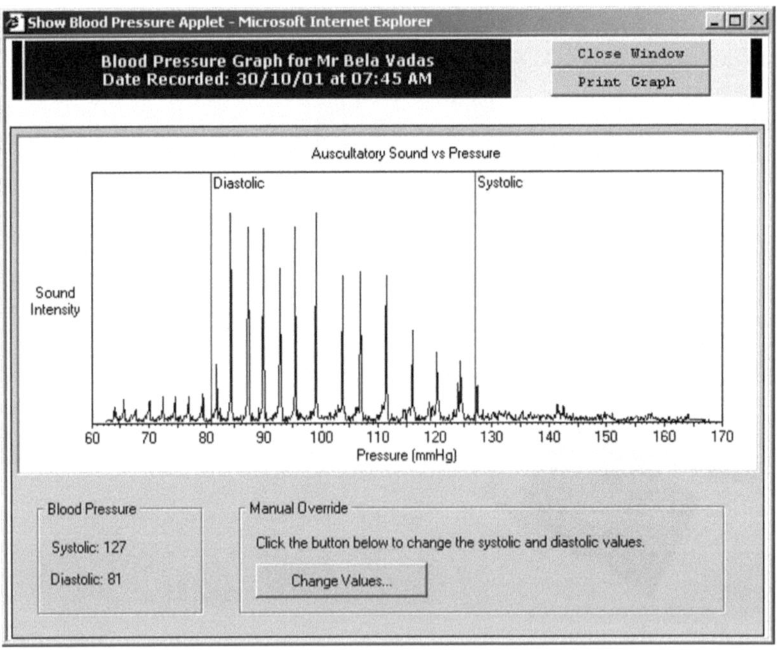

Figure 4: Clinicians can click on some measurements individually to enable them to scrutinise each measurement for accuracy and errors. This is available for blood pressure, ECG and spirometry.

Data is automatically sent from the client's monitor over the internet, usually overnight, to a central server maintained by TeleMedCare. If the client does not already have internet access this is established by the connection of the RPM unit to the telephone line in the home. A number of telephone line adaptors are available to ensure that other services that may depend on the telephone line are not interrupted. Broadband is utilized if the client already has it installed. Using broadband makes the transmission of data much faster, but because this project has not used the RPM units as emergency devices and has relied predominantly on routine overnight transmission of data, speed of data transfer has not been a problem.

The central server utilises Microsoft SQL server 2005, IIS Server, Apache cocoon and JBoss. The overall function of the server is to synchronise with the RPM units. This is done not only for the purpose of transmission of client data, but is useful to enable complete automatic software upgrades to keep the units up to date with current IT requirements. In addition the server can implement a remote support facility whereby non responding RPM units are automatically rebooted if they have not responded to the server for two consecutive attempts at synchronization. The server is also the means that allows decision support software to function. This software recognises data such as the blood pressure wave forms shown in Figure 4 and interprets this as systolic and diastolic blood pressure values.

Nurses gain access to the client's data transmitted from the server to their normal PC used in their workplaces. Each agency has specific passwords to access the website to view their own client's data. Staff at one agency cannot see the client data from other agencies. Nurses may use the operating systems of Windows (any version), Linux or Mac. The computer used needs access to a web browser, email services, Java, SVG Viewer and PDF reader.

Medical practitioners can also obtain their own password to view their client's data. Nurses can email or print out reports of the client's measurements for distributing to medical practitioners, placing on client files or giving to the clients. Currently the reports can be scanned into the GP's practice management systems, but are not automatically integrated into other IT applications. The system also supports HL7 messaging and full integration into practice management software may be developed in the future.

There are a number of features on the website that the nurses involved in this project have been able to use to assist with gaining data and management of their client's conditions. On first accessing the website nurses are able to view a list of client's names who they currently have access to. A status page can be viewed to give a quick indication of which clients RPM units have synchronized on that day and when the last data was received from each client. Details relating to each client such as name, record number, contact details are lodged on the system so that nurses can contact clients who have not submitted data as expected to check on their wellbeing or technical difficulties.

The measurements taken by the clients are presented to the nurse in graph and table form. Graphs are generated for each parameter in the form of applets. Each data point on the applet represents one measurement taken. Graphs can be viewed for various periods of time for the last 12 months of monitoring. Some of the parameters have data points that can be clicked on to enable the nurse to see the actual reading that was taken by the client. For example a blood pressure reading can be clicked on so that the actual reading of that particular blood pressure can be scrutinised (Figure 4) to determine if the values stated are completely accurate and not the product of artifact. Spirometry and ECG measurements can be viewed in detail in the same manner.

Reports of the measurements can be generated by the nurse for various periods of time for each individual client. Reports can show graphs of each measurement and/or tables of measurements and can be printed or emailed.

Nurses select the measurements that the clients perform by discussing this with the client and considering their medical needs. The measurement is scheduled by the nurse using the website accessed by the nurse's PC. Client reminders can be set whereby the RPM unit will chime and the screen will flash to indicate when measurements are due to be taken by the client.

The nurses in this project also used an educational links facility. This meant that a selection of internet links that were relevant to client health education could be made available to the monitored clients through their RPM unit. In effect the monitor can be used as a limited web browser. Browsing was by the use of the touch screen rather than a mouse or keyboard, so did not suit sites where typing was required. As most clients did not already have internet access this was a welcome additional feature.

A number of health monitoring and evaluative questionnaires were available to clients in this project. Those used most regularly were the short daily cardiac and respiratory questionnaires. The respiratory questionnaire contained items relating to difficulty of breathing, sputum amount, sputum colour, general wellness, presence of cold or flu, use of additional medications (inhaled, antibiotics and steroids) and additional use of oxygen. The cardiac questionnaire contained items relating to shortness of breath with activity, shortness of breath at rest, lightheadness, general wellness, ankle swelling, use of usual medications and alternations to diuretics.

Other features of the system that have been used to a lesser extent are the client health diary, the health carers journal and alerts. Clients have access to a health diary where they can select various health related activities that they may have engaged in. These activities were related to a variety of health care services that they may have accessed such as GP, medical specialist, community nurse, hospital outpatients, hospital emergency department or hospital admission. The reason for the use of the service could then be selected as: routine, management of a new health problem, management of an existing health problem or deterioration in health condition.

The health carers journal enables the health professional to type in entries that are designed for their use such as reminders of subsequent appointments and events, other assessment findings and plans for care. Although this journal is not integrated into any other patient management applications, the entries can be printed or copied and pasted into other word processed documents.

Implementation

As most previous deployments of RPM equipment had been implemented overseas, it was logical that LMHA looked for overseas suppliers of RPM devices. Several difficulties with overseas suppliers became apparent including difficulty with consultation, training and support. Communications with Telstra, Australia's largest telecommunication company, provided LMHA with an introduction to TeleMedCare, an Australian company that manufactures RPM equipment.

TeleMedCare Pty Ltd was established in 1992 to commercialise home telehealthcare technologies developed by the Biomedical Systems Laboratory at the University of NSW in Australia. It now has an operation in the United Kingdom (Austrade,2007).

The project management methodology utilized was related to that described by the Tasmanian Government (IAPP, 2005).This was selected because of it's relevance, ease of use and it's , comprehensive range of resources which are available online free of charge.

The governance of the project was undertaken by LMHA. A simple and straight forward governance structure (Figure 5) was decided upon in response to several challenges that became apparent including: large distances between stakeholders and the nature of the health care workforce involved in this project.

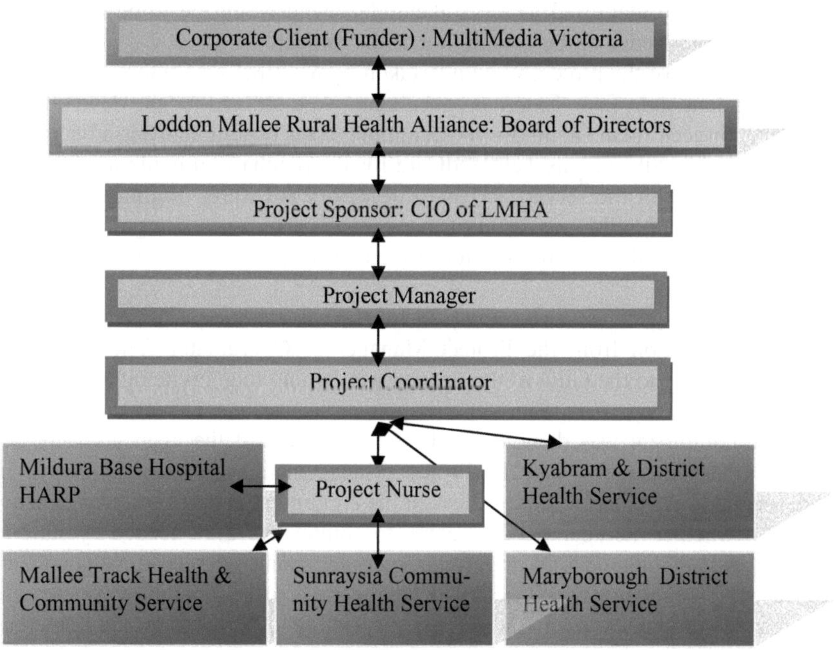

Figure 5: Organisational structure of *Connecting Clients ² Care*

A clear governance structure is necessary for any project in order to establish and maintain clarity about communications and responsibilies. The Corporate Client was MultiMedia Victoria who provided funding, received regular reports and encouraged public recognition of the project. LMHA Board of Directors oversee all activities undertaken by LMHA. The Chief Information Officer (CIO) is part of the Board and is also the Project Sponsor. The Project Sponsor takes ultimate responsibility for the project and who provides support, advocacy and advice from a senior level and ensures the necessary resources are available to the project. The Project Manager was appointed from LMHA and was a senior staff member with ICT and project management expertise. The Project Coordinator was a person with nursing, program development and evaluation expertise who was guided in project management by the Project Manager. The Project Coordinator recruited and led the Project Team composed of health care professionals from the five participating health care agencies where RPM was being implemented. A project nurse was appointed directly by the project to assist with the day to day issues at the three most distant agencies. The health care professionals at each agency were the main representatives of the project to the "business customers" who were the health care clients of the agency.

The Business Owner during the project was MultiMedia Victoria with title of the RPM equipment resting with LMHA. It was agreed during the project that ownership of the RPM devices purchased would transfer to the participating agencies at the conclusion of the project. The participating agencies and government departments were identified as the stakeholders who would be using the project outputs and knowledge at the completion of the project.

Quality audit of the project was undertaken by MultiMedia Victoria appointing an independent audit firm. External consultants were utilized for the development of legal contracts, financial audits and economic cost- benefit analysis advice. The main contractor utilized was TeleMedCare for the purchase of equipment, supply and maintenance of the server, access to necessary software, training of Project Team in the use of RPM, provision of manuals and provision of ongoing practical support. Occasionally, outside ICT technicians were contracted to assist with difficult installations.

Participating agencies were canvassed for their interest in participation by personal representation from the Project Manager or Coordinator. The initial approach was made to the CEO of the agency who would then invite other members of the agency management team to participate in discussions. During these discussions the equipment was demonstrated, and the views of the agencies were actively sought. The views that the Project Management were most interested in were related to the perceived usefulness of the equipment at that particular agency, and as to whether the agency could agree to commit the time needed by staff to training and ongoing use. Without the encouragement of senior management, clinical staff could not be expected to devote time to learning how to use and manage the equipment. While the project supplied funds for most of the resources required (including hardware, spare peripheral devices, data transmission, telephone parts, training, evaluation, most initial installations, project nurse support, project coordination and evaluation) it did not supply funds for back fill of nurses while they were trained, or supply funds for staff time involved in use of the data from the RPM units or in troubleshooting. Agency management and staff also needed to appreciate the time constraints of the project and adhere to deadlines.

One other agency that was initially approached to participate did not proceed. This agency recognized the usefulness of the equipment and supported the aims of the project but as they were going through a period of significant organizational change with the introduction of two other projects and a number of new staff, they decided not to participate in another new venture at that time.

A major challenge to project was also one of the main reasons for its initiation. This was the challenge of distance. Mildura Base Hospital and Sunraysia Community Health Service were both based in the rural city of Mildura which has a city population of 46,000, but services a catchment area of approximately 22,000 square km with a population in that area of approximately 80,000. Mildura is a five hour drive north from Bendigo (where the Project Manager and Project Coordinator were based). Mallee Track Health and Community Service is a part of the Mildura rural city area with it's own catchment area within it. It's main town is Ouyen, population 1380 located a one hour drive south of Mildura on the road to Bendigo. The part-time Project Nurse appointed by this project assisted nurses from these three services in smooth running of the RPM units, reallocation when necessary to other clients and assisted with evaluative data collection.

The other two services that participated in the project were Kyabram District Health Service and Maryborough District Health Service. Kyabram has a population of 7,100 and is located a 1.5 hour drive east of Bendigo. Maryborough has a population of 7,370 and is located a one hour drive west of Bendigo. Another campus of Maryborough District Health Service also participated and this was Avoca Health Service situated further west with a population of 1,220.

Although participating agencies were selected on the basis of rurality, distance, and having access to clients who may benefit from RPM, the distances involved were a challenge to communications, participation in the Project Team and monitoring of activity. Added to the challenge of distance was the fact that most of the nurses on the Project Team were part-time meaning that they were not as freely available for communications as may otherwise occur.

Not only were the participating agencies geographically spread but the type of services that were offered were different, and they represented the interests of different departments within their agencies. As the objectives of the project were to implement RPM and test it efficiencies, it was important to include a number of avenues of implementation to determine if RPM fitted into existing programs and work flow arrangements. Hospital Admission Risk Program- Chronic Disease Management was the department of Mildura Base Hospital that participated in this project. It offers: ongoing service coordination for clients with chronic or complex needs at risk of hospital admission, tertiary and secondary prevention, integrated comprehensive assessment and care planning, comprehensive discharge planning, embraces a self management approach and conducts home visits, office consultations and telephone support of clients. At the 12 month stage of the project

Mildura Base Hospital HARP had 650 clients registered with four FTE nurses. Other allied health professionals contribute to the HARP team. Mildura Base Hospital HARP deployed approximately 30 RPM units to client's homes.

A number of HARP clients from Maryborough District Health Service also received RPM units. HARP was in the process of being established at Maryborough and Avoca when this project became available to them. Maryborough and Avoca clients were also recruited from Avoca District Nursing and Breath of Fresh Air (pulmonary rehabilitation program) at Maryborough. District Nursing provides the services of community nursing, post acute care, hospital in the home, hospital to home care and palliative care. Maryborough and Avoca area received 10 RPM units.

Mallee Track Health and Community Service also allocated RPM units through District Nursing. District Nursing through this service also provided community nursing, post acute care, hospital to home care and palliative care over very large distances. Six monitors were deployed through this service.

Sunraysia Community Health Service, based in Mildura, provided a 12 month structured Chronic Disease Self Management Support Program. It emphasized self management strategies while using health coaching to supporting clients in being 'active' self managers, and to make lifestyle changes to improve their health outcomes and quality of life. It was a newly established program with 70 clients and 2.5 FTE nurses. This service deployed between 3-10 RPM units depending on the stage of the project and of their program.

Kyabram District Health Service deployed 10-14 monitors at different stages of the project through their Chronic Disease Management Coordinator. This team member worked with staff in the areas of diabetic education and pulmonary rehabilitation.

Communications with such a diverse Project Team were achieved by the following means:

- Group meetings at project initiation stage and at training,
- Regular onsite meetings with the coordinator in the first 12 months,
- Regular email and telephone communications, and
- Video conference meetings when personal meetings were not practical in the first 12 months.

During the initiation stage the predominant theme to emerge from the Project Team was that of time constraints. Although nurses recognized that RPM could potentially save them time they were concerned about how they were going to install and manage the equipment, have time to check on the RPM data and collect the data necessary for evaluation of the project.

In response to these concerns expressed at the initiation of the project strategies were instigated to alleviate the situation. These strategies included: providing assistance with installation, full training of staff, timely advice and support and the employment of the part-time Project Nurse to assist three sites. Meetings were also kept to a minimum. Quantitative evaluation methodology was designed to minimize the time required for nurses to spend on data collection. Most of the quantitative data was requested directly from the clients.

After participating agencies had agreed in principle to participate the setting up stage began. This stage included the development of a series of legal contracts. The first was a contract between LMHA and the supplier TeleMedCare. This contract covered the financial obligations and service agreement. The second document was an agreement between LMHA and each participating agency that explained much of the material in the LMHA/TeleMedCare contract including:

- purchase of equipment by LMHA,
- payment for data transmission and support by LMHA,
- payment for training and installations by LMHA,
- contingencies for data access in the event of technical difficulties,
- ownership of intellectual property rested with LMHA for evaluation and TeleMedCare for devices,
- ownership of equipment during and after the project rested with LMHA and may be transferred to the participating agencies at completion of the project,
- responsibility for clinical decision making was to rest with the agency, and
- duration of the project.

The final legal document prepared for the project was an "end user/ participating agency agreement". This explained to the client who was the user of the RPM unit, the nature of the project, the duration of the project, that the RPM was not an emergency device, and the responsibilities of the client, the agency and LMHA. The client was required to sign acceptance of these terms.

Two full days of training were provided at several sites to cater for all nurses involved in RPM. Training was conducted by staff from TeleMedCare and was conducted with a hands approach using RPM units and data from "dummy clients". Training included: unpacking and assembling the RPM units, connection to the internet, client education about taking measurements, receipt of RPM data via the website, responding to RPM data, troubleshooting, client selection, documentation for the project and evaluation methods to be used.

At the conclusion of training, planning commenced for installation of RPM units. Nurses were responsible for approaching clients who they thought would be suitable for RPM and who they also thought would benefit. The selection criteria used were consistent with those suggested by the American Telemedicine Association Home Telehealth Clinical Guidelines (2002). Specifically clients were required to:

- meet the inclusion criteria for the particular agency service being utilized,
- consent to having an RPM unit in their home and the terms of the "end-user/agency agreement",

- have a suitable location for the RPM unit that included access to electricity and a functional telephone line,
- have the capacity to understand and use the RPM unit,
- have the manual dexterity to use the peripheral devices, notably the blood pressure cuff,
- be able to read and understand enough English (or have a carer who could assist) so that the RPM screens could be read and telephone advice obtained when needed, and
- be within the physical parameters of the peripheral devices used, notably be under 150kg for weigh recordings (if required).

Nurses discussed the option of having an RPM unit installed with clients. Early in the project no particular visual aids were used for this discussion and some clients were not expecting devices that looked rather like computers. Nurses then started to show clients pictures of the RPM unit and this improved the clients understanding. TeleMedCare later produced a short video with an elderly client demonstrating the use of the device. This video was very useful in gaining client interest and acceptance of the technology.

Equipment was delivered direct to the participating agencies from the supplier. It was useful to notify the area that normally receives such deliveries in advance of this as the equipment is large and very valuable so will require good storage facilities and asset tracking.

After the client agreed to receiving an RPM unit, an appointment was made for installation. It was explained that this may take up to an hour and a half and would require the client to be available for education. Appointments for installation were initially scheduled very tightly and encountered numerous problems. Experience in this area has indicated that the following list are desirable points to include in an installation plan:

- Check equipment and connect to the internet before leaving for an installation. If there are any software upgrades that are required, allowing these to run before installation in the home will save significant time at the clients home.
- Take a range of telephone adaptors, extension cords, cable ties, documentation and spare parts. A mobile telephone for support during complex installations is invaluable.
- Make sure that the installer is familiar with the geography, has maps and directions.
- Confirm appointments with clients the day before, as some clients had unexpected appointments with other health care professionals etc.
- Make sure the client understands that a firm time for arrival is difficult to give as some installations take longer than planned.
- Estimate travel time between appointments generously, especially in remote areas.
- If within short distances, three installations per day is good progress, as the client needs to be adequately educated as well.

- The client's usual nurse should accompany the installer. This not only provide directions to the home, but facilitates rapport building and acceptance and comfort with the RPM unit. It should be the nurses responsibility to discuss with the client which measurements are needed and to educate the client about how to do these.
- The installer may be a nurse or a technician, but it was found that ICT technicians mastered the installation process admirably and dealt with more complex installations with ease. This allowed the nurse to focus on the client aspects of RPM use fully.
- Some clients were noticeably anxious if the installation process was difficult. As these clients have chronic illness or complex needs the nurse can play an important role by engaging them on more relevant matters until the difficulties are solved.
- Some clients were anxious about the use of the RPM unit. Effective steps to alleviate this included explaining that pressing the wrong button will not harm the unit, starting off monitoring with a small number of parameters, demonstrating taking the measurements then asking the client to return the demonstration to the nurse, ask the client to repeat the measurements after the installers and nurse have left the home, telephoning the client to reassure them that the data was transmitted, returning to the home within about one week to recheck their measurement technique and reassuring them that some clients feel daunted at first but that it does not take them long to adjust.

Once equipment was installed the task of managing the project became important. The components of the ongoing management fell into three areas: clinical management led by the nurses, ongoing project management led by the Project Coordinator and ongoing evaluation conducted by the Project Coordinator.

- Clinical management of the clients receiving RPM included:
- Continued encouragement and feedback from the nurses,
- Receipt of data from the clients so that the nurses could consider the data and respond appropriately,
- Developing a workflow that incorporated a systematic way of routinely checking the data,
- Follow up with clients who had not transmitted data as expected to determine their well being or if there were technical difficulties, and
- Finding a solution to technical difficulties.

A number of technical difficulties were encountered that could be summarized into the three areas of client difficulties, device/system difficulties and clinician difficulties. They are discussed here only as an indication of difficulties that may arise in RPM rather than as a full report of issues and risks.

The most common areas where clients had difficulties were: with blood pressure cuffs becoming twisted or poorly positioned, the arm being too large or too thin for the blood pressure cuff, not being able to stand still long enough while the scales recorded the weight or being too heavy for the scales. TeleMedCare have now introduced a more robust type of blood pressure cuff.

There were very few difficulties that required either the peripheral devices or the workstation to be repaired or replaced. The central server was non functional on one occasion only and a back up server was utilized within 24 hours. This did not result in the loss of any client data. Individual RPM units may loose their connection with the server. The usual remedy for this is to reboot the unit. If the server detects that a unit has not synchronized for two consecutive days the server will automatically reboot that unit remotely. This requires the unit to be left with the power on rather than turning it off as a response to it "not working".

Clinical difficulties that the nurses encountered were mostly related to questions about the accuracy of the data. Nurses could ascertain that the data was accurate by a number of means including:

- Adequate education of the client in the process of taking the measurements,
- Checking by telephone that the client had used the correct techniques,
- Revisiting the client to check technique and reinforce education,
- Using the applets and the "show recording" function described earlier to "drill down" and scrutinize the actual recording of blood pressure, ECG or spirometry in question. Some nurses sought advice on assessing the quality of these readings, but once the data was accepted as accurate the clinical response was the responsibility of the nurse and the clinical team.

Ongoing project management was important to ensure the smooth progress of the project after it had been initiated and to ensure that strengths were built upon and weaknesses identified and remedied in order to deliver the best outputs possible.

Stakeholder engagement was an ongoing requirement. Management at participating agencies needed to be kept informed of progress so that they could encourage staff and recognize their contributions. TeleMedCare as the service provider was in constant communication with the Project Coordinator and the Project Team in relation to issues, questions, requests for advice and suggestions for future product development. The Project Team needed to participate in regular discussions and emails to provide feedback and receive news

Risk management was an important activity in ongoing management. The main risks anticipated but that did not occur were: client misadventure associated with the RPM units, cost increases, significant equipment malfunction, significant lack of use, non realization of benefits, loss of project management staff and loss of evaluative data. The risk that is always identified and that *did* occur was delay leading to an approved extension of the project from one year to two years.

Issues were tracked to ensure that the many small details that prevent risk from occurring are recorded and followed up in the best time possible. Issues tracking related highly to the financial aspects that needed to be attended to, the management of human resources and the management and tracking of assets. Information resources needed to be considered in terms of document control and back up and back-up and storage of the clinical data that was generated.

The LMHA Board was kept informed by monthly reports and the Sponsor and Project Manager were consulted with weekly. MultiMedia, as the funding body, received quarterly status reports describing progress, challenges and achievements.

Appropriate closure to this project is vital to ensure that its benefits are long lasting. The effects of an inadequately planned closure could include: wastage of infrastructure, wastage of skills developed in health care professionals, loss of enhanced productivity of health care professionals and a return to the previous care environment where transmittable, continuous, comprehensive and easy to use monitoring could not be undertaken by clients in their own homes.

Although project closure was the final stage of the projects life, the preparation for this stage began in the initiation stage. The duration of the project was defined in the contracts as being for 12 months, but this was later extended to 24 months. It is important for stakeholders at all levels to understand when the benefits of the project will cease so that plans can be made for continuation under other arrangements if desired. Importantly clients using the RPM units needed to know from the outset how long they could use the units for under the project which supplied them free of charge to agencies and clients.

Arrangements were made for the transfer of assets, acceptance of responsibility for payment of service fees for units that are required to be continued and acceptance of follow on actions which included unresolved issues and risks.

Stakeholders wanted to know what the overall benefits of the project were revealing and what the cost benefit analysis was showing. To build the best and most accurate case for continued use, the final results of the evaluation will consider the maximum use of evaluative data that is collected over the maximum time permissible. This means that there will be a short period of time between presentation of the final analysis and closure of the project where the issue of continuation will reach a climax.

Continuity of service after the closure of the project is now the most pressing issue. Just as there was an obvious need for the implementation of this project at the start, because the project has been successful, there remains an obvious need for continuation. However, projects have a defined life span and this has almost been reached at the time of writing this chapter. Although not usually a part of project management, the Project Coordinator and Manager have put proposals forward to cater for the continuation of the service. If these proposals are successful it will ensure a smooth transition from project status to integration in normal service delivery in the areas where it is currently used. Significantly, it should result in a seamless continuance from the client's point of view with no interruptions to the service.

Evaluation

To date, this is the largest deployment of RPM in Australia. Other Australian deployments have included a randomized controlled research trial of RPM undertaken at the Austin Hospital, funded by DHS, using approximately 24 monitors. Results of this trial are not available as yet.

The LMHA initiative covered a wider area, engaged more agencies, used more monitors and had a greater emphasis on implementation and usage. Lessons learned relate to the realistic implementation of technology in health care: avoiding delay, engagement, building in evaluation, building in contingencies and choosing partners wisely.

Clients, carers and nurses have reported improvements in quality of life: clients experience a greater sense of independence and security, more regular connection with the health service, reduced feelings of isolation and vulnerability and increased confidence in managing their condition.

For the agencies, improvements have included: decreased number of routine nursing visits, decreased travel by nurses to visit clients and increasing the reach of agencies to cater for clients that would not otherwise have been catered for. The Mildura HARP has experienced increased capacity to service clients associated with the introduction of RPM. The average number of clients per nurse (EFT) when RPM was introduced was 114. After 12 months of use of RPM, the average number of clients per nurse is 162, an increase of 48 clients per nurse. This represents 42% efficiency in terms of nurse to client ratios. Additionally, the health care systems gain efficiencies as clients tend to use the primary care system more appropriately, with a consequent drop in use of the acute sector.

The use of this system has enhanced integrated care management for clients with chronic disease or complex physical conditions in the region. The clients and carers are reporting that they feel much more reassured and "connected" to the agencies providing their health care stating repeatedly that they are aware that the nurses observe their data and respond to it when appropriate. They discuss with their nurse, which measurements to take and how often. The clients are taking ownership of this process and watch their measurements on the graphs on the monitor. As a result of having access to this information for the first time, clients are making positive changes to their health behaviour because they understand that the measurements are indicators of underlying changes in their health. In addition, knowing that the nurse can monitor a client's compliance with their measurement regime adds an incentive to be compliant. The appended case studies provide actual evidence of this.

The nurses who view the data online are able to make clinical decisions based on the up-to-date information they now have. The system provides accurate clinical data, as frequently as the nursing staff requires to effectively manage their client's condition. The cost of nurses visiting a client to perform an ECG, spirometry, blood pressure reading or weight measurement are high, but by using RPM even clients in remote locations may receive these services easily. Access is determined by the client having a functional telephone line and electricity and the nurse having access to a computer linked to the internet.

Various cost efficiencies were demonstrated in situations where there was a clear need for monitoring. Three levels of cost efficiencies related to reduced nursing visits have been identified. These are: moderate efficiencies, high efficiencies and expanded reach efficiency. These will be described here in turn.

Moderate efficiencies were found when a number of clients could be maintained with reduced nursing visits. The numbers of clients with these efficiencies varies, but if for example, five actual clients in the Mildura area are considered, a clear cost reduction is demonstrated with these clients using RPM. Previously, the five clients had required a total of seven routine visits per week. Due to their location this took 3.6 hours in travel time and 2.3 hours for the actual visits, resulting in the time used being 5.9 hours. This would cost $212 per week in wages and on costs and $73 for the 130km (Woods, 2008) that needed to be travelled. This results in a total cost of care for these five clients as $285 per week, or $7,410 if this situation persisted for six months.

The same five clients were allocated RPM units and are using them effectively. This has resulted in only one routine nursing visit per week to one of these clients. The others are all maintained without routine nursing visits, but the nurse is able to visit if the need arises. The travel time is now 20 minutes per week, for eight kilometers, and the nursing time for the visit is approximately 20 minutes. This results in a cost of $28.24 per week for these five clients being maintained with RPM. If this persisted for six months the total cost would be $734.

The comparison of costs for these five clients before and after RPM is $7,410 vs $734, a cost reduction of $6,676 over a six month period. In this situation the current annual service fee is 75% of the cost reduction of this six month projection. Hence in cases where visits are reduced to this degree, the RPM units could be said to pay for their own annual service fee in less than six months, as well as contributing to an enhanced quality of life for the client and improved workflow for the nurses.

High efficiencies in terms of dramatic cost reductions have been evident with higher needs clients who live further from their health care service. For example the client in Case Study 2 with COPD lives 40 km from the service. At the commencement of monitoring he required District Nurse visits three times per week. After a month of monitoring his visits were comfortably reduced to weekly. This reduced the hours the nurse spent in travel and visits by 135 hours per year, or $4867 in wages and on costs. The saving on travel was 8320 km per year or $4687 (Woods, 2008) totaling $9554 per year savings. With RPM being available to this high needs client the savings are approximately double the purchase price of equipment. Annual operating costs are about one fifth of the total amount saved. This indicates that RPM is a very cost effective intervention in high needs clients who are motivated to use the system.

Expanding the reach of the health care service, and thereby increasing efficiency, has been another aspect of cost benefit analysis. However this is more difficult to calculate valid cost figures for as the clients were not receiving these nursing visits in the first place. RPM has enabled nurses to monitor clients who would not have received any visits at all from them. In the Mildura area there were at times 10 clients who lived in areas too far from the service to be visited on an ongoing basis. In addition, clients who lived over the nearby state boundary could be registered with the program but could not receive nursing visits. These clients previously received telephone advice from the nurses and only received face to face attention when the client visited Mildura hospital for services such as Pulmonary Rehabilitation or doctors visits.

A number of these clients had high needs. Many benefits were observed in these clients. One younger client lived in a remote area that was a three hour drive from Mildura. His nearest doctor was a 1.5 hour drive from his home on the family farm. At the time of the project Australian farming communities were suffering much hardship due to a prolonged drought. The client's condition would have added to their hardship. After being diagnosed earlier as having a significant cardiac condition the client and his family were understandably very anxious and the client was inclined to be inactive on the farm and in general. By using RPM on a daily basis and keeping in regular telephone contact with the nurse and with continued support of the cardiologist this client's quality of life was transformed. He was much more optimistic, with improved mood being evident when nurses did see him and he resumed farming work and sporting activities.

A comprehensive evaluation, examining previous and current health care utilisation rates, quality of life, levels of anxiety/depression, and ability to cope with specific disease states is being conducted. It compares monitored clients with an unmonitored group at three points over a 12 month period. Process evaluation and a series of case studies from a client perspective and from a project perspective are additional aspects of the evaluation. A summary of the quantitative evaluation may be seen in Appendix C. Data has been collected from clients to contribute towards the cost benefit analysis. This data will provide a demographic profile and as well as a comparison of health care utilization before RPM was used and during the use of RPM. It asks for information related to following items:

Demographics

- Age and gender
- Postcode and living arrangements
- Size of community
- Ethnicity
- Primary diagnosis
- Diagnosed co-morbidities

Health Care Utilisation

- Amount spent on pharmaceuticals by client
- Amount spent on travel for health visits
- Total distance travelled for health visits
- Nursing visits
- Time spent on nursing visits, including travel
- Number of client visits to or from:
    - General practitioner
    - Medical specialist
    - Hospital Emergency Department
    - Days as a hospital inpatient
    - Pathology or imaging services
    - Allied health
    - Community or outpatient services
    - Domiciliary care

Conclusion

This chapter has described "*Connecting Clients* [2] *Care*", a deployment of RPM units in the Loddon Mallee Region of Victoria Australia. This has been the largest deployment of this technology to date in Australia. Due to the preliminary evaluation of this project being so positive and because of the strong logic supporting the need for this technology in health care, it is hoped that this is an area for future expansion in Australia. Benefits to date indicate that remote client monitoring is an effective and viable part of addressing the problems of geographic isolation, distance and workforce problems whilst delivering health services to those with chronic illness in their own homes.

Acknowledgements:

This project was funded by the Victorian Department of Innovation, Industry and Regional Development: Multimedia Victoria. Equipment was purchased from and serviced by TeleMedCare Pty. Ltd

The project was authorized, governed and encouraged by the LMHA Board of Directors and CIO Bruce Winzar.

The participation and support of management and staff of the partner agencies was a key point of success of this project. These were: *Mildura Base Hospital*: Michael Krieg CEO, Amanda Jones, Mandie Hayes, Andrea Bock, Craig Millard, Kylie Harry, Marina Lloyd, Raelene Gibson, Julie Galbraith. *Kyabram District Health Service:* Neil Cowen CEO, Di Roberts, Wendy Pogue. *Maryborough District Health Service:* Peter Appledore CEO, Michael Coleman, Robin Jensen, Heather Bucknall, Raylene Liddicoat. *Mallee Track Health and Community Service:* John Senior CEO, Sue White, Jagit Dahliwal, Glenis Barnes, Barb Nunn, Margaret Prentice. *Sunraysia Community Health*: Craig Stanbridge CEO, Shelley Faulks, Jackie Reddick, Jennifer Rudkin, Jackie Cesco.

We would like to acknowledge the contribution of all clients and their carers who were patient and enthusiastic while staff learnt to install and use the equipment, who diligently completed evaluation surveys and who provided descriptions of their experiences to illustrate their experiences, especially Vicki Cosson and Bob and Thelma Herbertson.

References

ABS 2006 Census QuickStats: Loddon-Mallee (Statistical Region) (2007a), http://www.censusdata.abs.gov.au/ (Accessed, 14 September 2008)

ABS 2006 Census QuickStats: Victoria, Statistical Region (2007b), http://www.censusdata.abs.gov.au/ (Accessed, 14 September 2008)

American Telemedicine Association, Home telehealth clinical guidelines (2002), http://www.atmeda.org/ICOT/hometelehealthguidelines.htm (Accessed, 14 September 2008)

Austrade (2007), http://www.austradehealth.gov.au/TeleMedCare-Pty-Ltd/default.aspx (Accessed, 14 September 2008)

DHS, Nurses in Victoria, A Supply and Demand Analysis, 2003-04 to 2011-12, Service and Workforce Planning, Department of Human Services, Melbourne (2004)

DHS, Victorian Burden of Disease Study Mortality and Morbidity in 2001, Public Health Group, Rural and Regional Health and Aged Care Services Division, Department of Human Services, Melbourne (2005)

IAPP Inter Agency Policy and Projects Unit, Tasmanian Government Project Management Guidelines, Version 6. Government Information and Services Division Department of Premier and Cabinet, Tasmania (2005), http://www.egovernment.tas.gov.au/themes/project_management/tasmanian_government_project_management_guidelines (Accessed, 14 September 2008)

Wood, D.: The cents in driving. Royal Auto. Royal Automobile Club of Victoria, 50–55 (July 2008)

Appendix A: Case Study One
Technology helps Vicki take control of her health

Having a Remote Patient Monitor at home has given kidney disease client Vicki Cosson, an Aboriginal woman from Mildura, added motivation to seek a second chance at life.

When Vicki was diagnosed with end stage kidney disease in late 2006 she admits the future looked fairly bleak.

Like many Aboriginal people she was at greater risk of developing kidney disease than other Australians, and faced further health complications, regular dialysis and a shortened lifespan.

But after being given a remote patient monitor 12 months ago by Craig Millard, a care coordinator with the Hospital Admission Risk Program (HARP) at Mildura Base Hospital, Vicki found the determination she needed to dramatically alter her future by changing her diet, losing weight and preparing for a kidney transplant.

What RPM does

Since late 2006, more than 30 patient monitors have been distributed across Mildura and Robinvale in north-western Victoria, to people with chronic illnesses such as heart and lung disease, diabetes or kidney disease.

The technology is provided to HARP, via Loddon Mallee Rural Health Alliance with funding from Victorian Government agency for information and communications technology, Multimedia Victoria.

In Vicki's case the monitor is hooked up using an ordinary telephone line, which she uses once a day to measure her blood pressure, heart rate, body weight and blood sugar levels. The data is then transmitted overnight to a central database, via the internet, which Craig can access remotely.

How it works

"I use the monitor every morning before breakfast for about 20 minutes," explained Vicki who has the machine in pride of place in the kitchen.

"It was a little bit hard to remember what to do at first but its part of my daily routine now and it's really very easy to use. It makes me feel more in control of my health because it gives me a chance to see how my blood pressure and sugar diabetes is going."

The benefits

Since using the monitor Vicki's kidney function has stabilised and her overall health has significantly improved. She has also avoided dialysis which was originally expected within three months.

"When I was first diagnosed I was very concerned about my weight and my blood pressure but I didn't know what to do. The monitor has given me the focus I needed. Before my kidney trouble I weighed about 115 kilograms but now I'm down to 94 kilograms," said Vicki.

Successful weight loss has also reduced Vicki's blood sugar levels. "My sugar diabetes used to be high all the time but now it's down to almost normal."

Vicki said taking her own readings on a daily basis had given her a better understanding of her own health and more motivation to eat healthily. “I’ve gone off a lot of stuff, especially dairy products and I feel a lot better in myself. I just didn’t care that much before but now I make sure I eat healthy every day including fruit and vegies and not too much sugar.”

Knowing Craig was keeping an eye on her results also provided an extra incentive.

“He makes sure everything is ok with me. If my blood pressure is up he always checks I’m ok and we talk about what’s been going on.” Instead of seeing Craig every week, Vicki now sees him every two or three months, although they are in regular contact over the phone.

Vicki’s family are calling in more often to see how she’s going too. “And I can’t tell lies any more about what’s been happening because it’s all there on the machine.”

Future opportunities

Although Vicki’s kidney function has stabilised, over time it will gradually diminish so she is currently on the waiting list for a kidney transplant operation. The operation is only performed on clients who look after their health to give themselves the best possible chance of success.

“My husband has offered to donate one of his kidneys to me, which is incredible, but we can’t go ahead until we both lose a bit more weight. My goal is 85 kilograms which I’m determined to reach in a few months. I’ll get there.”

This Case Study was commissioned by MultiMedia Victoria with fully informed and written consent of the client. It is reproduced here with permission of MultiMedia Victoria.

Appendix B: Case Study Two
Monitor helps Bob stay at home longer

Remote patient monitoring has given heart disease client Bob Herbertson more time at home with his wife Thelma and significantly improved his quality of life.

Without a monitoring device in their home Bob and Thelma Herbertson, who live on an isolated property about 40km from Avoca, would not have felt confident to manage Bob’s day-to-day health needs.

Bob, who suffers from Chronic Obstructive Pulmonary Disease, was one of the first clients in the region to receive a monitor in late 2007, which enables Thelma to keep a close eye on her husband’s health and seek advice from local district nurse, Heather Bucknall.

The technology is provided by the Loddon Mallee Rural Health Alliance (LMHA) which represents the ICT interests of 16 hospitals and 65 health agencies across the Loddon Mallee Region, including the Avoca campus of Maryborough District Health Service. Funding is provided by Victorian Government agency for information and communications technology, Multimedia Victoria.

What RPM does

Since late 2007, five remote patient monitors have been distributed across the Avoca region, mostly to people with chronic illnesses such as heart and lung disease, diabetes or kidney disease.

In Bob's case the monitor is hooked up using an ordinary telephone line, and Thelma – a retired nurse – uses it once every couple of days to measure her husband's blood pressure, heart rate, body weight, oxygen saturation and lung function. The data is then transmitted overnight to a central database which Heather can access remotely from Avoca.

"Because we are 40km from a hospital or a doctor, I can judge by the results and by conversations with Heather how well Bob is and whether we can continue to manage at home or if we need to bring his doctor's appointment forward or go to hospital," explained Thelma.

How it works

Thelma said the monitor was very easy to use and required virtually no training. "It has a touch screen, which prompts you every step of the way."

"I take readings every second day unless there is a change in Bob's blood pressure or oxygen levels, and then I do it more often and discuss the findings with Heather over the phone," said Thelma.

She said one of the great things about the system was the reassurance of knowing someone else was looking at the results. "You need that backup because it's an emotional situation when you're looking after someone with a life threatening disease."

The benefits

Thelma said the major benefit of the monitor was keeping track of Bob's health on a daily basis. "It's great for monitoring his oxygen levels, which is very important because he is on an oxygen machine a lot of the time, particularly at night."

Before having the monitor Thelma used a hand-held digital device to keep track of Bob's blood pressure and heart rate but had no way of monitoring his oxygen levels or lung function, which meant he was at risk of developing chest infections and other associated conditions.

"It's given us a much better quality of life. I think without it there's no doubt Bob would be in a hospital or nursing home by now. We're so far away from everything that without this backup, we couldn't have managed," said Thelma.

Having the monitor has also relieved some of the financial burden of regular visits back and forwards to the doctor and to hospital. "We don't need to go to the doctor as often for the simple reason Bob is kept under constant observation here. We only go when there are abnormalities, which has really helped us financially."

Since using the monitor, fortnightly doctors' visits have been reduced to once every four or five weeks, district nurse visits have been cut back to once a week instead of three and Thelma suspects they may have avoided three unnecessary trips to the hospital.

"It's made a huge difference for us," explained Thelma. "Bob is an old fashioned man who's far more comfortable at home. He can sit on the front veranda and see the kangaroos and the birds all around. He has a much better life here than he would in hospital."

Future opportunities

After using remote patient monitoring for several months, Thelma hoped it could be made available to more people. "It's the continuous contact between you and the district nurse that's so important. It just provides that extra confidence you need."

This Case Study was commissioned by MultiMedia Victoria with fully informed and written consent of the client. It is reproduced here with permission of MultiMedia Victoria.

Appendix C: Summary of Quantitative Evaluation Methods Used in RPM Project

Summary of Quantitative Evaluative Tools being used in *Connecting Clients* [2] *Care:* Remote Patient Monitoring

	Nurse's Survey	Client Survey	SF36	K10	Living with heart failure questionnaire	Chronic respiratory disease questionnaire	Diabetes Questionnaire (derived from DIMS)
Who uses it	Nurses for all RPM clients and controls	All clients on RPM and controls	All clients On RPM and controls	All clients on RPM and controls	Clients on RPM and controls with heart failure	COPD clients on RPM and controls with COPD	Diabetic clients on RPM and controls with diabetes
When it is completed	Baseline 6 months 12 months	Baseline 6 months 12 months	Baseline 6 months 12 months	Baseline 6 months 12 months	Baseline 6 months 12 months	Baseline 6 months 12 months	Baseline 6 months 12 months
Time it takes	10 min	10 min	10 min	5 min	15-20 min	15-25 min	15-20 min
What it measures	Diagnoses. Past nursing time used Past other health care utilisation	Demographic and economic variables	Physical Social Emotion Mental health Role Pain General health Vitality Role	Anxiety depression	Physical Social Emotion (anxiety, depress) Mental (memory, control, burden)	Dyspnoea Fatigue Emotional Mastery	Symptoms Confidence in self management of diabetes

Abbreviations used in this chapter

ABS	Australian Bureau of Statistics
CEO	Chief Executive Officer
CIO	Chief Information Officer
DHS	Department of Human Services
ECG	Electrogrardiogram
FTE	Full Time Equivalent
GP	General (medical) Practitioner
HL7	Health Level 7
ICT	Information and Communication Technology
IIS	Internet Information Service
LMHA	Loddon Mallee 1 Health Alliance
PDF	Portable Document Format
RPM	Remote Patient Monitor
SQL	Structured Query Language
SVG	Scalable Vector Graphics

A Home-Based Care Model of Cardiac Rehabilitation Using Digital Technology

Mohanraj Karunanithi (a), Antti Sarela (b)

(a) The Australian E-Health Research Centre, Brisbane, Australia, +61 7 32533623, mohan.karunanithi@csiro.au
(b)The Australian E-Health Research Centre, Brisbane, Australia, +61 7 32533612, antti.sarela@csiro.au

Abstract Cardiovascular disease (CVD) is the number one cause of death globally. There already exists a structured guideline to cardiac rehabilitation for CVD patients as a means of preventing recurrence(s) of any cardiac events and return to an active, healthy and satisfying lifestyle. Despite the availability of cardiac rehabilitation programs, utilisation among eligible patients has been less than 20%. The barriers to this underutilisation have been factors relating to patients, services, and professionals. An alternative approach is a home-based cardiac rehabilitation has shown some improvements in the patients' uptake of these services. Recent developments in physiological monitoring, information processing, and communication technologies have shown potential to enable a home-based cardiac rehabilitation program for better uptake and adherence and coordination between a team of multidisciplinary carers. One approach has been to use communication technologies such as mobile phone platform to help improve the carers' ability to give multimodal feedback to the patients regularly and enable the use of other multi media formats.

Table of contents

K. Yogesan et al. (Eds.): Handbook of Digital Homecare, BIOMED, pp. 329–352.
springerlink.com

1 Introduction

Cardiovascular disease (CVD) is the leading chronic disease and the number one cause of death globally [1]. The World Health report in 2005 estimated 17.5 million people died from various forms of CVD, which represents 30% of global deaths. Coronary artery or heart disease (CHD) is the most common of the CVD that results in conditions of sustainable disability, recurrence of cardiac events, and the loss of productivity, in particular with the ageing population. Most of these are preventable through management of major primary risk factors such as unhealthy diet, physical inactivity and smoking. To prevent such conditions, agencies such as the American Heart Association (AHA), American Association of Cardiovascular and Pulmonary Rehabilitation (AACVPR) (USA), Heart Foundation of Australia (HFA), and National Heath Service (NHS) Centre (UK) have set guidelines for a structured cardiac rehabilitation (CR) programs, as an essential part of secondary prevention, to manage patients with CVD. Patients that are recommended for CR are those with angina (chest pain), coronary artery disease (blockages in the coronary arteries), heart attack (myocardial infarction (MI)), heart failure (reduced pump function or cardiomyopathy), coronary arterial bypass graft (CABG), and stent or angioplasty procedures. Other patients may include post transplant, valve replacement, patients at high risk and those with arrhythmias.

Cardiac rehabilitation programs consist of 3 phases. The first phase is an inpatient evaluation program prior to hospital discharge. Both the second and third phases follow hospital discharge. The second phase is an outpatient program designed to assist patients to return to normal activities. The third phase is a maintenance program for regular exercise and control of risk factors. While the first phase is conducted in acute care, following a cardiac procedure, the second and third phase CR occurs in an outpatient clinic within the hospital infrastructure with a multidisciplinary team comprising of hospital staff. The demand on the hospital to provide these services has become unsustainable because of the increases in healthcare costs [2] and increased prevalence of CVD, in particular with the ageing population [3]. More importantly, the programs provided by this traditional model of the hospital-based CR have resulted in many barriers to patient referrals, patient uptake, and adherence [4]. Geographical location of CR programs is often a major contributor to barriers relating to patient uptake and adherence.

To alleviate the barriers contributing to the patient uptake and adherence barriers, alternative models have been to move CR programs to the community to manage patients from their homes. In addition to these CR barriers, adherence to performance measures aligned with the national guidelines of a CR program becomes challenging for a coordinated multidisciplinary team to manage patients from their homes in a community. The focus of this article is to explore how recent developments in information, communication, and technology can address and enable a structured CR approach in a home-based care model.

2 Components of a Comprehensive Cardiac Rehabilitation/Secondary Prevention Programs

Core components outlined for a comprehensive model of cardiac rehabilitation program by the HFA [7] and AHA/AACVPR [7] are: patient assessment, nutritional counselling, weight management, blood pressure management, lipid management, diabetes management, tobacco cessation, psychological management, physical activity counselling, exercise training, use of preventative medications, and data collection for CR.

The patient assessment comprises of 2 levels:

- Initial assessment reviewing current and prior CV medical and surgical diagnoses, co-morbidities, delineation of CV symptoms and risk profile, and the perceived status of health. Physical examination and 12-lead resting ECG is standard for this assessment.
- Assessment of the interventions planned during the course of the CR program such as goals outlined for risk reduction strategies and pharmaceutical management. This includes the interactive communication of the treatment and follow-up plans with patient and family members/partners in collaboration with the primary health provider.

Other components can be categorised into lifestyle/behavioural risk factors and management, biomedical risk factors/medical management, pharmacological management, and psychosocial factors and assessment.

The lifestyle/behavioural risk factors and management comprises of nutritional counselling, weight management, tobacco cessation, physical activity counselling, and exercise training. Nutritional counselling relies on first obtaining the patients baseline daily caloric intake, dietary content, their eating habits, alcohol consumption, before commencing education and counselling towards targeted dietary goals and individualised dietary modifications. Weight management is considered because obesity is a risk factor of CVD. This is monitored and assessed through measurements of body mass index (BMI) and/or waist circumference for establishing both short- and long-term weight goals relative to patient's specific CVD condition and risk factors. These weight goals are combined with diet, physical activity/exercise and behavioural programs. In physical activity counselling, activity levels and exercise of daily living, the readiness to change physical activity behaviour, and barriers to increasing physical activity are assessed, before advice and support and referral to an exercise program are arranged. Normal recommendations are for a minimum of 30 to 60 minutes of moderate physical activity, preferably on each day of the week, with strategies aimed to integrate into their daily living activities. Exercise training is often an individualized exercise prescription for those with possible risk of cardiovascular complications of exercise. For this, symptom-limited exercise testing is performed prior to enrolment into an exercised-based cardiac rehabilitation.

The biomedical risk factors/medical management comprises of blood pressure management, lipid management, and diabetes management. The blood pressure management encompasses the diagnosis and management for hypertension, and also orthostatic hypotension. The components of the lifestyle risk factors is also assessed in association with the management of hypertension such as physical activity, weight management and low -salt and -fat intake in the diet. In general, goals for blood pressure are <140/90mmHg for normal, <130/80mmHg for more stringent (for high risk patients), and <120/80mmHg for those with ventricular dysfunction. Management of hypertension includes blood pressure management that may be associated with renal disease risk which can be ascertained from urine (protein) analysis. Lipid management through pharmacotherapy has been incorporated in CR for the assessment and regulation of levels of fasting measures of total cholesterol, high density lipoprotein cholesterol (HDL-C), low-density lipoprotein cholesterol (LDL-C), and triglycerides. While counselling on lipid management involves dietary recommendations by a dietitian, provision and monitoring of the pharmacotherapy would require coordination with the patient's primary provider or cardiologist. Diabetes management is considered as an essential part of CR because both diabetes mellitus and impaired fasting glucose are associated with adverse long-term cardiovascular outcomes. Following assessment of the patient's diabetic condition, education is provided regarding exercise and self-monitoring skills for unsupervised exercise, because physical activity has been shown to reduce insulin resistance and glucose intolerance [9].

Pharmacological management involves assessment, education and counselling on the importance of adherence to preventive medications that are prescribed by the healthcare provider. This is a process of ongoing communication with the primary healthcare provider and/or cardiologist with regard to changes to medications. The preventive medications include drugs that are blood-thinners, anti-arrhythmic, blood-pressure lowering, cholesterol lowering, etc, depending on the cardiac symptoms or events undergone by the patient.

Psychosocial factors and assessment encompasses the identification of depression, anxiety, anger or hostility, social isolation, family distress, sexual dysfunction, and substance abuse which are significant risk factors following acute cardiac events. These are managed with identified psychotropic medications, individualised education or counselling.

3 Traditional Cardiac Rehabilitation

Traditionally, CR has been conducted in hospital-based settings in outpatient clinics. Most of these CR programs concentrated on low-risk patients who have had MI [10] despite benefits shown in moderate to high risk cardiac patients in previous clinical trial studies [10]. The majority of CR programs have been exercise-based, with group-based exercise sessions 1 to 3 times a week for 6 to 12 weeks [6]. In 2001, the Cochrane Database review of trials on exercise-based rehabilitation found exercised-based CR effectively reduced all-cause mortality, death rates, and relative risk from cardiovascular causes [13]. Despite the many randomized, controlled trials of CR, including those with exercise training, only a few studies provided evidence of statistically significant coronary risk [14]. The lack of evidence in the other studies was a result of insufficient numbers of subjects to reach adequate statistical power and subject dropouts and crossovers [16].

Despite the effectiveness of CR programs, there have been many barriers to traditional CR that has resulted in low referral, uptake, and adherence. A recent review published on the literature across studies of CR barriers [5] reported referrals varying from 9% to 74%, uptake/enrolment varying from 11% to 69%, and among the patients enrolled, adherence rate ranged from 53% to 88%. In USA and Australia, eligible patient participating in CR programs were found to be below 20%. The contributing barriers to this underutilisation of CR programs have been factors related to professional, patient, and service aspects.

Professional factors have varied from clinicians' lack of beliefs and judgements on the effectiveness of CR for patients (at the time of hospital discharge) to clinicians' eligibility criteria for patients being biased on the proximity of CR programs available or on the lack of awareness of program availability [6]. While these factors remain partially amenable to changes in better awareness of programs, practice guidelines and improvement through healthcare delivery systems and policies within the hospitals, it does not guarantee full cooperation and participation of patients in CR.

Patient factors are several and include work or domestic commitment, lack of interests in rehabilitation or a reluctance to change their lifestyle, a dislike of groups, functional status, patient depression, living in rural setting, and lack of support from the family. Lack of women participation, in particular married women, in CR has been mainly due to competing demands of domestic commitments [4]. Similarly, for patients that return to work, the demands of work commitments also conflict with attendance to CR programs. Uptake from the elderly is often hampered by the lack of motivation caused by their status of functional decline which is also compounded by any anxiety and depression that results from significant cardiac events. The lack of uptake from ethnic minorities in CR have been language barriers, poor experience of health during the acute cardiac event, religious insensitivity and attribution of the health problem to stress and worry, such that exercise is not relevant [17]. The low uptake in patients from low socio-economic groups, on the other hand, have been from the lack of education, causing misconceptions of CR, and lack of affordability to the CR program, particularly when it comes to fee for services, as in the USA. The lack of affordability to the CR programs among eligible CR patients is often a major issue due to the lack of reimbursement provided for CR services [5].

Service factors are related to the inadequate service provision caused by: absence of services especially in smaller and rural communities, long waiting lists, appropriateness of the CR program, poor communication leading to delays, and facilitating factors that prevented patients accessing services when they most need it [18]. The absence of services was the result of a lack of commitment and investments in CR services in the past. The long waiting list was an inevitable consequence of the limited CR services capability. Appropriateness of CR services in the delivery of education and exercise in a group setting differs between participants (i.e. stressed socially, lacked privacy, etc).The poor communication was due to the lack of proper communication systems, standardised information and poor understanding of CR services by the healthcare workers. The facilitating factors pertain to deficiencies in the public health services. In a recent review article that explored similar barriers to CR with respect to women's lack of participation, various changes were recommended for referrals, enrolment and uptake of CR programs [5]. The recommended change to the enrolment process was to implement health policy measures with a standard quality indicator for CR. In addition, automating the referral process with a requirement to document reasons for not referring a patient would eliminate the majority of referral barriers pertaining to prescriber biases. The review also recommended practice innovations to CR settings through programs with flexibility in service delivery such as home-based CR, personalising the treatment plan to individuals needs, and heightening psychosocial support.

4 Requirements of CR services

The role of cardiac rehabilitation and position statements for the comprehensive secondary prevention of cardiovascular events have been widely documented, endorsed, and promoted by a number of health care organizations and agencies but have overlooked minimum performance standard measures for the referral and delivery of CR programs to ensure better utilization CR services. It was only recently that the AACVPR/AHA Cardiac Rehabilitation/Secondary Prevention developed these performance measures [19]. This was initiated by the formation of the Writing Committee, comprising of members from latter organizations, convening in 2005 and collaborating to design these performance measurement. These developed performance measures were based on existing guidelines established by the ACC/AHA Task force on Performance Measures and found to provide scientific and other supporting evidences. The outcome of the performance measurement sets are:

1) referral of eligible patients to an outpatient CR program and, 2) delivery of CR services through multidisciplinary CR programs. These performance measures were designed to enable health professionals to potentially identify, correct and action on structure- and process- based gaps in CR services.

The AACVPR/AHA CR performance measures have the potential to remove some of the barriers relating to professional and service factors by making both healthcare systems and its providers accountable for the referral of eligible patients and also, ensure a standard of CR services is met through the CR programs. Through implementation of these measures, healthcare providers' beliefs and judgments towards the effectiveness and lack of awareness of CR programs, and non-referral of eligible patients could be eradicated. Patient related service factors related to patients with regard to inappropriateness and delays to their enrollment in CR programs could also be addressed in these performance measures. However, these performance measures do not address the major barrier relating to patient factors such as CR program uptake due to work or domestic commitment, lack of interests in rehabilitation or reluctance to change their lifestyle, a dislike of groups, functional status, patient depression, living in rural setting, and lack of support from the family. In addition, even the geographical barriers of service provision of CR is unmet by these measures. This was mainly due to the performance measures being designed around inpatient and outpatients settings of CVD care and therefore, targeting measures for 3 specific settings 1) hospital settings, 2) office (physician's) practices, and 3) CR programs. Most of the barriers that remain unmet by these performance measures can be overcome only by the option of an alternative care model such as a home-based CR program. Despite the limited application of these performance measures to a home-based CR, they are still relatively new and needs to be tested for its effectiveness in meeting their objectives for the existing inpatient and outpatient settings. These objectives are for:

1. appropriate referral of eligible patients to an early outpatient CR program from: all hospitalized patients prior to discharge and all outpatients with a qualifying CVD event within the past year (by their healthcare provider)
2. an optimal structure measure of the provider and multidisciplinary team responsible for the CR program and care, process measures of assessment, evaluation and documentation of patient CVD risk factors, and also provide evidence of a plan to monitor response and document on the program effectiveness.

Once this model of performance measures evolves with the current inpatient and outpatient settings, it is then feasible to transfer these tested methods to a home-based care models of CR services.

5 Home-Based Cardiac Rehabilitation

In the mid-1980s, the provision of aerobic exercise in the home for post-MI patients began as an equally safe option as that of supervised exercise in traditional CR, to achieve functional improvement [20]. The goals set for these exercise-based CR at home were intensities according to targeted heart rates, which the patients monitored with portable heart rate monitors. These home-based CR programs were limited to only low-risk patients with uncomplicated MI. These initial programs also provided only minimal CHD risk reduction but gradually over the next 8 years, smoking cessation [22], blood pressure control and diet modification [23], together with education and counselling, were included [25]. By the 1990's, these programs evolved to become a physician-directed, nurse-managed, home-based CR program aimed at the reduction of CHD factors. One of first programs to achieve this was called the MULTIFIT system. This system focussed on active patient participation as the key to change their lifestyle as a need for establishing a successful

CHD risk management. To achieve this, the MULTIFIT system enrolled patients after acute MI, angioplasty or CABG surgery with a nurse case manager assigned to each patient to manage their CHD risk reduction remotely [27]. The remote facilitation of the program included a computer-based nutritional counselling, serum lipid management, and as for those patients free of cardiac complications, home-based aerobic exercise was prescribed. Another program known as the Stanford Coronary Risk Intervention Project (SCRIP) aimed at a more comprehensive reduction of CHD risk factor management through a large scale randomized controlled study over 4 years. This study was successful in demonstrating highly significant reductions in major CVD risk factors using both intensive lifestyle management plus cholesterol lowering medications on the progression and regression of coronary atherosclerosis and clinical cardiac events in men and women with established heart disease [28].

In a recent a systematic review and meta-analysis that explored the effectiveness of home–based CR compared with supervised centre based CR through mortality, health related quality of life, and modifiable CHD risk factors [29], only 6 out of the 18 randomised control trials compared home-based with comprehensive supervised centre-based CR programs. These 6 trials, however, were among patients with low risk of cardiac events without significant ischemia, arrhythmias or heart failure, and not high risk patients.

In four of the trials that measured adherence, either as an objective measure or self-report, the home-based CR group reported higher levels of adherence to exercise session than that of centre-based CR group. Meta-analysis of exercise capacity, systolic blood pressure, and total cholesterol as three outcome measures for CR was only reported in one of the trials. No significant differences were found between the home and centre-based CR for these outcome measures. Two studies that reported health related quality of life as an outcome measure found significant improvement in physical and mental health summary measure and greater perception of social support in the home-based CR group. Sickness impact profile, as health related quality life measure, was similar in both home-based and centre-based CR groups.

In view of patient preferences to CR services, a small survey study in Canada reported that work committed cardiac patients, regardless of age or gender, were likely to prefer home-based CR services [30]. In another study, adherence rate of participation in medically directed home-exercise was high as 72% at 6 months and 41% at 4 years [31].

6 ICT for Home-based Care

The alternative, home-based care model for CR programs has shown evidence of patient preferences and alignment towards the needs to overcome majority of the barriers faced by the existing models of traditional CR services (as discussed in Section 1.3). Previous studies/trials of home-based CR have demonstrated the use of monitoring and communication technology, such as heart rate monitors and internet, respectively, to enable the process. While the home-based CR programs were predominantly exercised-based CR, only a few attempted to manage CHD risk factor reduction, as part of the comprehensive CR program outlined by AHA/AACVPR guideline. The rapid advances in sensor, information, and communication technologies over the last decade; however, has wide potential to address the many barriers and offer a range of services that is expected and outlined by the comprehensive CR services from a distance. As discussed in section 1.5, home-based care initiatives have attempted distance communication via electronic media (internet-based) and heart rate monitoring technology to provide some CHD risk management strategies and exercise-based, respectively, for CR programs.

Apart from the initial patient assessment that requires referral from hospital discharge or that from physical examination by a health care provider to determine the type of CR program, other components of comprehensive CR services are able to be delivered from home using the digital technology. The continuous ongoing assessment of patients' physiological parameters can be effectively monitored with commercially available physiological monitors and sensor technologies, which are currently in research and development and waiting to be adopted in healthcare.

For the lifestyle/behavioural risk factors and management of CR, physiological/ wellness monitors are available commercially for example weight scales that measure BMI and activity monitors that measure physical activity levels. For weight management, weight scales such as in the precisionTech from Taylor [32] (for example, Model no. 7507) has algorithm to calculate the BMI with electronic entry of ones height, and these are readily available in department stores. For physical activity monitors, there are commercial activity watch monitors such as IST Vivago [33] and ActiWatch [34], which are based on motion sensors such as accelerometers. Recently, clinical research on accelerometer based ambulatory monitors to extract levels, trends and classification of physical activity, specifically for CR, have been conducted by the author's research group [35] (See next section 1.7 for more details).

Similar commercial physiological monitors for blood pressure and diabetes management and other biomedical risk factors/medical management of the comprehensive CR component, have been widely used over a number of years. These include ambulatory BP monitors from major vendors such as Omron healthcare [36] and Welch Allyn [37]. Similarly, the management of diabetes through monitoring of blood glucose levels using glucometer kits, from major vendors such as AccuCheck [38], have been used widely by diabetic patients over the last decade. One of the limitations of these physiological monitoring technologies has been the lack of standard protocols to integrate to a communication platform which can then send data to an information portal. Current activity of a consortium of major technology vendors such as Intel, Microsoft, Cisco system, and medical industries such as Philips Medical Systems, General Electric, is the Continua Health Alliance [39]. Their objective is to develop design guidelines for interoperability of sensors, home networks, telehealth platforms and health and wellness services to establish a product certification program.

Other core elements of the comprehensive CR components are predominantly the multidisciplinary teams' interaction with the patients, specific to their clinical domain of care management. Most of these belongs to tasks that require education, counselling and guidance/mentoring services, such as in exercise training, adherence to medication, diet, etc. which are recommended to patients throughout the course of the CR program. In view of the advances communication technology, most services could be easily deployed through telehealth using a multimodal approach (voice, text and video). With increasing speed of the internet technology and broadband or mobile network, simultaneous videoconferencing, text messaging, and audio communication would become increasingly feasible for either education, counselling or mentoring. Another important factor to consider for the ICT for home-based CR is the useability criteria of patients ability to interact with the communication platform/technology, in particular, those with severe cardiac events presenting psychological disorders. Other limiting factors are in the communication's technology capacity to provide sufficient network speed and reliability to operate in a healthcare and/or critical need environment. One of the most recent advances in the digital technologies has been the mobile phone over 3G networks, and the similarity in the capacity to provide internet technology as that of a standard home personal computer. The discussion in section 1.8, describes the concept of applying this mobile phone and the internet technology in a CR service model to enable a home-based care model.

7 Clinically relevant measurements and measures for CR from ambulatory monitoring

Physical exercise is one of the key elements in a CR program. The goal is to return the individual to an appropriate level of functional capacity (FC), improve the quality of life, and modify the risk factors [40]. Exercise can also improve mental health outcomes in depressed and socially isolated patients [7]. It also affects autonomic nervous systems regulation of the heart by improving heart rate recovery [41] and increasing heart rate variability [42]. To achieve these outcomes, the current CR guidelines target an accumulation of 30 minutes moderate level physical activity each day. Telemonitoring tools are a viable method to measure, quantify and evaluate the exercise levels and heart function remotely to assess patient's adherence to the guidelines in a home-based CR model. The information measured continuously from patients' free living environment can additionally provide more physiologically representative information than snapshot data measured at the hospital setting or collected via questionaries.

Inexpensive ambulatory accelerometers and heart rate monitors have been widely used in research projects related to patient monitoring in home-based care models. Body movements and postures can be measured by using accelerometers attached to the body. Ambulatory ECG monitors have been used to measure heart rate and other cardiac functionality. These measurements produce large amounts of physiological data that needs to be translated into clinically relevant information that describes the patient's condition continuously and can be used to assess the patient against CR guidelines.

Recently, research projects conducted at the Australian E-Health Research Centre (AEHRC) developed algorithms and used commercially available tools for ECG analysis (First Beat Pro, Jyväskylä, Finland) to derive measures from ambulatory accelerometer and ECG signals to be used in CR programs [35]. These derived measures include:

Accelerometer based measures:

- Metabolic expenditure
- Activity/Inactivity ratio
- Total daily walking duration
- Walking speed
- Frequency of daily walking
- Walking control through gait characteristics
- Sit to Stand transition duration
- Adverse events such as falling

ECG based measures:

- Heart Rate distribution
- Heart Rate Variability (RMSSD)
- Respiratory rate

Some of these measures have technical or physiological limitations that restrict their use in practice. For example, motion artefacts from ambulatory monitored ECG significantly disturb the ECG based respiratory rate measures. Medication effects on heart rates will need to be accounted for when using Heart Rate Variability (HRV) analysis to determine physiological changes.

The metabolic expenditure measures describing the patient's general physical activity and measures of walking were more reliable for practical use because they directly compared with the established CR exercise program and performance of individual patients. This is depicted as an example in Fig 1.7.1 a) which shows a 24 hour plot of minute by minute energy expenditure of a patient that attended the exercise CR program. The graph indicates that the patient performed a 30 minute walk at a moderate level, as recommended by CR guidelines, around 6am in the morning. This information can provide important understanding of a patient's behaviour for the clinicians to motivate the patient to achieve their activity goals. The Activity/Inactivity ratio graph shown in Fig 1.7.1 b) depicts the progress of the patient's overall activity during the course of the CR program. The patient is shown here to become more active towards the end of the 6-week CR program, indicating that the program was beneficial in regaining functional capacity. This information can enable personalised care in home-based CR.

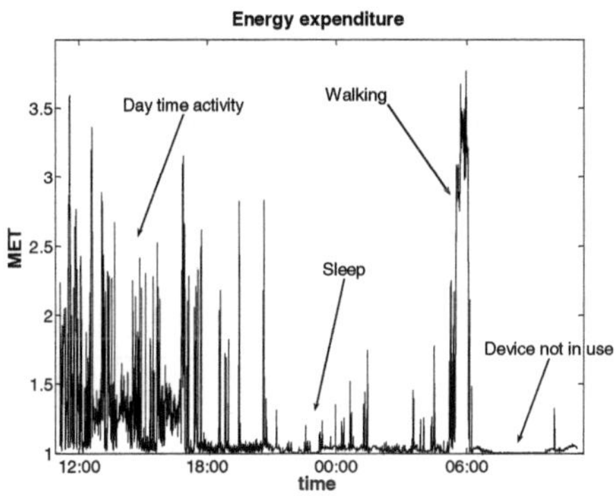

Fig 1.7.1. a) 24 hour energy expenditure

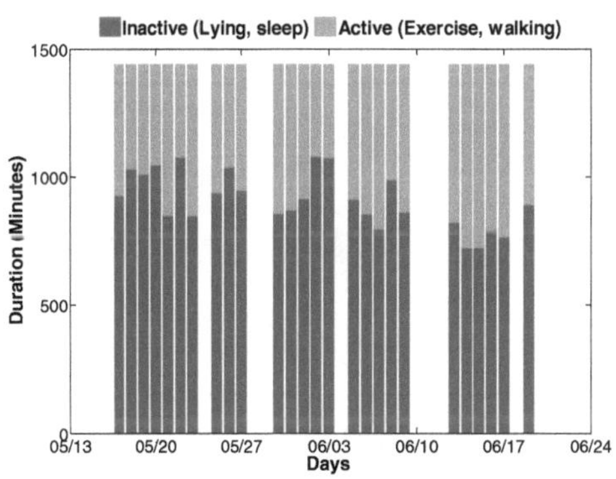

Fig 1.7.1.b) Activity/Inactivity ratio during CR

Current research on ECG and HRV analysis indicates that increased resting HRV describes improved heart regulation. Combined use of ECG and activity data could potentially separate the exercise effect on heart regulation from the psychological or emotional effects. This is a fertile field for future research in determining the correspondence of ECG and HRV measures to coronary risk factors such as lipid levels, blood pressure, anxiety, and depression.

8 Communications technology and infrastructure for home-based outpatient care

Current telecommunication networks and internet services provide a number of features which can be used to efficiently support outpatient cardiac rehabilitation and home care processes. The development of smart mobile phones which are capable of collecting and displaying advanced multimedia information and affordable personal computers and home-care devices, offer a cost effective infrastructure without special purpose technology. Mobile phones have been found to be suitable tools for wellness management [43] and health related web-portals are becoming increasingly popular. By combining these two modalities, it is possible to set up a basic communication system to support home-based care models to provide interventions in remote settings. An illustration of such a system model is shown in Fig 1.8.1.

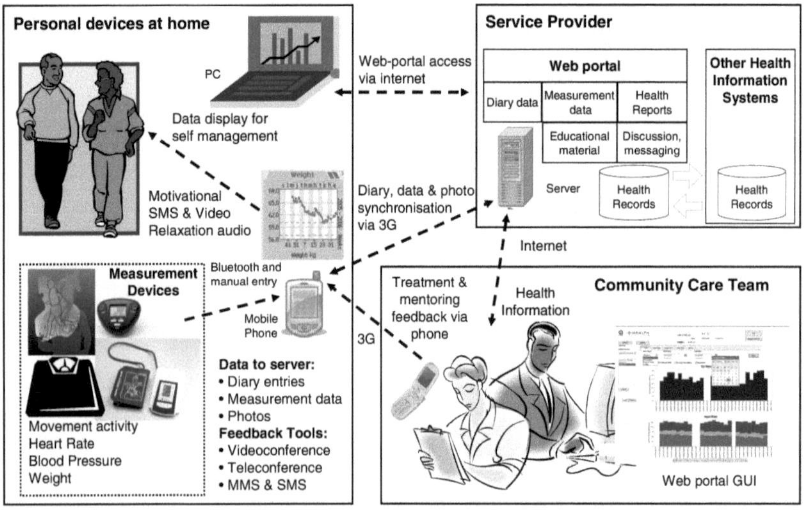

Fig 1.8.1. Technology infrastructure for home-based care models.

The setup consists of personal devices, software used by the patients, and a server with a web-portal that provides comprehensive detail of a patient's information. Because physical exercise is one of the core components of CR, an essential part of the technology setup requires the measurement of movement activity.

This can be measured and quantified with an accelerometer and additionally, heart rate monitor to provide a measure of exercise intensity. Important risk factors such as weight and blood pressure can be measured with weight scales and blood pressure-cuff monitor, designed for home care. The mobile phone is used as a personal hub to collect all the measurement data and transfer it to the server via 3G, WLAN or other available networking technology. The standard features of the mobile phones and 3G networks can be used to support the care model, which will be described in detail in Section 1.8.1.

Both the clinicians and patients can securely access the web-portal by using a standard web browser on their personal computer. The server application includes interface services to enter and upload data from devices and other external systems, view the relevant information, and create reports. The business logics include analysis modules to extract clinically relevant information from the data. The data services provide a Database to store and access all the collected information and an interface to share data with other information systems.

8.1 Use Cases of using a tele-health system in cardiac rehabilitation

Three main high level use cases can be identified from the system:

1. Treat and mentor the patients at home.

   Community Care Team wants to contact the patients to give coaching and education remotely.

2. Collect health and wellness data.

   – Community Care Team wants to collect and view objective measures of patient's health status and progress at home and use the information to give personalised feedback.

3. Self management of wellbeing.

   – The patients want to actively manage their own health and wellbeing, set goals and follow their progress and health status, discuss with health professionals and find information on their condition.

The following system modalities can be used to support the use cases.

8.1.1 Use Case 1: Treat and mentor the patients at home

Modality: Videoconferencing

Current mobile phones with inbuilt cameras using fast 3G networks have good quality person to person videoconferencing capability. No special equipment is needed and the conference can be held anytime and anywhere. Videoconferencing may substitute face-to-face communication at the hospital.

Modality: Teleconferencing

Normal phone calls can be used for short status check-up. The patient may also initiate a call to the health mentor.

Modality: SMS (text messages)

SMS messages can be sent to the patients as reminders, for example, to start physical exercise or give positive motivational feedback based on their progress.

Modality: MMS (multimedia messages)

MMS messages can be used to deliver educational material on the symptoms, background and treatment of the disease. They may contain combined speech, video, animations and text.

Modality: Messaging and discussion through the web- portal.

The web portal discussion and messaging tools can be used as a secure and confidential method to ask personal questions and exchange more detailed information on the patient's condition.

8.1.2 Use Case 2: Collect health and wellness data

Modality: Home monitoring devices and data transfer through the mobile phone to a server.

Physiological data such as weight, blood pressure, movement activity, heart rate, and ECG can be measured, entered in the phone either manually or automatically via Bluetooth, and transferred to the web portal. The measurement information on the portal can be viewed by the health professionals to objectively assess the patient's condition and progress. The phone may also contain in-built measurement functions such as a "step counter" for physical activity.

Modality: Diary application software on the mobile phone and web portal.

The diaries can be used to collect self measured data and observations on health and wellbeing. The mobile phone diary may include questionaries, numerical data entry, and scoring tools such as perceived intensity of exercise.

Modality: Digital photos.

Photos taken with the mobile phone can be uploaded to the web-portal. Photos of the patient's meals can be used to assess their dietary habits. Qualitative nutritional feedback can be given based on the photos. Photos can also be used to make assessment of visible medical conditions e.g. the healing of scars/wounds, skin problems, etc..

8.1.3 Use Case 3: Self management of the wellbeing

Modality: Pre installed media content on the mobile phone.

Mobile phones have sufficient memory capacity to hold pre-installed multimedia content that the patient may view and listen to, anywhere and anytime. Such multimedia may be audio files for relaxation and/or video files of educational material on heart attack.

Modality: Web portal.

Educational content material on the patient's disease, information on healthy lifestyle, and links to additional supporting web-content, can be accessed via the personal computer or the mobile phone.

Modality: Mobile phone and web portal diary applications for storing and viewing physiological data from home.

The diary data can be used for self management of patient's own health. By observing and entering data, the patient will become more aware of his/her own behaviour, which may facilitate change. In addition, feedback through observation of graphical trends and patterns of his/her own physiological signals and other data, may provide the patient with a better understanding of his/her own condition.

9 Case scenario

The technology setup should fulfil requirements arising from the specific care model guidelines. Outpatient cardiac rehabilitation programs have well documented guidelines such as in [40]. The main elements of CR programs should include:

- Individual assessment, review and follow-up
- Low or moderate level of physical activity
- Education, discussion and counselling targeting behaviour modifications in inactivity, weight, diet, smoking, stress, hypertension and psychological issues.

Mobile communication technologies and web-services can efficiently provide these main elements in a home-based setting for patients who do not travel to the community care facility, and therefore, loose normal face-to-face interaction with the community care personnel. The following case scenario illustrates the practical use of the described system in a comprehensive CR program.

Introduction:

This example describes how the clinicians managing and the patient referred to, a phase 2 CR program could use the information and communication technology (ICT) tools and system, described above, in a practical home-based care process. Assuming the patient is a post-MI, 55 year old female who has undergone CR phase 1 and has been discharged from the hospital with a referral to a community care, home-based CR phase 2 program.

Pre-assessment:

Initially the patient is referred to the CR phase 2 program and she arrives at the community care centre or hospital for enrolling and pre-assessment. The personnel enters the patient's demographic data into their information system which automatically creates a new patient also in the web-portal. A software tool is used by the clinicians to collect the patient's baseline data that is relevant to the CR program. The patient's previous medical history such as their demographic data, diagnosis, procedures, and prescribed medications may be already available in the Hospital Information System (HIS) from previous visit(s) to the hospital. This data can be fetched into the software tool automatically. The clinicians perform the measurements and fill in the questionaries required by the program guidelines. The pre-assessment results are recorded in the software tool and stored in a database. A baseline report summarising the patient's current health status and other relevant information is generated and uploaded to the web-portal.

The clinicians then give her basic training in using the mobile phone handset to receive video calls, listen to the audio files, watch the videos, take photos and use the diary application, web portal and the measurement devices. The home exercise program schedule is also planned with the patient. The patient sets her own exercise and lifestyle modification goals with the clinician for the following week.

Home program, description of a daily routine

The patient follows a schedule that was developed with the clinician. The program is also stored in her mobile phone's calendar. She starts her day by measuring her blood pressure and weight. She enters the data manually in the Diary software installed on the mobile phone. She also enters the length and quality of sleep in the Diary software. The data is automatically uploaded to the web-portal.

In the morning she receives an educational multimedia message on how to cope with heart disease. She views the message immediately. At noon, she receives a text message reminding her to start the home exercise program. She wears a heart rate monitor and goes for a walk, carrying the mobile phone with her. The phone measures and records her step count, intensity and energy expenditure during the course of her walk. The heart rate monitor recordings are transferred automatically to the phone. In a steep uphill incline the phone sounds a beep alerting her to slow down, because her heart rate had exceeded the maximum limit set by the clinician. After arriving home she wants to do the stretches and work out that was instructed to her. She views a video clip on her mobile phone that shows the correct work out moves and performs them, accordingly. She eats lunch and takes a photo of the meal and sends it directly to the web-portal. In the afternoon she receives a video call from her health mentor at the hospital who talks to her about how to achieve her exercise and other goals. The health mentor, having reviewed her data on the portal, provides feedback on how she has started to improve in terms of walking at higher intensity than before but still within safe heart rate limits. The mentor also reminds her to relax in the evening. In the evening she listens to a relaxation audio file stored on the mobile phone. She also logs onto the web-portal with her PC and types a few questions to her health mentor for discussion at the next videoconference. Before going to sleep, she opens the diary application on the phone and records her mood by answering a questionary related to tiredness, depression and stress.

Post-assessment:

The patient has completed her 6-week CR program and in the last videoconference the health mentor congratulates her on achieving the exercise levels. The health mentor also provides feedback on how her other risk factors such as blood pressure and weight had improved. The patient travels to the community care centre for post-assessment. The clinicians use the software tool to record her condition and health status for the end of the program assessment. The tool fetches relevant data from the portal database and creates a report addressing all the core components in the CR program guidelines. The report is stored in a database of the web-portal and a summary print-out is given to the patient. The patient is encouraged to continue using the mobile phone diary and web portal for the next few months follow-up period for her own self-observations and discussion with the health mentor, accordingly.

10 Issues and Limitations for the uptake of tele-health technologies

There are several barriers related to services and technologies that have been identified to limit the extensive use of tele-health systems despite promising results and extensive research in the field. Complete care specific integrated solutions for outpatient care are still rare. The implementation of these systems requires special expertise, which is not usually available within health care organisations. Commercially ready devices, system components and partial solutions exist, but there is a lack of service providers offering complete turn-key solutions for health care. There is also a lack of evidence in terms of health outcomes and cost-benefit analysis that would demonstrate the benefits of home-based technology enabled care solutions. Tele-health solutions often require simultaneous changes to care models and processes to be efficient. It is extremely slow to change health care processes, which restricts the penetration of new tele-health technologies and systems [44].

Barriers related to the tele-health technologies limit the uptake in addition to the problems in service provision and system integration. The missing standards for tele-health equipment and software, especially related to the communication protocols, has led to a situation where device and system vendors offer proprietary solutions. The lack of interoperability between the devices and software limits the possibilities to set up working solutions. Current systems have also been favouring large amounts of sensor data over processed summary results making the tele-health systems difficult and time consuming to use [45].

11 Summary

Cardiovascular disease is the leading chronic disease globally, accounting for 30% of global deaths. There is an increased prevalence of CVD with the ageing population. Cardiac rehabilitation has become a secondary prevention program, not only for patients with CVD, but other major chronic diseases such as COPD. The CR program is a comprehensive, structured approach with core components of patient assessment, lifestyle risk factors of CVD, biomedical risk factors of CVD, pharmacotherapy, and psychosocial factors management. Despite the availability of CR programs, there have been barriers to the utilisation of these services. These barriers are contributed by factors related to professional, service and patient. It begins with the inconsistency in professionals approach to patient's eligibility and enrolment to CR programs to patient's lack of uptake and adherence to the program, which is mainly a result of geographical distance from programs, sensitivity to a group setting, competing demands from family and work commitments, socio-economic/ethnic background, costs and the lack of reimbursement within public healthcare service model (in particular, USA). One alternative approach has been to move the CR program to the community in which patients are managed from homes. This has been predominantly an exercise-based CR program and very little of CVD risk factor reduction. The rapid advances in digital technology have improved immensely, the sensor technology in physiological monitoring, information processing of large volume of data, and more importantly, the capacity of the communicating technology. In particular, the internet technology and the mobile platform has transformed the way people communicate in business but also certain areas of acute healthcare services, such as diagnostic radiology imaging. With the increasing capacity of broadband and mobile network, mobile phone can be integrated as the communication platform between patient monitoring devices and information processing/storage retrieval, web-portal computer. Such integration for a home-based CR services could overcome the many barriers relating to the geography, patient preference and uptake, flexibility with other commitments and yet provide a co-ordinated multidisciplinary team-patient interaction. A proven model of this IT supported home-based care will provide patients with a lifestyle, self-management, and better quality care management.

References

[1] World Health Organisation. Cardiovascular diseases (2007), http://www.who.int/cardiovascular_diseases/en/ (Accessed 3/12/2007)

[2] Oldridge, N.B.: Comprehensive cardiac rehabilitation: is it cost-effective? Eur. Heart J. 19(suppl. O), 42–50 (1998)

[3] Nadar, S., Lip, G.Y.: Secular trends in cardiovascular disease. J. Hum. Hypertens 16(10), 663–666 (2002)

[4] Cooper, A.F.: Factors associated with cardiac rehabilitation attendance: a systematic review of the literature. Clin. Rehabil. 16(5), 541–552 (2002)

[5] Parkosewich, J.A.: Cardiac rehabilitation barriers and opportunities among women with cardiovascular disease. Cardiol. Rev. 16(1), 36–52 (2008)

[6] Scott, I.A., Lindsay, K.A., Harden, H.E.: Utilisation of outpatient cardiac rehabilitation in Queensland. Med. J. Aust. 179(7), 332–333 (2003)

[7] Reducing Risk in Heart Disease 2007. In: National Heart Foundation of Australia (2007)

[8] Balady, G.J., Williams, M.A., Ades, P.A., Bittner, V., Comoss, P., Foody, J.M., Franklin, B., Sanderson, B., Southard, D.: Core components of cardiac rehabilitation/secondary prevention programs: 2007 update: a scientific statement from the American Heart Association Exercise, Cardiac Rehabilitation, and Prevention Committee, the Council on Clinical Cardiology; the Councils on Cardiovascular Nursing, Epidemiology and Prevention, and Nutrition, Physical Activity, and Metabolism; and the American Association of Cardiovascular and Pulmonary Rehabilitation. Circulation 115(20), 2675–2682 (2007)

[9] Thomson, P.D., Buchner, D., Pina, I.L., Balady, G.J., et al.: Exercise and physical activity in the prevention and treatment of atherosclerotic cardiovascular disease: a statement from the Council on Clinical Cardiology (Subcommittee on Exercise, Rehabilitation, and Prevention) and the Council on Nutrition, Physical Activity, and Metabolism (Subcommittee on Physical Activity). Circulation 107(24), 3109–3116 (2003)
[10] Campbell, N.C., Grimshaw, J.M., Rawles, J.M., Ritchie, L.: Cardiac rehabilitation in Scotland: is current provision satisfactory? J. Public Health Med. 18(4), 478–480 (1996)
[11] Thompson, D.R., Bowman, G.S., Kitson, A.L., de Bono, D.P., Hopkins, A.: Cardiac rehabilitation in the United Kingdom: guidelines and audit standards. National Institute for Nursing, the British Cardiac Society and the Royal College of Physicians of London. Heart 75(1), 89–93 (1996)
[12] Campbell, N.C., Grimshaw, J.M., Ritchie, L.D., Rawles, J.M.: Outpatient cardiac rehabilitation: are the potential benefits being realised? J. R. Coll Physicians 30(6), 514–519 (1996)
[13] Jolliffe, J., Rees, K., Taylor, R., Thompson, D., Oldridge, N., Ebrahim, S.: Exercise-based rehabilitationfor coronary heart disease (Cochrane review). The Cochrane Library 2, 1–58 (2001)
[14] Hämäläinen, H., Luurila, O.J., Kallio, V., Knuts, L.R., Arstila, M., Hakkila, J.: Long-term reduction in sudden deaths after a multifactorial intervention programme in patients with myocardial infarction: 10-year results of a controlled investigation. Eur. Heart J. 10(1), 55–62 (1989)
[15] Kallio, V., Hämäläinen, H., Hakkila, J., Luurila, O.J.: Reduction in sudden deaths by a multifactorial intervention programme after acute myocardial infarction. Lancet. 24(2(8152)), 1091–1094 (1979)
[16] Squires, R.W., Hamm, L.: Exercise and the Coronary Heart Disease Connection. In: Ma, W. (ed.) AACVPR Cardiac Rehabilitation Resource Manual. Human Kinetics Europe Ltd, Champaign (2006)
[17] Jolly, K., Greenfield, S., Hare, R.: Attendance of ethnic minority patients in cardiac rehabilitation. J. Cardiopulm Rehabil. 24, 308–312 (2004)
[18] Tod, A., Lacey, E., McNeill, F.: I'm still waiting..':barriers to accessing cardiac rehabilitation services. J. Adv. Nurs. 40, 421–431 (2002)
[19] Thomas, R.J., King, M., Lui, K., Oldridge, N., Piña, I.L., Spertus, J., Bonow, R.O., Estes, N.A., Goff, D.C., Grady, K.L., Hiniker, A.R., Masoudi, F.A., Radford, M.J., Rumsfeld, J.S., Whitman, G.R.: AACVPR, ACC, AHA, American College of Chest Physicians, American College of Sports Medicine, American Physical Therapy Association, Canadian Association of Cardiac Rehabilitation, European Association for Cardiovascular Prevention and Rehabilitation, Inter-American Heart Foundation, National Association of Clinical Nurse Specialists, Preventive Cardiovascular Nurses Association; Society of Thoracic Surgeons. AACVPR/ACC/AHA 2007 performance measures on cardiac rehabilitation for referral to and delivery of cardiac rehabilitation/secondary prevention services endorsed by the American College of Chest Physicians, American College of Sports Medicine, American Physical Therapy Association, Canadian Association of Cardiac Rehabilitation, European Association for Cardiovascular Prevention and Rehabilitation, Inter-American Heart Foundation, National Association of Clinical Nurse Specialists, Preventive Cardiovascular Nurses Association, and the Society of Thoracic Surgeons. Journal of the American College of Cardiology 50, 1400–1433 (2008)

[20] Debusk, R.F., Haskell, W.L., Miller, N.H., Berra, K., Taylor, C.B.: Medically directed at home rehabilitation soon after clinically uncomplicated acute myocardial infarction: a new model for patient care. Am. J. Cardiol. 55, 251–257 (1985)
[21] Miller, N.H., Haskell, W.L., Berra, D., DeBusk, R.: Home versus group exercise training for increasing functional capacity after myocardial infarction. Circulation 107(4), 645–649 (1984)
[22] Krumholz, H.M., Cohen, B.J., Tsevat, J., Pasternak, R.C., Weinstein, M.: Cost-effectiveness of a smoking cessation program after myocardial infarction. J. Am. Coll. Cardiol. 22(6), 1697–1702 (1993)
[23] Fletcher, B.J., Dunbar, S.B., Felner, J.M., Jensen, B.E., Almon, L., Cotsonis, G., Fletcher, G.F.: Exercise testing and training in physically disabled men with clinical evidence of coronary artery disease. Am. J. Cardiol. 73(2), 170–174 (1994)
[24] Green, K., Lydon, S.: Home health cardiac rehabilitation. Home Healthc Nurse 13(2), 29–39 (1995)
[25] Heath, G.W., Moloney, P.M., Fure, C.: Group exercise versushome activity habilts. J. Cardiopulm Rehabil. 7, 190–195 (1987)
[26] Lewin, B., Robertson, I.H., Cay, E.L., Irving, J.B., Campbell, M.: Effects of self-help post-myocardial-infarction rehabilitation on psychological adjustment and use of health services. Lancet. 339, 1036–1040 (1992)
[27] DeBusk, R.F.: MULTIFIT: a new approach to risk factor modification. Cardiol Clin. 14(1), 143–157 (1996)
[28] Haskell, W.L., Alderman, E.L., Fair, J.M., Maron, D.J., Mackey, S.F., Superko, H.R., Williams, P.T., Johnstone, I.M., Champagne, M.A., Krauss, R.M., et al.: Effects of intensive multifactor risk reduction on coronary atherosclerosis and clinical cardiac events in men and women with coronary artery disease: The Stanford Coronary Risk Intervention Project. Circulation 89, 975–990 (1994)
[29] Jolly, K., Taylor, R.S., Lip, G.Y., Stevens, A.: Home-based cardiac rehabilitation compared with centre-based rehabilitation and usual care: a systematic review and meta analysis. Int. J. Cardiol. 111(3), 343–351 (2006)
[30] Grace, S.L., McDonald, J., Fishman, D., Caruso, V.: Patient preferences for home-based versus hospital-based cardiac rehabilitation. J. Cardiopulm Rehabil. 25, 24–29 (2005)
[31] Burke, L.: Adherence to a heart-healthy lifestyle-what makes the difference? In: Wenger, N.K., Smith, L.K., Froelicher, E.S., et al. (eds.) CArdiac rehabilitation. A guide to practice in the 21st century, pp. 385–393. Marcel Dekker, New York (1999)
[32] Taylor. Taylor, Consumer Products, `http://www.taylorusa.com/consumer/scales/precisiontech.html` (Accessed, 14 September 2008)
[33] IST International Security Technology. Vivago Active Personal Wellness Manager, `http://www.istsec.fi/index.php?k=8458` (Accessed, 14 September 2008)
[34] Respironics. Actiwatch, `http://actiwatch.respironics.com/` (Accessed, 14 September 2008)
[35] Bidargaddi, N.P., Sarela, A.: Activity and heart rate based measures for outpatient cardiac rehabilitation. Methods Inf. Med. 47, 208–216 (2008)
[36] Omron Healthcare. Blood Pressure Monitor, `http://www.omronhealthcare.com/product/default.asp?t=192` (Accessed, 14 September 2008)

[37] WelchAllyn Inc. Blood Pressure Management, http://www.welchallyn.com/apps/products/product_category.jsp?catcode=BPM (Accessed, 14 September 2008)
[38] AccuCheck. Accu-chek Glucometer Review, http://www.accucheckglucometer.com/ (Accessed, 14 September 2008)
[39] Continua Healthcare Alliance, http://www.continuaalliance.org/home (Accessed, 14 September 2008)
[40] Outpatient Cardiac Rehabilitation. In: Health, Q. (ed.) Best practice guidelines for health professionals (2004)
[41] Kukielka, M., et al.: Cardiac vagal modulation of heart rate during prolonged submaximal exercise in animals with healed myocardial infarction: effects of training. Am. J. Physiol. Heart Circ. Physiol. 290, 1680–1685 (2005)
[42] Myers, J., et al.: Effects of exercise training on heart rate recovery in patients with chronic heart failure. American Heart Journal 153(6), 1056–1063
[43] Mattila, M., et al.: Mobile Diary for Wellness management – Results on Usage and Usability in Two User Studies. IEEE Transactions on Information Technology in Biomedicine 12(4) (2008)
[44] Haux, R.: Health information systems - past, present, future. Int. J. Med. Inform. 75(3-4), 268–281 (2006)
[45] Labb, F., Gagnon, M.P., Lamothe, L., Fortin, J.P., Messikh, D.: Impacts of telehomecare on patients, providers, and organizations. Telemed. J. E. Health 12(3), 363–369 (2006)

Acknowledgements:

We would like to thank Dr. Niranjan Bidargaddi for his contribution made in the examples included for the derived clinically relevant measures of accelerometer-based ambulatory monitoring. We would also like to thank the rehabilitation coordinators of the Northside Health Service District, Queensland Health,Queensland, Australia for gathering patient accelerometer data for the latter derivation of the clinical measures.

Role of Nano- and Microtechnologies in Clinical Point-of-Care Testing

Jason Y. Park[†] and Larry J. Kricka[*]

*Author for correspondence: Center for Biomedical Micro & Nanotechnology, Department of Pathology & Laboratory Medicine, University of Pennsylvania School of Medicine; Philadelphia, Pennsylvania, USA; (Fax: + 1-215-662-7529; E-mail: kricka@mail.med.upenn.edu).

†Department of Pathology. Johns Hopkins University School of Medicine; Baltimore, Maryland, USA.

Abstract There is increasing interest in point-of-care diagnostic testing in hospitals and within homes. Advances in engineering and innovation in diagnostic technologies are enabling miniaturized devices (e.g., lab-on-a-chip) at the micro or nanoscale and these devices may eventually provide most if not all of the current range of central laboratory clinical tests at the point-of-care. Specific benefits for miniaturized devices include integration of all steps in a clinical test in single device), replicate analysis for enhanced reliability, portability, low cost, implantability (e.g., in vivo devices), and simplified operation. However, often the true potential of these new technologies cannot be readily assessed because there is inadequate validation with real samples in a clinically relevant environment. It is important to know how common interfering substances (e.g., bilirubin, lipids, hemoglobin, drugs) present in some biological samples may affect a detection technology. Even if a technology can successfully negotiate these hurdles, it must be formatted or packaged to meet the essential requirements of point-of-care testing. This chapter explores the scope of micro and nanotechnologies in the context of point-of-care testing and discusses issues relevant to their implementation.

Table of Contents

K. Yogesan et al. (Eds.): Handbook of Digital Homecare, BIOMED, pp. 353–362.
springerlink.com

1. Introduction

Within healthcare, there is an increasing interest in point-of-care (POC) diagnostic testing in hospitals and within homes. This interest is built on the significant success of patients self-administering tests at home for the evaluation of blood glucose, as well as pregnancy and fertility hormones [1]. The success of patients self-administering tests can be measured by improved morbidity, mortality and overall reduction in healthcare dollars [2-5]. Advances in engineering and innovation in diagnostic technologies increasingly enable miniaturized devices (e.g., lab-on-a-chip) at the micro or nanoscale and these devices may eventually provide most if not all of the current range of central laboratory clinical tests at the POC [6]. This chapter explores the scope of micro and nanotechnologies in the context of POC testing and discusses issues relevant to their implementation.

2. Clinical need for miniaturized devices

One of the central tenets of POC testing is that immediately providing the results of a clinical test will lead to rapid medical intervention or the promotion of well-being. For example, relatively simple medical intervention can quickly correct a low or high glucose revealed by POC testing. Likewise, POC blood gas testing is valuable for maintaining the correct ventilator settings for intubated patients, and POC pregnancy tests provide rapid testing for patients prior to radiologic imaging studies or surgical procedures that might harm a fetus. Various scenarios support a wider implementation and broader scope of POC testing. Currently, hospital-based POC testing is the largest and most diverse enterprise (Table 1.1).

Table 1.1 Typical profile of a POCT service in a health system

Staff trained for POC testing	>4000 Nurses, Perfusionists, Respiratory therapists, Certified nurses assistants, Medical assistants
Number of test	>1 million tests/year
Menu of test	Glucose, Coagulation, Occult blood, Urinalysis, Urine hCG, Hemoglobin, Blood gases/ electrolytes/hematocrit, Co-oximetry, Strep A, pH, Gastric occult blood, Neonatal bilirubin
Meters for POC *testing*	>100

Hospital-based POC necessitates the training and monitoring of the performance of thousands of staff [7]. In such a large operation, essential POC testing requirements include: robustness (i.e., usable any time of day by many different operators), ease of use, self-calibration, restricted access via lock-outs to prevent unauthorized use of POC analyzers or use when quality control (QC) has failed, and connectivity for data downloads to a laboratory information system. The latter is particularly important in the context of tele-health applications.

Home testing represents the other major site of POC testing. Indeed, home pregnancy testing and home glucose monitors are a significant financial portion of the success of the POC device industry (http://www.roche.com/irp170505diausrc.pdf). In the context of home testing, some intriguing POC testing scenarios are emerging that involve the coupling of testing and communication technology such as mobile phone technology or Wi-Fi. A prime example is the T+Medical glucose program based on a cell phone that incorporates a glucose meter which provides real-time data transfer and intensive medical feedback to the user (www.tplusmedical.com)[8]. Another device that exploits wireless transmissions is the Guardian REAL-Time System. This is based on an in vivo glucose sensor that connects directly to a local transmitter which wirelessly sends 24-hour glucose data to a portable data collection device (www.minimed.com). A more expansive system, the Viterion 100 TeleHealth Monitor, has been specifically designed for use by patients in the home after a hospitalization (www.viterion.com). The Viterion monitor is a tele-health system that is intended to supplement in-home visits by providing communication and recording capabilites of parameters such as blood pressure, blood oxygen, blood sugar, body weight, and body temperature, peak flow. The monitor is designed to facilitate increased communication between the patient and healthcare worker.

These devices may represent the beginning of an important trend towards remote and continuous monitoring of patient diagnostic information. Not only will patients have real-time and on demand information of their health, but this same information can be instantaneously transferred to a knowledgeable healthcare professional or stored as information in the patient's electronic medical record. In particular, the miniaturization of wireless communication devices is particularly promising for the creation of an individualized network of devices which may be embedded in a person to monitor and respond to changes in not only analytes in the blood, but also cardiovascular status, infection, and mental alertness.

3. Reliability of POC tests

POC testing technology has evolved rapidly from the early tests based on reagent tablets to dipstick-type tests to the current one-step tests that just require addition of a sample. Qualitative tests have used visual inspection of color formation as an end-point and quantitative tests have employed hand-held meters that provide a quantitative result. Ensuring test reliability, removing operator dependence and meeting regulatory compliance are key considerations in any new or candidate POC testing technology.

An important consideration for any POC test is ensuring that it is reliable, easy to use, and foolproof. To this end, many tests now include positive controls, and end-of-test and invalid test indicators. These mechanisms provide feedback to the operator on the operation and success of the test. Further improvements have removed ambiguity in result interpretation by designing a test to give a simple "plus" or "minus" result or to give a direct text message to the operator (e.g., "pregnant" or "not pregnant")(ww.unipath.com/ClearblueDigital.cfm). A challenge for POC testing is that it must be appropriate for multiple users with varying education levels and minimal experience with technologies. The end user of a POC testing device may have educational levels ranging from high school to post-doctorate. Thus a reasonable starting point, even for technologies destined for the hospital or doctor's office, would be to design the device for use in the home.

4. Micro and nanotechnology

Different types of microtechnologies (e.g., lithography, laser ablation, micromolding, reactive ion etching) have been used to fabricate a variety of analyzers and analytical devices. These types of devices are frequently referred to as "Lab-on-a-chip" or "micro total analysis systems" (Table 1.2) [9-11]. At a much smaller scale, nanotechnology (1-100 nm scale) is providing both nanomaterials and nanodevices that have analytical potential (Table 1.2) [12].

Table 1.2 Miniaturization technologies with potential applications in POCT

Microtechnology		
	Microfluidic chips	
		Capillary electrophoresis microchip
		Cell separation microchip
		Flow cytometer microchip
		Liquid chromatography microchip
		Polymerase chain reaction microchip
	Bioelectronic chips	
	Microarray chips	
		Antibody microarray
		Antigen microarray
		cDNA microarray
		Oligonucleotide microarray
Nanotechnology		

Nanoarrays
Nanocantilevers
Nanodisks
Nanoelectronics
Nanoparticles
Nanoprisms
Nanoribbons
Nanorods
Nanorobots
Nanoshells
Nanotubes
Nanowires

Specific benefits for miniaturized devices in the clinical testing realm include: integration of all steps in a clinical test in single device (e.g. sample processing, analytical reaction, data manipulation, result reporting), analysis of specimens in duplicate for enhanced reliability, portability, low cost, implantability (e.g., in vivo diagnostic devices), and simplified operation. Also, these simplified devices have a specific niche for the lay consumer as well as non-laboratory oriented healthcare workers.

5. Barriers to implementation

A common criticism of the current scope of analytical miniaturization technology is that there is a need for researchers to focus on developing novel technologies to meet the demands of the marketplace rather than developing novel technologies that aim to create their own demand [6, 13]. Generally, technological development of miniaturized analytical devices continues to be rapid, but there are few examples of the marketplace welcoming these types of innovations. Indeed, devices such as microfluidic chips (CD-based, silicon wafer based) have had limited impact on the clinical laboratory market. It appears that the number of new generations of miniaturization and novel analytical techniques outpaces the willingness of the market to accept them.

Generally, the clinical laboratory is extremely cautious when implementing new technologies and this is due in part to the special needs of POCT in a hospital setting and the hurdles imposed by clinical laboratory regulatory agencies such as the Food and Drug Administration (FDA), Joint Commission on the Accreditation of Healthcare Organizations (JCHAO), and the College of American Pathologists (CAP) [14, 15]. For example, the College of American Pathologists' Commission on Laboratory Accreditation has an extensive checklist of requirements which must be fulfilled by any laboratory that desires accreditation to perform POC testing [16]. This checklist covers numerous aspects of training, proficiency testing, quality control and quality management. A list of specific regulatory requirements are listed separately (Table 1.3).

Table 1.3 Regulatory requirements for POCT by United States laboratory accreditation agencies (adapted from reference 14, Bennett et al 2000).

Policy and procedure manual
- Up-to-date documentation of approved policies and procedures
- Testing assay protocols
- Analytical measurement range
- Clinically reportable range
- Reference range

Quality assurance and Quality control (QA/QC)
- Description of metrics used and corrective actions
- Reporting of quality measures
- Setting quality control limits and results

Proficiency testing program
- Documentation of proficiency testing results
- Specific action taken to address deficiencies at proficiency testing

Correlation studies
- Comparison of POCT device results versus a reference method
- Comparison of POCT devices with each other

Personnel requirements and records
- Job description of device users
- Orientation of new device users
- Resumes
- Diplomas, credentials and certificates documenting education and training
- Results of periodic proficiency testing of each device-user

Instrument maintenance records

Document retention

Depending on the complexity of the technology, the federal government has varying degrees of oversight depending on the complexity of the technology. In the case of low complexity technologies such as glucose meters, patients are allowed to test their own specimens. However, the very same low complexity technologies that can be used by patients in their homes with minimal quality control may require significant quality control when used in a healthcare setting such as a hospital or doctor's office. Although complying with clinical laboratory accreditation in the prototype phase of a new device may be premature; being aware of the eventual hurdles is critical in even the earliest phases of development.

In the case of high complexity technologies, the regulatory requirements are significantly greater. A further complication is that the regulatory environment continues to become more complex. For example, the FDA recently issued a draft guidance for industry addressing the expanded role of the FDA for in vitro diagnostic assays with multiple variables or analytes (http://www.fda.gov/cdrh/oivd/guidance/1610.pdf)[17]. POC tests that utilize multianalyte analyses (e.g., microarrays) will be affected as much as any clinical laboratory assay. In the near future, increasing oversight and intervention by regulatory agencies can be expected.

In addition, devices that are implanted into humans require FDA approval; thus it is foreseeable that any implanted POC devices may be evaluated by stringent standards that have not yet been foreseen in standard clinical laboratory testing [18]. The standards for regulation of implantable diagnostic devices that assess analytes will likely be based on some form of the standards which currently exist for implantable cardiac defibrillators and pacemakers.

6. Technology development

Many technologies continue to emerge from current research in micro and nano-scale miniaturization that may have application in POC testing. These include technologies that facilitate miniaturization of the device (e.g., lab-on-a-chip type devices, nanorobots) and technologies that facilitate assays that are faster, easier to perform or have higher sensitivity (e.g., nanowires, nanoparticles, nanoarrays) (Table 1.2). However, often the true potential of these new technologies cannot be readily assessed because there is inadequate validation with real samples in a clinically relevant environment. It is important to know, at an early stage, how common interfering substances (e.g., bilirubin, lipids, hemoglobin, drugs) that may be present in biological samples will affect a candidate detection technology. Even if a candidate technology can successfully negotiate these hurdles, it must be formatted or packaged to meet the essential requirements of hospital POC described above.

7. Future directions in testing

The overall direction of point-of-care testing is increasing personalization; the endpoint of this is likely implantable monitoring devices. The first steps to implantable analytical devices have already been taken. Thus far there are two major types of implantable devices which have implications for clinical testing. The first is a FDA-cleared human-implantable radio frequency identification (RFID) microchip (VeriChip™) intended for infant protection, wander prevention, and patient identification applications (www.verichipcorp.com). The second are a new generation of implantable glucose monitors that provide continuous monitoring of glucose values (19). This new generation of implantable glucose monitors is particularly exciting because they can be coupled with the infusion of drugs; indeed, the monitoring of glucose with the infusion of insulin in response to glucose levels exemplifies a closed-loop model of a therapeutic response to a monitored analyte with minimal user intervention.

Some have foreseen that the development of implantable or wearable devices will facilitate the formation of personalized wireless networks. In some models, these wireless local area networks (WLAN) or body sensor networks (BSN) are coordinated wireless devices which monitor multiple functions in a patient including: heart rate, blood pressure, serum biomarkers and toxins [20, 21]. This coordinated and personalized network can constantly update the patient's permanent electronic medical record as well as link the patient's health status to service providers including routine primary care physicians as well as emergency responders. For example, in the care of patients at risk for myocardial infarction, a POC device implanted in the heart may detect biomarkers at the first instance of ischemia which may be minutes to hours faster than any of the current biomarkers which rely on peripheral blood sampling. Another example may be implantation in novel sites for uses such as tumor or infection monitoring at a previous surgical site; rather than having patients scheduled for recurring visits to their oncologist or surgeon, a POC implanted device may constantly update the patient to their tumor or infection status. Indeed, POC devices may enable true 'personalized healthcare' with each patient having an assortment of biologic sensors which provide continuous monitoring and testing of each patient's serum markers and physiology. With continuous monitoring a patient or their physician can follow trends or minute changes in the patient's health over long periods of time. Indeed, patients may become more invested in their healthcare if they can see immediate and continuous changes in the multiple analytes within their blood. Akin to managing a stock portfolio, a patient could monitor their changing health and have speedy access to trends and worrisome changes and thereby seek early expert advice or intervention.

The ultimate extent of nanotechnology offers futuristic nanosized analyzers with multiple diagnostic and therapeutic capabilities that would circulate freely within the body - usually referred to as nanorobots (www.nanorobotdesign.com) [22, 23]. The precursor to these nanorobots may lie in more simplistic passive devices which are used for diagnostic purposes; indeed, nanoparticulate imaging agents which undergo changes when subjected to different environments may be the foundation of future nanorobots. However, the technology underlying these nanorobots is still speculative and the regulatory issues for a freely mobile diagnostic/therapeutic device have yet to be identified and resolved.

Many people envision a world in which POC testing is widespread. This belief seems feasible with the current pace of technological development in micro and nanotechnology [24-26]. However, the clinical environment will be a demanding environment for these new technologies. We propose that from the inception of a new POC technology, consideration should be given to the marketplace, end-user and regulatory requirements. These are not functions that every laboratory can adequately model and predict, but with appropriate foresight and collaboration many future obstacles can be anticipated and overcome.

8. References

1. Price, C.P., St. John, A., Hicks, J.M. (eds.): Point of Care Testing, 2nd edn. AACC Press, Washington, DC (2004)
2. Van den Berghe, G., Wilmer, A., Hermans, G., et al.: Intensive insulin therapy in the medical ICU. NEJM 354, 449–461 (2006)
3. Noffsinger, R., Chin, S.: Improving the delivery of care and reducing healthcare costs with the digitization of information. J. Healthcare Informat. Manag. 14, 23–30 (2000)
4. Paxton, A.: Nearing high tide on low blood sugars. CAP Today (March 2006)
5. Jahn, U.R., Van Aken, H.: Near-patient testing—point-of-care or point of costs and convenience? Br. J. Anaesth. 90, 425–427 (2003)
6. Kricka, L.J., Park, J.Y.: Prospects for nano- and microtechnologies in clinical point-of-care testing Lab Chip, p. 547 (2007)
7. Jacobs, E., Hinson, K.A., Tolnai, J., et al.: Implementation, management and continuous quality improvement of point-of-care testing in academic health care setting. Clin. Chim. Acta 307, 49–59 (2001)
8. Farmer, A.J., Gibson, O.J., Dudley, C., et al.: A randomized controlled trial of the effect of real-time telemedicine support on glycemic control in young adults with Type 1 diabetes (ISRCTN 46889446). Diabetes Care 28, 2697–2702 (2005)
9. Cheng, J., Kricka, L.J. (eds.): Biochip Technology. Harwood, Philadelphia (2001)
10. Kricka, L.J., Wilding, P., et al.: Microchip PCR. Anal. Bioanal. Chem. 377, 820–825 (2003)
11. Kricka, L.J., Wild, D.: Lab-on-a-chip, micro- and nanoscale immunoassay systems. In: Wild, D. (ed.) The Immunoassay Handbook, 3rd edn., pp. 294–309. Elsevier, Amsterdam (2005)
12. Fortina, P., Kricka, L.J., Park, J.Y., et al.: Beyond microtechnology-nanotechnology in molecular diagnosis. In: Liu, R., Lee, A.P. (eds.) Integrated Biochips for DNA Analysis Landes Bioscience, Austin, TX, pp. 186–197 (2007)

13. Van Merkerk, R.O., van den Berg, A.: More than technology alone. Lab Chip. 6, 838–839 (2006)
14. Bennett, J., Cervantes, C., Pacheco, S.: Point-of-care testing: inspection preparedness. Perfusion 15, 137–142 (2000)
15. Anderson, M.: POCT regulatory compliance: What is it and how does it impact you? Crit. Care Nurs. Quart. 24, 1–6 (2001)
16. http://www.cap.org/apps/docs/laboratory_accreditation/checklists/point_of_care_testing_october2005.pdf
17. McDowell, J.: FDA begins regulating multivariate assays. Clin. Lab News 32, 1–4 (2006)
18. Medical devices; general hospital and personal use devices; classification of implantable radiofrequency transponder system for patient identification and health information. Final rule. Fed Register 69, 71702–71704 (2004)
19. Halvorson, M., Carpenter, S., Kaiserman, K., et al.: A pilot trial in pediatrics with the sensor-augmented pump: Combining real-time continuous glucose monitoring with the insulin pump. J. Pediatr. 150, 103–105 (2007)
20. Ng, S., Po, C., Dagang, G., et al.: MEMSWear – Biomonitoring – Incorporating sensors into smart shirt for wireless sentinel medical detection and alarm. In: J. Phys. Conference Series, vol. 34, pp. 1068–1072 (2006)
21. Gyselinckx, B., Van Hoof, C., Ryckaert, J., et al.: Human++: Autonomous wireless sensors for body area networks. In: Proceedings of the Custom Integrated Circuits Conference, Proceedings of the IEEE 2005 Custom Integrated Circuits Conference, pp. 12–18 (2005)
22. Haberzettl, C.A.: Nanomedicine: destination or journey? Nanotechnol 13, R9–R13 (2002)
23. Bansal, R.: Stranger than fiction? IEEE Microwave magazine 8, 26–28 (2007)
24. Fortina, P., Kricka, L.J., Surrey, S., et al.: Nanobiotechnology: the promise and reality of new approaches to molecular recognition. Trends Biotechnol. 23, 168–173 (2005)
25. Kricka, L.J.: The hitchhikers guide to analytical microchips. AACC Press, Washington (2002)
26. Kricka, L.J., Park, J.Y., Li, S.F.Y., et al.: Miniaturized detection technology in molecular diagnostics. Exp. Rev. Mol. Diagn. 5, 549–558 (2005)

Author Index

FSC
www.fsc.org

MIX
Papier aus verantwortungsvollen Quellen
Paper from responsible sources
FSC® C105338

If you have any concerns about our products,
you can contact us on
ProductSafety@springernature.com

In case Publisher is established outside the EU,
the EU authorized representative is:
Springer Nature Customer Service Center GmbH
Europaplatz 3, 69115 Heidelberg, Germany

Printed by Libri Plureos GmbH
in Hamburg, Germany